DATE DUE

DE 9'02		
DE 2 02		
AP 24 03		
SE 7 03		
OC 2 0 08		
NO 11 08		

NURTURING CHILDREN

A HISTORY OF PEDIATRICS

A. R. COLÓN,
with *P. A. Colón*

GREENWOOD PRESS
Westport, Connecticut • London

Library of Congress Cataloging-in-Publication Data

Colón, A. R.
    Nurturing children : a history of pediatrics / by A. R. Colón with
P. A. Colón.
      p. cm.
    Includes bibliographical references and index.
    ISBN 0–313–31080–7 (alk. paper)
    1. Pediatrics—History. I. Colón, P. A. II. Title.
    [DNLM: 1. Pediatrics—history. WS 11.1 C719n 1999]
    RJ36.C65   1999
    618.92′0009—dc21
    DNLM/DLC
                                       99–25000

British Library Cataloguing in Publication Data is available.

Library of Congress Catalog Card Number: 99–25000
ISBN: 0–313–31080–7

First published in 1999

Greenwood Press, 88 Post Road West, Westport, CT 06881
An imprint of Greenwood Publishing Group, Inc.
www.greenwood.com

Printed in the United States of America

∞™ The paper used in this book complies with the
Permanent Paper Standard issued by the National
Information Standards Organization (Z39.48–1984).

10 9 8 7 6 5 4 3 2 1

Copyright Acknowledgments

For material reproduced in this book, the following publishers are gratefully acknowledged:

Figures

Figure 1.1 reproduced by permission from *Lancet* (1995), vol. 345, page 757. Copyright © 1995 by The Lancet Ltd.

Figure 1.3 reproduced by permission from the November 1989 issue of *National Geographic*. Copyright © 1989 by The National Geographic Society.

Figure 1.5 reproduced by permission from *The Archaeology of York: The Medieval Cemeteries*. Copyright © 1984 by The York Archaeological Trust for Excavation and Research Ltd.

Figure 2.1 reproduced by permission. Copyright © 1951 by Brill.

Figure 6.4 reproduced by kind permission of the Royal College of Surgeons of Edinburgh.

Figure 7.1 reproduced by permission from *Lancet* (1996), vol. 348, page 902. Copyright © 1996 by The Lancet Ltd.

Figure 8.5 reproduced by permission from M. J. Waserman, "Henry Coit and the Certified Milk Movement," *Bulletin of the History of Medicine*, vol. 46 (1972): 359–90. Copyright © 1972 by The Johns Hopkins University Press.

Text

The *passim* quotations from G. F. Still, *The History of Pediatrics*, are reproduced with permission from Oxford University Press. Copyright © 1931 by Oxford University Press.

For three remarkable professors of pediatrics:

THOMAS E. CONE,
extraordinary chronicler of American Pediatrics,

FRANK A. OSKI,
scholar and advocate of legislation guarding the welfare of children,

BENJAMIN SPOCK,
who restored maternal confidence and instincts,

and

for my pediatric colleagues, whose work and devotion to their profession have rendered an anachronism the observation made by Petrus Toletus:

Hactenus infantes multi periere dolore
Ignoto, haud aderat qui dare posset opem.

[Till now the babes oft died with ills unknown,
For none there was with skills to succour them.]

—Introduction to *Libellus de Egritudinibus Infantum*
Bagellardus of Padua, 1472 (Lyon edition, 1560)

Contents

Illustrations

Introduction

Were the question "What is a pediatrician?" put to me, my response, clearly influenced by the wit and prose of Ambrose Bierce, would be that a pediatrician is a doctor who, with distractions and tickles, cajoles voiceless babes and wary toddlers into making audible their woes.

After more than thirty years of treating infants and children—and a good number who have passed the age of adolescence—and of teaching pediatric medicine to newly qualified physicians, my work continues to be absorbing as well as rewarding and has kindled in me a passionate interest in the history of children's medical treatment in the past.

Cicero defined the value of studying history in general and in the process used a metaphor quite suited to a history of pediatrics:

Not to know what has been transacted in former times is to continue always a child; if no use is made of the labors of the first ages, the world must remain always in the infancy of knowledge. (*de Oratore* 2.34)

Moreover, historian Edwin Ackerknecht's (1906–1988) belief that "a man can be a competent doctor without a knowledge of medical history, but an acquaintance with medical history can make him a better doctor"[1] supported my thesis that pediatric history is an important adjunct topic that students and pediatric residents should know. I also believed that the general public would find it a fascinating saga to read about the extent of the impact that medical care (or lack of it) has had on the world's history. In the case of children, it seemed to me an especially captivating topic since it relates to the most vulnerable and least independent members of our species.

Whereas taking a child to a pediatrician is routine today, the concept and reality of physicians especially trained to treat sick children and to prevent sickness in well children are very modern phenomena. In a world that can trace its historical roots back several millennia, the notion of doctors for children did not begin to be formulated until the nineteenth century.

In the corpus of Western medical writing that has survived the ages, certain documents did offer advice and treatment regarding diseases and medical conditions of childhood.[2] None, however, acknowledged the need for disciplined and systematic forms of treatment designed specifically for children's unique physiology and susceptibility, although rudimentary aspects of the discipline of pediatrics in the West traditionally are said to be found in four incunabula published during the fifteenth century.[3]

The physiological differences in infants, young children, adolescents, and adults that necessitate different diagnostic and treatment modalities, unrecognized in the past, seem so obvious now. As a result, medical care—as it existed—was rendered with no appreciation of the vital significance in outcome when age-based physiological differences of patients is a clinical consideration. There were some renowned physicians who understood and readily admitted their inadequacy in treating children, acknowledging ignorance and expressing fear of caring for the *infans*—the voiceless—but their reticence did not lead to any useful insights regarding child care.[4]

For countless centuries, women and children were perceived conceptually as single entities in a series of associations: pregnancy and birth, breast feeding and the newborn, maternal nurturing and child growth, and so on. Few dared to isolate the child from this biological axis. High mortality further reinforced the notion of the fragility of infant life and the prevailing wisdom of the futility of efforts to master the subtleties that now are known to be prerequisite for the diagnosis and treatment of children.

With the rate of infant mortality so extreme and life expectancy so poor, the care of infants generally was left to midwives, who blended wisdom gleaned from experience with magic, superstition, and ritual. A strong feature of *all* medical treatment in the past, in fact, included a liberal dose of magic. Healers, shamans and priests, and charlatans commonly were (and in many places still are) appealed to by the sick and by their families for the spells and incantations that were (and are) believed to cure sickness and relieve pain.

Childhood itself is arguably a modern concept, one that some believe did not begin to emerge until the mid-seventeenth century. In primitive, ancient, medieval, and emerging industrial societies, children's value to the family was viewed from the perspective of survival. Among the wealthy, children were resources that contributed to dynastic economies. In impoverished families—the majority—children were commercial assets to be sold, indentured, and pressed into labor at what we now regard as sinfully young ages.

These factors, conjoined with children's vulnerability to disease that led to sickness and early death, determined individual and societal attitudes about children and certainly determined the focus and attention of physicians in Western societies, who had all they could do to help patients attain what used to be a very short life expectancy. There were no incentives to persuade doctors that study, energy, and time committed to treat and cure little *merdeaux* would meet with success, let alone professional and emotional satisfaction.

For the most part, parents and society in general were helpless in the face of epidemics that decimated both adult and child populations. Smallpox, plague, cholera, and childhood diseases such as diphtheria, measles, and whooping cough took a common toll. Added to this doleful reality were malnutrition and starvation—commonplace consequences of war, pestilence, famine, ignorance, and sometimes neglect. Infanticide and child abandonment, rooted in desperation and despair, were widespread and were countered by inadequate attempts to salvage the innocents that too often exacted their own tragic toll. The foundling homes that were established were often breeding grounds for infectious diseases that led to death; children placed in church institutions and in servile positions in private homes too often were abused and in general ill-treated, and they too succumbed, victims of long and arduous work, poor nutrition and brutality.

Healthier, more stable, and more prosperous populations became a possibility from about the time of the industrial revolution, and the advances in economics, agriculture, science, and medicine gave societies opportunity to rethink and reevaluate attitudes and relationships—an alliance, if you will, was formed between compassion and economic advantage and a newly discovered luxury of hope that promised bright futures. In this milieu the health and care of children became a stronger concern to all, and physicians began in earnest to focus on the medical needs of children.

In this book, I have allowed myself two liberties. First, I assume that the reader understands that pediatric medicine is a late-vintage development; therefore, I chose to apply the term *pediatrics* to all child care, whether ancient or modern, to facilitate the narrative flow. Second, each chapter begins with a little "time table," and I incorporate some discussion of historical events and cultural environments because both, of course, are major factors contributing to the health status of societies. Often child care is colored not so much by what the doctor dictates but rather by what the culture or the mother allows. Working within this constraint constitutes part of the "art" of pediatrics.

The use of some medical terms has been unavoidable, and some simply have been used for facility and economy of expression. For these reasons a glossary can be found in the text. The extensive bibliography acknowledges the scholarship of historians and translators—guardians all of the historical past whose efforts preserve ancient wisdom for our times and for the future; and I am particularly beholden to John Ruhräh, George Frederic Still, and Thomas E. Cone for their excellent histories of pediatrics. I also gratefully acknowledge the staff of the History of Medicine section of the National Library of Medicine, which provided nearly all the primary sources I used.

I also am indebted to my university colleagues, Drs. Charlotte Barbey-Morel, Joseph Kadlec, S.J., Margit Hamosh, Thomas Reichmann, and Wei Yee Chan for their generous and enthusiastic assistance with difficult translations of text.

NOTES

1. Ackerknecht, 1982, p. xix.

2. A large body of Eastern medical literature dedicated to child care was well known and consulted in the West, but it was not incorporated into the Western medical literature. Chapter 4 fully examines the importance of the pediatric contributions to the West by Eastern medicine. As chapter 2 reveals, however, the ignorance with respect to pediatrics in the Orient was total.

3. Louffenburg's *Versehung des Leibs* (1429), Bagellardus's *De Infantium Aegritudinibus et Remediis* (1472), Metlinger's *Ein Regiment der Jungerkinder* (1473), and Roelans' *Buchlein* (Latinized: *Libellus Aegritudinum Infantium*) (1483). See chapter 5.

4. "[F]or which Reason, several Physicians of the first Rank have openly declared to me, that they go very unwillingly to take care of the Disease of Children, especially such as are newly born, as if they were to unravel some strange Mystery" (Walter Harris, *De morbis acutis infantum*, 1689).

"I have heard an eminent physician say, that he never wished to be called in to a young child; because he was really at a loss to know what to order for it. Nay, I am told, that there is nothing to be done for children when they are ill" (George Armstrong, *An Account of the Diseases Most Incident to Children*, 1808).

Chapter 1

Archaeological Pediatrics

	B.C.	
2,000,000	Taung Baby
1,600,000	Turkana Boy
500,000	Evidence of longhouses
100,000	Neanderthal man
40,000	Last ice age begins
28,000	Bering Strait land bridge
20,000	Art of Lascaux, Altamira
7,000	Walled city of Jericho

To begin an examination of the history of child health care, rooting through fossils may seem a fruitless effort. After all, the soft semicartilaginous endoskeleton of a newborn is a poor matrix for fossilization. Therefore, extant prehistorical child specimens are rare. There have been findings of lithopedions,[1] or "stone babies." These are not, in the strictest sense, fossils but examples of an exceedingly uncommon phenomenon of fetal calcification either in utero or ectopically (figure 1.1). This occurrence probably is mediated by aberrant lymphocytes that produce excessive bone morphogenic protein, as can be observed in a rare disease called fibrodysplasia ossificans progressiva,[2] in which a child's injured soft tissues turn into bone.*

---

*A lithopedion described in 1853 strongly suggests this mechanism of calcification: ". . . a post mortem examination was held . . . on the body of the widow of Amos Eddy . . . age 77 years, and to the utter astonishment of all present, a full-grown child was found, which she had carried for the term of 46 years. It was encased in a sort of bony or cartilaginous structure, except for one leg and foot, and one elbow, which were almost entirely ossified" (Bernard, 1947, p. 377).

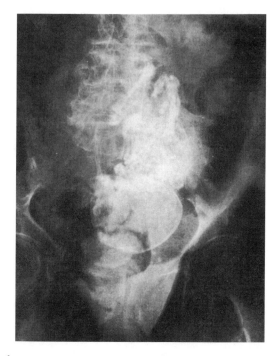

Figure 1.1 A lithopedion (*Lancet* 1995; 345:757).

A study of child health in prehistory assumes that care and nurture were qualities of life. The notion is challenged vigorously by some scholars, despite evidence to support this position.[3] Utilizing paleopathology methods on fossil records yields diagnoses of conditions in which survival would have been inconceivable without parental or community support. The archaeological finds of burial sites laden with artifacts of a caring and symbolic internment, suggesting mourning and loss, also bespeak care, lending additional weight to this theory.

There are, all the same, only a few prehistorical pediatric records. Anatomically normal remains tell us nearly as much as abnormal ones. Of the former, there are the "Taung baby," the "First Family," and the "Turkana boy." All of these are remains of apparently healthy children who likely met a sudden traumatic demise. The skull of the Taung baby is that of a three-year-old *Australopithecus* (figure 1.2) found in 1924 in South Africa, the site then called Bechuanaland. Cast in limestone, it was in a remarkable state of preservation, showing a full set of deciduous teeth and an erupting second molar. It was deposited with bones and detritus of bats, rats, tortoises, and crabs, suggesting that some 5 to 2 million years ago, this baby was snatched into the air by a flying bird of prey and taken to the bird's lair for consumption.[4]

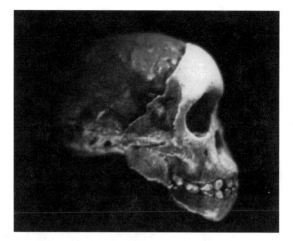

Figure 1.2 Head of the Taung baby, a three-year-old *Australopithecus*. Note the well-preserved endocast of the brain vault revealing vascular and commissure structures. COURTESY DEPARTMENT OF LIBRARY SERVICES, AMERICAN MUSEUM OF NATURAL HISTORY.

The First Family find consisted of thirteen members in a cluster—four of them under five years of age—who apparently died suddenly, en masse, in one catastrophic event. They may have been huddled together seeking shelter from a storm, and were engulfed by a flash flood.[5] We cannot be certain, but there do not appear to be carnivore marks on the bones or evidence of trampling or of diseased bone.

The Turkana boy is a much more complete record of a 12-year-old *Homo erectus* (figure 1.3) with all the physical characteristics of a healthy, growing preadolescent. How he died remains an unanswered question, but there was no evidence of obvious trauma, poor nutrition, or disease.

None of these specimens reveals traces of articulation defects, infection, or fractures. They all showed normal growth plates and fusion lines. By implication all these children were cared for and nourished and functioned in a biological unit. They are early hominid specimens, but there are several ancient *Homo sapiens* and Neanderthal burial finds of children that also reveal clues to us about age of death, nutrition, disease, and care. Moreover, burial sites often display traces of vermilion or mercuric sulfide, both of which serve as bone preservatives.[6] They are further evidence of careful interment.

Abnormal fossil records, such as those with congenital malformations, afford an opportunity to speculate on epidemiology and frequency of occurrence, as well as on care. Newborn records are exceedingly rare in general. The fact that specimens have been found of older children, even adults, with malformations suggests two scenarios: the defect was not life-threatening or

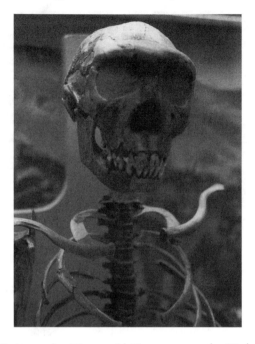

Figure 1.3 Skeleton of a 12-year-old *Homo erectus*, the "Turkana boy" found in Kenya. COURTESY NATIONAL GEOGRAPHIC SOCIETY EXPLORERS HALL, WASHINGTON, DC.

the newborn or child received care and attention from a social unit or community, perhaps in the guise of a healer, shaman, *curandero*, or village herbalist. Given the fact that early mortality was so commonplace, finding congenital lesions in toddlers, latent children, and even adolescent specimens bolsters the hypothesis that nurturing care took place. An examination of 173 upper Paleolithic period specimens, gathered from various regions (Europe, Africa, Asia, and Middle East), revealed that, based on bone age at death, 68 percent died under the age of one year. Only three fossil records were older than 50 years.[7]

About 40 percent of congenital malformations are skeletal and therefore can be identified readily in bony records. The remaining 60 percent are soft-tissue lesions, some of which produced recognizable secondary osseous defects allowing for diagnosis. Others can be found in late prehistorical mummified specimens, where soft tissues have "survived." Some we come to recognize from depictions rather than actual specimens; other conditions we recognize from combined sources.

An example of the latter is achondroplasia. The dwarf, or achondroplastic, is a victim of a dominantly inherited gene in which the long bones grow abnormally while the skull, face, and a few small bones generally proceed

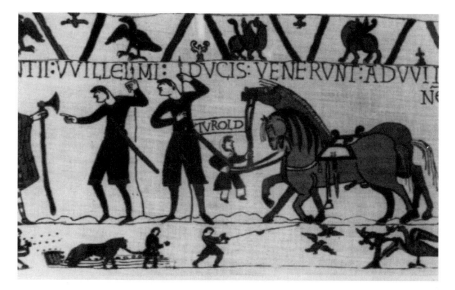

Figure 1.4 Turold in the Bayeux tapestry (Fowke, 1898, plate II).

normally. The incidence is about 1 per 25,000 births, and in the nonthana-tropic variety, survival is common—unless infanticide or abandonment claims its victims. In the first year of life, common heart and lung failure, secondary to the small chest cavity, are threatening. After the first year, survival and maturation generally can be anticipated. The common existence of both prehistoric and historic records of dwarfs attests to, at the very least, community support in the first year of life.

There are extant prehistorical specimens from Paleolithic Italy, predynastic Egypt, and Neolithic England and North America.[8] The child dwarf may have been the recipient of special care and privilege in many cultures, as evidenced by the many artistic representations of adults. The Egyptian god Phtha, or Bes, was depicted as a dwarf, and dwarfs and their families were rendered in funerary statuary. In recorded history, the Roman emperors[9] Tiberus, Alexander, Severus, and Mark Antony had achondroplastic advisers and augurers, as did William of Normandy, whose dwarf Turold (figure 1.4) was depicted in the Bayeux tapestry.[10] The French king Charles IX received a gift of nine dwarfs from the Polish monarchy.

Of other congenital bony disease, two diagnoses of lethal infirmities have been made from bone remnants: an Egyptian XXI Dynasty infant with osteogenesis imperfecta and an anencephalic mummy from Hermopolis.[11] Osteogenesis imperfecta is characterized by abnormal bone formation leading to fragile, brittle bones that break and distort with facile frequency, resulting in a malformed, "bestial" torso. The anencephalic infant is born without a brain and cranial vault, a lesion obviously incompatible with life. Today the child with osteogenesis imperfecta can survive into adulthood with continuous medical attention, but it is conceivable that in pre- and late history, both these conditions resulted in infanticide. The anencephalic in later cultures represented the archetypical demon's child—the changeling—and would have been particularly vulnerable to infanticide. It is not unreasonable to speculate that that would have been the case in the prehistoric world.

Spina bifida is a bony lesion of the lower spine in which there is incomplete fusion of the vertebral bodies, resulting in a cleft. The more severe forms leave the spinal cord exposed and subject to fatal infections, but the milder forms may be undetectable and consequently are called spina bifida occulta. The child of antiquity born with overt spina bifida (cystica) would have died shortly after birth, from catastrophic meningitis or infanticide. The occulta form, however, generally is compatible with a normal life span. The many extant bony records of spina bifida in prehistory and antiquity indicate these children grew up, along with their siblings, as part of their households.

There are other bony defects recorded in burial specimens that insinuate that they received attention, defects that in themselves are not life-threatening but require parental and communal support and care. Club foot, congenital hip dislocations, scoliosis, and cleft palate are all examples of these congenital skeletal anomalies. *Primary* abnormalities, they are obvious on examination of the archaeological record.

There is a category of bony abnormalities and nutritional consequences that is *acquired*. Some *soft-tissue congenital* malformations result in *secondary* recognizable bony anomalies. Hydrocephalus is an extraordinary and dramatic example. The brain of the hydrocephalic child is enlarged by fluid-containing spaces or ventricles, with increased pressure. The brain rapidly enlarges, causing the entire cranial vault to grow. The head becomes disproportionately big and occasionally grotesque. The defect is immediately evident in a skeleton. Hydrocephalus is more commonly an acquired lesion that generally occurs in the first six months of life. Most cases spontaneously arrest in progress between 9 and 24 months, but the child requires continued special attention. Most examined specimens are from the first millennium. One recent find, however, dates to approximately 2500 B.C. It shows anomalous femoral development suggestive of palsy.[12]

Down's syndrome, a common chromosomal trisomy defect, produces a universally characteristic facial appearance regardless of the child's ethnic extraction. The skull assumes a relative shortening, with flattened occiput by the time of latency, and therefore is not recognizable in archaeological studies of infant remains. The remains of older children with this condition have been identified—in my view, implying nurture. The same conclusion is derived with respect to cretinism or newborn hypothyroidism. Many records, mostly European, of all these have survived.

Blood, too, can run anomalously. Abnormal red cell lines associated with hemolytic anemias in time can mark the bones, leading to porotic hyperostosis, or enlarged, porous trabeculated bones. Many examples have been identified in Neolithic specimens.[13] Digital clubbing, or hypertrophic osteoarthropathy, is often referred to as "drumstick fingers" because of the peculiar appearance of the ends of the fingers. It is generally associated with diseases that result in chronic hypoxia, such as chronic lung or heart disease. The process leaves recognizable bony remodeling, evident in several Meso-American specimens from as early as 2000 B.C.[14]

There are *acquired soft-tissue* conditions that also leave a diagnosable bony lesion. These can be infectious in nature, such as mastoiditis, or nutritional, such as rickets. In mastoiditis a purulent middle ear infection erodes into the air pockets of the mastoid skull just behind the ear. The resulting infection is commonly fatal if it extends into the brain or does not drain exteriorly. Many specimens are known. Other infections that have left bony landmarks include syphilis, with osteomyelitic "sabre shin," along with dental anomalies of notched incisors and multicrowned molars, leprous sinusitis and digital loss,[15] and tuberculosis with spinal Pott's disease. One recent study actually documented *Mycobacterium tuberculosis* infection in a 12-year-old pre-Columbian female through DNA typing from vertebral material.[16]

A final category of soft-tissue infections can be identified in desiccated tissues, mummified either through geoclimatic preservation or through controlled mummification. These include pneumonias, appendicitis, parasitoses, and even smallpox. One particular Egyptian mummy of a ten-year-old boy revealed infection with trichuris, ascaris, and schistosoma.

Of the nutritional defects, rickets is the most readily recognizable. Rickets commonly results from a lack of vitamin D, generally due to combined dietary and sun-exposure deficiencies. (Sunrays convert skin ergosterol into vitamin D.) Paleolithic findings from Meso-America, Egypt, and other sunny lands reveal no records of rickets—but Neolithic northern European specimens abound. The disease leads to bent or deformed bones; a classic example is evident from burials at St. Helens on the Wall (figure 1.5). Another nutritional deficiency, scurvy, results from a lack of vitamin C. Bones are surrounded with a membrane called the periosteum, and vitamin C deficiency results in bleeding under this membrane. Subperiosteal hemorrhages lead to new bone formation in any bone but particularly around the orbits and jaws. This bony reaction to bleeding has been identified in several pediatric specimens both in the Americas and in Europe.[17] Iron deficiency anemia is

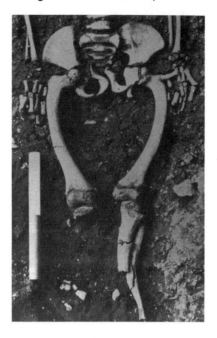

Figure 1.5 Skeleton of a child with rickets, showing severe femoral bowing.
COURTESY YORK ARCHAEOLOGICAL TRUST FOR EXCAVATION AND RESEARCH LTD.

hypothesized to be the cause of cribra orbitalia or small apertures in a bony plate above the eye sockets[18] evident in skulls ranging in age from 6 months to 12 years. This appears to be a transient hyperostosis phenomenon and in the same milieu; those surviving beyond 20 years of age show no evidence of disease.[19]

Childhood malnutrition during periods of famine also can be assessed by studying Harris lines—radiological lines of arrested growth evident as transverse densities in the long bones.[20] Harris lines occur only during growth and therefore are particularly valuable for the study of children. Additionally, enamel hypoplasia or dysplasia evident in tooth records can contribute to the study of prehistoric child health. The majority of enamel defects occur at weaning time and will be variable depending on cultural elements[21] or periods of famine. A study of middle Pleistocene hominids found that hypoplasia was most commonly evident in the canines of one- to seven-year-olds with a frequency of 40 percent.[22]

One final prehistoric product aiding the study of disease is the coprolite, or fossilized feces. Analysis of these biological remnants reveals evidence of fibers, seeds, pollen, and even parasite eggs, enabling us to learn about seasonal migration patterns as well as eating and living habits. Speculation on nutrition is possible, depending on fiber and seed content and on health depending on a parasitic load. For example, Southwest Native American coprolitic analyses reveal a pattern of parasitic infections that indicates that hunter–gatherer groups had fewer infections than agricultural groups had. This is consistent with the common fecal-oral contamination cycles of most intestinal parasites.[23]

In summary, there is evidence of congenital and acquired childhood diseases in prehistory, including bony and soft-tissues lesions, as well as metabolic, infectious, and nutritional processes involving many organ systems. There is, of course, no direct evidence of children's doctoring, but strong inference for care and attention is assumed.

NOTES

1. The oldest known extant specimen is from the American Southwest and is about 3,100 years old. *Am J Obstet Gynecol* 1993; 169:140–41.
2. Roush, 1996, p. 1170.
3. Dettwyler, 1991, pp. 875–84.
4. Holden, 1995, p. 1675.
5. Johanson and Edey, 1981, pp. 213–16.
6. Martin-Gil, 1995, pp. 759–61.
7. Janssens, 1970, pp. 60–63.
8. Roberts and Manchester, 1995, p. 33.
9. Warkany, 1971, p. 771.
10. Denny and Filmer-Sankey, 1966, p. 12.
11. Roberts and Manchester, 1995, pp. 34–35.
12. Richards and Anton, 1991, pp. 185–200.
13. Hershkovitz et al., 1991, pp. 7–13.
14. Martinez-Lavin et al., 1994, pp. 238–41.
15. Boocock et al., 1995, pp. 483–95.
16. Arriaza et al., 1995, pp. 37–45.
17. Soren, 1995, pp. 13–42.
18. Cribra orbitalia of Welcher are small apertures in the lamina cribosa ossis ethmoidalis that render a porotic appearance and are thought to channel veins from the diploë to the orbit.
19. Mittler and Van Gerven, 1994, pp. 287–97.
20. Wells, 1967, pp. 390–404.
21. Roberts and Manchester, 1995, pp. 133–34.
22. Bermudez de Castro and Perez, 1995, pp. 301–14.
23. Reinhard et al., 1987, pp. 630–39.

Chapter 2

Ancient Pediatrics

Fossils, bones, and funerary artifacts provide evidence for social anthropologists to ponder the evolution of prehistoric communities and physical anthropologists to speculate on health and disease. When written records began to appear, these conjectures ceased.

By all extant evidence, writing initially was conceived for accounting and business purposes and followed the pictographic writing of the ice ages. Accounting tokens first appeared in the Mesopotamian valley about 8000 B.C., followed by Sumerian clay tablets (3300 B.C.), Egyptian hieroglyphics (3100 B.C.), Indus script (2500 B.C.), and linear A (1800 B.C.).[1] Such a useful tool as writing ultimately was deemed to have better uses, so symbols gradually evolved that expressed thoughts and ideas. Prayers to multiple gods, letters to countless lords and masters, titles accorded personages, records of achievements, and epitaphs for all manner of folks came first, then the "texts"—and among them a corpus of works dedicated to recording methods of diagnosis and healing.

With no absolute claims to which came first but simply because a beginning must be made, the medical records of Mesopotamia will be examined first.

MESOPOTAMIA

Mesopotamia, from the Greek, meaning "between the rivers" (Tigris and Euphrates), was located in what is now southeastern Iraq and was one of the four great river civilizations: Egypt and the Nile, the Indus valley and Hindus River, China and the Yellow River were the other three. The Sumerians first settled Mesopotamia sometime near 5000 B.C., followed by the Semites, who founded Assyria and Babylonia around 2300 B.C. "History," it has been said, "begins in Sumer,"[2] no doubt because an early written record of nearly 150,000 clay tablets incised in cuneiform is extant, as is the Babylonian Code of Hammurabi, a set of laws that gives us evidence of a societal attempt to regulate behavior and interactions.

There is evidence in the Code of equitable attention to children and therefore, by inference, to their health. It is known that the Code regulated medical fees for adults,[3] and presumably this was so for children since there are multiple records with prognostications for infants and children. The Code's control of child welfare, however, was partially based on *lex talionis*, which did not always auger kindly for the child, as the following examples show.

192: If a son of a NER.SE.GA, or the son of a devotée, say to his father who has reared him, or his mother who has reared him: "My father thou art not," "My mother thou art not," they shall cut out his tongue.

193: If the son of a NER.SE.GA, or the son of a devotée identify his own father's house and hate the father who has reared him and the mother who has reared him and goes back to his father's house, they shall pluck out his eye.

195: If a son strike his father, they shall cut off his fingers.

(Code of Hammurabi, translation of Harper, 1904)

TABLE 2.1
**SOME OF THE KNOWN MESOPOTAMIAN DEITIES
RESPONSIBLE FOR ILLNESS**[10]

Illness (to)	Demon/God
Neck	Adad
Breast	Ishtar
Throat	Utukku
Chest	Alu
Hand	Gallu
Skin	Rabisu
Epilepsy	Labasu
Newborn	Labartu
Wasting	Ashakku
Fever	T'iu

Medicine in Mesopotamia centered around deities and the *asu** and his pharmacopeia. *Asu* was the term for physician[4] and meant "the man who knows water" implying either divination by water[5] or diagnosis by urinoscopy. Since deities and demons were believed to cause illness, an intermediary called the *ashipu*, a genre of witch doctor or exorciser,[6] worked together with the *asu* to suppress or assuage the supernatural powers responsible for disease and to invoke healing gods. The pantheon of Mesopotamian gods[7] consisted of triads: Anu, the great god of heaven; Enlil, the god of earth; Ea, the god of water; Shamash, the sun god; Sin, the moon god; and Ishtar, the *mater magna* and the mother-goddess (commonly depicted seated, nursing), who nurtured all. Ninib was the god of healing, and his consort was Gula (also known as Bau and Ninisinna).[8] There were also many demons responsible or sickness (table 2.1), among them Labartu, who threatened newborns and was depicted with a serpent in each hand and swine at her breast.[9] Nergal, the demon of pestilence, was presciently depicted in the form of a fly.

Astrological events were considered causative or prognostic, as shown by the following examples from the many divinations:[11]

---

*Herodotus (484–?425 B.C.) contended that the Babylonians had no doctors: "They bring out all their sick into the streets, for they have no regular doctors. People that come along offer the sick man advice . . . no-one is allowed to pass by a sick person without asking what ails him" (I, 199). Herodotus, however, traveled widely and broadly, and most scholars contend that he observed this custom in the countryside, where physicians probably were few.

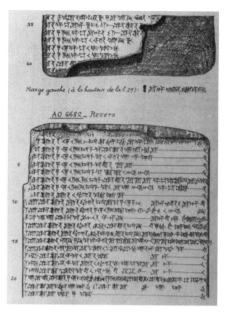

Figure 2.1 Illustration of fragments of the TDP, from Labat (Leiden: Brill, 1951).

If an eclipse of the sun occurs on the twenty-ninth day of the month of Iyyar, there will be many deaths on the first day.

If a halo surrounds the moon and if Regulus stands within, women will bear male children.

Our knowledge of Mesopotamian medicine stems from a number of tablets executed over some five hundred years. One tablet from Nippur is dated to about 2200 B.C., but most tablets are Akkadian, originating during the Babylonian era, 1900 to 1600 B.C. They survive primarily as copies from Ashurbanipal's library at Nineveh.[12]

Surviving medical texts fall into two major categories: symptom descriptive and pharmacopoeia, or prescriptive. The aphoristic contents of these texts generally invoke the name of a god after an omen or clinical statement. Sources include the British Museum Assyrian medical text, the Berlin Babylonisch-assyrische Medizin, the Sultantepe tablets at Ankara, the Keilschrifttext, and the Akkadian diagnostic and prognostic tract (TDP) (figure 2.1), which in particular holds our pediatric interest.[13] The French Assyriologist Rene Labat translated and compiled the TDP texts, which include those addressing the child. Both appendix A and the examples that follow are from his translations of the old Akkadian.[14] Five major parts are designated.[15] Part 1 consists of two tablets and contains omens based on signs encountered on the way to examine the patient. For example:

If the ashipu sees either a black dog or pig, the patient will die.

Part 2 has twelve tablets grouping symptoms by organ and body parts.

If his [the patient's] brow is white and his tongue is white, his illness will be long, but he will recover.

If blood flows out of his penis: [it is] hand of Shamash.

Part 3 contains ten tablets and consists of prognostications based on disease duration.

If having been ill 4 days, he keeps putting his hand on his belly and his face is overcast with yellow, he will die.

Part 4 originally had ten tablets but is mostly lost. What remains is very damaged and, in some instances, unintelligible. Part 5, however, has six tablets relating specifically to pregnancy, the newborn, and the child.

A Sumerian woman, safely delivered of a healthy baby, prayed to the midwife Belitile and to Mama, the goddess of the young. Both goddesses were absorbed into Ishtar. Since a higher power had a predestination over a baby, infants were used for divination (along with hepatoscopy and astrology), and their numbers and appearance were frequently recorded as birth omens. Twinning and malformations carried particular significance.

If a woman gives birth to a boy and a girl, ill luck will enter the land, the land will be diminished.

If a woman gives birth to two girls, the house will be destroyed.

If a woman gives birth to three well-developed girls, the land of the ruler will be enlarged.

If a woman gives birth to a child and the right ear is small, the house of the man will be destroyed.

If a woman gives birth to a child and the left ear is small, the house of the man will be enlarged.

If a woman gives birth to a child and both ears are small the house of the man will be overthrown.

While some of the prognostications on pregnancy are simply superstitions, others presciently appear to auger a valid clinical outcome. Some prattle nonsense; others suggest keen observations. Regardless of the nature of the text, the touchpoints are defects of the newborn, survival of the newborn, and the death of both newborn and mother. For example:

If the nipples of a pregnant woman are yellow, that which is within her womb will be miscarried.

If the womb of a pregnant woman lies on her stomach, she will bear a deaf child.

If the womb of a pregnant woman is thrown down upon the right side of her stomach, she has conceived a man-child.

If the pregnant woman keeps vomiting, she will not bring to completion.

If the pregnant woman discharges matter from her mouth, she will die together with that which is within her womb.

A set of Babylonian tablets from the British Museum records congenital malformations of conjoined twins, with references to twins with common internal organs and those sharing thorax (ribs) or spine.[16]

There are over 120 entries of pediatric texts translated by Assyriologist Rene Labat. Many make no clinical sense, but a few seem almost pathognomonic. Most are simplistic and repetitious in description. All blame some demon or god. Although they begin with the intonation, "If a baby," it is clear that some texts refer to toddlers and older children. Many are incomplete and have missing text, denoted here by (. . .). There are entries that invoke the supernatural or serve as omens:

20. If a baby at the mother's breast is always afraid and sick; if crying and fever remain constant, evil prayers [a spell] have seized him.

110. If a baby at 1 or 2 months, while nursing, has a fit and his hands and feet are spastic: hand of god . . . at his feet, either his father or his mother will die.

111. If a baby has a fit, the kind with spastic hands and feet, and his eyes are fogged with tears: at his feet, the house of his father shall collapse.

Some offer practical and useful advice, such as changing the wet nurse or medicating the breast as a means of delivering medicine to the baby.

36. If a baby, while nursing, his flesh becomes flabby, even though his wet-nurse has milk, when offered the breast does not eat [suck]; if he rejects the breast change to the other for his healing [get a new wet nurse].

39. If a baby suffers from cough, grind and mix im-kal-gug with honey and fine fat [light oil]; the baby will absorb it in fasting; if he will not take it himself, place it on the mother's nipple and he will take it at the same time he nurses: thus, he will recover.

Some, predicting prognoses, give thorough descriptions that enable the modern clinician to speculate on specific diagnoses.

10. If a baby has a hot head, if his body is not feverish . . . he does not sweat, hand and feet do not move, if he drools, cries a lot, keeps no food down and vomits: if his teeth fall out; after 15 or 20 days he will experience a painful period and will be prostrated.

The clinical symptoms of a child who is irritable, with bone or joint pain, mouth sores, gum inflammation, gastric distress, and a prolonged illness and debilitation suggest a generalized, infectious vasculitis. A differential diagnosis of scurvy might be considered.

45. If a baby . . . his head is loose the kind of which the skull is dilated; he will die.

This is probably hydrocephalus.

48. If a baby vomits all he eats, if he has diarrhea, if his hands and feet are paralyzed: you shall petition Sin.

Could this be enteric poliomyelitis?

62. If a baby extends his thumb, his abdomen, his hands and does not stop laughing, if his flesh has a disease [rash]: he shall know the flaccidity of flesh and die.

Is this child posturing or opisthotonic with risus sardonicus and mottled hemorrhagic skin? Does he have meningococcemia?

63. If a baby, his intestines are always full [constipated] and his eyes drowsy: hand of god; he will recover.

Does this baby have botulism?

96. If a baby, his bowels are blocked and his body is yellow, he has been seized by the bad smell; Hand of Gula.

Was this sepsis or perhaps cholestatic necrotizing enterocolitis, jaundice with gangrene of the bowel?

These few examples indicate the general flavor of the Akkadian texts. Labat's entire translation from the cuneiform of the pediatric texts appears in appendix A.

Several pharmacopoeia or prescriptive texts date back to before 2200 B.C. and deal with ingredients and methods of delivery. Topical applications (poultice, bathing) or systemic compounds (potions, enemas, inhalation) were employed, consisting of herbs, plants, minerals, oil, and salt, and often mixed with milk or beer for imbibition.[17] Some, such as the following Sumerian example, employed agents with known pharmacologic activity. Unfortunately, the prescription carried no indications and what "nignagar" was remains a puzzle. "Pulverize the seeds of the *nignagar*-vegetable, myrrh, and thyme; put in beer, let the man drink."[18]

Both frankincense and myrrh are aromatic conifer products, resins collected from scattered, uncultivated trees that grow in Somalia and the Arabian peninsula. They have been used for millennia to treat a wide array of ailments.[19] The Ebers papyrus (c.1500 B.C.) recommended frankincense for wounds, the Syriac Book of Medicine (c.400 A.D.) suggested its use for colic, and Avicenna used it to treat urinary tract infections. Myrrh's antibiotic effects recommended its use in cough mixtures, antidiarrheals, antifungals, and on fresh-cut umbilical cords (see Louffenburg's *Ein Regiment*). Its anesthetic effects also helped to soothe sore throats. The seventeenth-century herbalist Nicholas Culpeper employed it to treat stomach ulcers, and today some cultures still use it as a cough remedy. The Hebrews believed that, when mixed with wine, myrrh numbed all pain. In the New Testament of the Bible, Christ was offered this mixture at his crucifixion.[20]

Thyme provides an aromatic antiseptic and antibacterial called thymol. Today it still is used in common cold preparations and as a meat preservative. The alcohol in the beer vehicle, presumably somewhere between 2 to 5 percent by volume, served as a diuretic.

Babylonian texts describe the standard fees of some surgical procedures, primarily abscess drainage. There is no evidence that surgery was done on children, and circumcision was not part of the Mesopotamian culture.[21] The texts clearly address dysentery and liver abscess (both amebic?), tuberculosis (pulmonary and meningitic), epilepsy, gangrene, and even heartburn or gastroesophageal reflux:

If a man's stomach is greatly distended and he regularly returns food and drink through his mouth, he must overcome the condition by his own efforts. . . . Cakes of finely-ground flour he should bake, and these he should eat frequently without honey, fats or leban. Every three days he should not eat onions, garlic, dill seeds, cress seed and aniseed; also he should not bathe. So he will recover.[22]

In addition to the medical tablets, there are letters that provide insights into the care of children. Letters from the Babylonian province of Mari frequently made references to physicians and special requests being made. One particular letter, sent around 1800 B.C. to the king of Mari on the Euphrates says:

To my Lord say this: thus speaks I Aquim-Addu, thy servant. A child who is with me is ill. From beneath his ear, an abscess is discharging . . . would my Lord, dispatch his physician to me . . . or an expert physician, that he may examine the disease of the child, and treat him.[23]

Whether this was otitis media, mastoiditis, or scrofula is not as noteworthy as the care and concern evoked by the letter.

Letters from Nippur suggest that it was a busy clinical center:[24]

Your servant Mukallim: I am ready to die for my Lord.

The daughter of Ayaru was feeling well during the first watch of the night and fell asleep after midnight. . . . Nobody has touched the dressing which they always put on her at night. . . . Although she was feeling very well before, she does not feel well now. I shall try to learn more about the situation, will see [how she feels] and then send my messenger.

Mukallim wrote the following epistle as well. It suggests endemic leishmaniasis or tuberculosis:

Your servant Mukallim: I am ready to die for my Lord. The same disease has now affected the girl Etirtu.

The daughters of Kuru and of Ahuni are fine, their health is good. Should my lord so order, they can both leave and attend school again.

The abscesses of the daughter of Mustalu are healed. She does not cough any more. . . . The abscess of the daughter of Ili-ippasra, which persisted, has now formed a scab, and her nostril has become better.

The . . . nape of the neck of the woman Bitti hurts her. . . . The abscesses on the ribs of the daughter of the woman Babati persist, and she is also coughing.[25]

Letters from the *asu* Arad Nana (c.675 B.C.) in Nineveh relate the progress made in treating a child with difficult epistaxis:

Hearty greetings to the King's son. The treatment which we prescribed for him is to be given every two-thirds of a double hour during the day.

In regard to the bleeding of his nose . . . there was much bleeding, those dressings are not properly applied; they have been placed upon the alae of the nose, obstructing the breathing, while at the same time the blood flows into the mouth. Let the nose be plugged up to the back so that air will be held off and the bleeding will cease.[26]

In ending this short review of Mesopotamian medicine, it is evident that although infants and children were for the most part addressed *in passim*, they did feature in the corpus of general medical care. The awareness of their value to their society as the "heritage of the future" is reflected best, however, in a curse directed at the city of Agade (c.2300 B.C.) by the gods of the Sumerian pantheon:

You butchered sheep—may you butcher your children instead.
Your poor—may they be forced to drown their precious children.[27]

EGYPT

Whereas the historian Herodotus claims the Mesopotamians had no doctors, he is on record about various medical specialties of the Egyptian physician, or *swnw*:

The practice of medicine they split up into separate parts, each doctor being responsible for the treatment of only one disease. There are, in consequence, innumerable doctors, some specializing in diseases of the eyes, others of the head, others of the teeth, others of the stomach, and so on; while others, again, deal with the sort of troubles which cannot be exactly localized.[28]

There appears to have been no swnw dedicated to children, but the Egyptian pantheon of healing deities (table 2.2) included gods that rallied to children's causes. Meskhenit appeared vigilantly at the child's cradle, and Rannut assured nursing and proper nutrition. Survival, however, was under the control of Seshat, the goddess of numbers, who determined the predestined longevity of each at the moment of birth. Other gods were petitioned in invocations recited each morning while a protective amulet was tied to a child's arm:

The crown of your head is the crown of *Re*, oh my sturdy child, the back of your neck is that of *Osiris*, your forehead is the forehead of *Satis*, ruler of Elephantine, your hair is the hair of *Neith*, your eyebrows are those of the Mistress of the East, your eyes are the eyes of the Lord of the Universe, your nose is the nose of the

TABLE 2.2
SOME OF THE KNOWN EGYPTIAN GODS OF HEALING

Eye diseases	Thoth
Childbirth	Neith
Near-death	Isis
All illness	Ra
Epidemics	Seth
Gynecology	Sechmet

Teacher of the Gods, your ears are the ears of the Two Cobras, your forearms are those of the Falcon, one of your shoulders is the shoulder of *Horus* and the other belongs to *Seth.*[29]

There are several references pertaining to the healing of children—magical treatments, for the most part. Swarms of mice appeared after the annual Nile floods and were believed to generate spontaneously from the deposited silt. Mice became an Egyptian symbol of life. A life-giving mouse was used to insufflate breath back into a dying child. Mouse bones were placed in a little bag, tied with seven knots, and placed around an infant's neck as an amulet.[30] One formula prescribed that a mother consume a mouse before nursing her baby. Evidence of skinned mice also have been found in the stomachs of children buried in the early Nagada cemetery epoch (4500–3100 B.C.).[31]

Some cures employed charms coupled with recitations. A string of three beads—lapis lazuli, jasper, and malachite—was hung around a newborn's neck with the following incantation: "The voice of the *Re* calls for the wpt, because the stomach of this infant whom *Isis* has borne, is sick."[32]

Most references are pharmacological, as in the Ebers papyrus. It was copied around 1550 B.C. in hieratic script. Several elements can be dated back to 3400 B.C. The Ebers is one of three surviving principal papyri pertaining to medicine. It was found in a tomb in Thebes together with the so-called Edwin Smith papyrus, which referred mostly to surgery and broken bones. The third, the Kahun papyrus, contains gynecological data. Several minor medical papyri also have been found (table 2.3), of which only one, the Erman papyrus (c.1600 B.C.) specifically touches on the subject of children, childbirth and infants (figure 2.2). This document consists entirely of

TABLE 2.3
EGYPTIAN MEDICAL PAPYRI[33]

Name	Date B.C.	Contents
Kahun	1900	women's diseases, pregnancy
Smith	1600	surgical
Ebers	1550	medical
Hearst	1550	prescriptive
Erman	1550	childbirth, infants, children
London	1350	prescriptive
Berlin	1350	prescriptive and pregnancy
Beatty	1200	proctologic

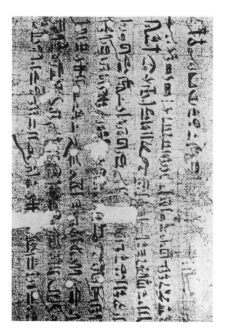

Figure 2.2 Fragments of the Erman papyrus (Berlin: Preuss Akademie der Wissenschaften, 1901).

incantations invoking gods to promote the health of the child (such as the two prayers listed above).

The materia medica of the Ebers document consist of a pharmacopoeia melange of herbal elements, incantations, and superstitions. There are a few curious entries that apply to children. Under the category "Diseases of Women" one prognostication ominously states:

> At birth if a child cries *ni*, it will live.
> If a child cries *ba*, it will die.[34]

What reactions this prediction elicited can only be imagined. Did the parents abandon a child who cried *ba*, or did they merely delay naming the child, fearfully awaiting a fatal outcome? Another omen found in a Ramesseum fragment offers a prognostic recipe: "Give a piece of its placenta rubbed in milk; if it vomits, it will die."[35]

The Egyptians considered maternal milk pharmacological and omnipotent as well as the basis of nutrition. One prescription reflects a method to increase breast milk supply: "To get a supply of milk in a woman's breast for suckling a child: warm the bones and fins of a Xra-fish (Nile perch) in oil and rub her back with it."[36]

Maternal milk to be used as remedies was stored in jars shaped like Isis suckling Horus. If it was the milk of a mother who had borne a male, it was considered particularly potent and was used to treat colic and eye infections.[37] Some cultures even today apply two drops of freshly expressed milk into each eye four times a day to treat uncomplicated conjunctivitis.[38]

A remedy cited to relieve a colicky baby would have appealed to sleep-deprived parents despite the apparent contradiction of the remedy's claim of instant relief that took four days to effect:

> Pods of the poppy plant
> Fly dirt which is on the wall
> Make into one, strain, and take for four days
> It acts at once![39]

The use of the poppy, from which morphine and heroin are derived, would have provided relief from the painful cramps experienced by babies with colic, and fly dung may have acted as an emulsifier.

Worthy of note is the following recipe for breasts sore from nursing, a combination of both the sound and the curious:

> Calamine, gall of ox, fly's dirt, yellow ochre. Mix together, and rub the breast therewith for four days.[40]

The ox bile made the compound miscible. The ointment contained two active ingredients: zinc (calamine) and iron (ochre). The fly's dirt and the prescription of four days' use may have been the touches of magic or *Dreckapotheke* the ancients relied on. (*Dreckapotheke* called for ingesting or applying foul and disgusting substances to repel evil spirits. Dung of various species was commonly compounded into prescriptions.)

Microscopic examinations of Egyptian child mummies reveal that children commonly suffered from the *heft*worm (*Ascaris*, or the common round worm), *pend*worm (the flatworm, *Taenia*), and probably a form of parasitic anemia attributable to hookworm, or *Ancylostoma*, called *uha* disease, marked by painful body swelling or anasarca (*uxedu*). An infusion made from the bark and roots of the pomegranate was used as a vermifuge.[41] Other documented parasites include schistosoma (*aaa* disease?), *sa*worm (filariasis), and amebiasis.[42] Nonparasitic infective diseases included granular conjunctivitis or trachoma, which today still is prevalent in Egypt and the Levant as a major cause of blindness. Polio is assumed to have been present based on an Eighteenth dynasty stele that now resides in the Carlsberg Ny Glyptothek in Copenhagen. The stone depicts a man with a withered right leg.

There was an eczema-like skin ailment (*neshu*). Toothache was blamed on the *fenet*worm, which reached under the teeth by way of the *metw* and gnawed at the tooth.[43] In fact, most toothache probably was due to the grinding of teeth down to the pulp. The windblown silica sand of the desert was ubiquitous, and silica was used by flour grinders. Inevitably, silica would be in the flour used for bread making and for cooking in general.[44] Dental skeletal records from ancient Egypt reveal this bruxism to have been widespread.

Tonsilar infections and lymphadenopathy were treated with poultices. Interestingly, analyses of bones from neighbors to the south, the Sudanese Nubia, show tetracycline fluorescence at levels that suggest therapeutic intent. Grain products contaminated with *Streptomyces*, a moldlike bacterium that produces tetracycline and comprises nearly 70 percent of the bacterial flora of the Sudanese desert would have been the source.[45] It is reasonable to assume that the Nubians discovered the therapeutic value of consuming these grains during febrile periods. Perhaps the Egyptians accomplished the same ends with *ht-w3*, or moldy "rotten wood" that was ground into a formulary.[46]

The Ebers papyrus had several entries promoting diuresis in children. The number of references is remarkable since this generally is an uncommon medical need in children. At first glance one dismisses one diuretic prescription as mere superstition:

An old book cooked in oil
Smear it on his body.[47]

On second look, however, a micturition action would have occurred, stimulated by the lead in ink made from red oxide lead and honey that was used for writing on papyri—the "old books." The lead mixed with oil would have been absorbed by the skin, possibly poisoning the proximal kidney tubules. Presumably, a child so treated urinated excessive phosphorus, glucose, amino acids, and water (Fanconi syndrome?). If the speculation on how the remedy worked is accurate, with lead poisoning the mechanism, then the child also would have developed anemia in the process, and possibly encephalopathy and high blood pressure.

Other diuretics were less challenging to the body. The following prescription has a touch of whimsy but owes its efficacy to the alcohol content of the concoction:

Blossom plucked from the nebat plant mixed in sweet beer. A girl should drink it from a cool flask, a boy should drink it from a henna-vessel [0.465-liter capacity].[48]

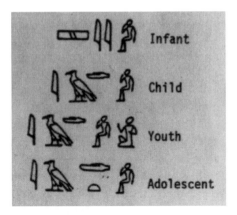

Figure 2.3 Hieroglyphics of children: infant, toddler, child, adolescent.
DRAWING BY AUTHOR.

Another reveals an intuitive understanding of how breast milk transports ingested and imbibed substances to the infant during nursing:

Xentgrain pills given to the child with his nourishment or the wet-nurse who must nurse the baby for four days or the nurse warm it in her mouth and spurt it into the child's mouth.[49]

The entries suggested a dosage schedule in treating children of different sizes as well as different methods of drug delivery. There are separate hieroglyphics for infant, toddler, child, and adolescent (figure 2.3).

In the pharmacopeia of ancient Egypt there were nearly 700 items devoted to defecation and micturition. This seeming preoccupation with diuretics and cathartics was grounded partially in the endemic presence of schistosomiasis in the Nile basin and was a feature in the treatment of true organic disease. It also responded to the belief that a fecal contaminant called *ukhedu* or *whdw* should be eliminated from the body.[50]

Whdw was thought to be carried and spread through vessels, or *metw*, which coursed through and around vital organs, including the anus and bladder, carrying blood, air, urine, feces, and tears.[51] The ancients considered *whdw* to be an etiologic or causative agent that adhered to feces, precipitating rot. They feared that, if it was absorbed by the gut, it would cause coagulation followed by suppuration and putrefaction. The Egyptians treated all prodromal stages of disease with purgatives and diuretics, since urine and *whdw* were blamed for putrefaction in the bladder and bowel. The number of diuretics specifically suggested for the treatment of children indicates that the ancients may have believed that the young were particularly sensitive to *whdw*. Embalmers, too, feared the destructive properties of *whdw* on the body. To further retard the body's deterioration, therefore, Egyptian mummifiers began their work with rectal disembowelment and dissection, thereby removing first the *whdw* toxin.

Schistosoma is a water-borne parasite that produces liver and bladder scarring, or fibrosis. Pathological examination of mummies have documented the infestation in ancient times. A recent study, using sensitive immunological tests, confirms the diagnosis of schistosomiasis in tissues of an adolescent male weaver—Nakht, from Thebes (1198–1150 B.C.)—and an unnamed predynastic adolescent (3200 B.C.).[52] Other studies have documented the infection in children as young as one to two years.[53] One, that of a fifteen-year-old male mummy (c.1200 B.C.), is a textbook case of the number of diseases, including intestinal and liver schistosomiasis with cirrhosis, that led to an early demise among the Egyptians. This unfortunate boy, in addition to the diseases mentioned, was afflicted with pulmonary anthracosis (deposits of inhaled black pigment hydrocarbons from polluted air), the common roundworm, *Ascaris*; *Taenia* flatworm from eating measly meats; and *Trichinella* from eating pork. Pork was a totem animal of the great god Osiris and was forbidden throughout the year. On the feast of Osiris, however, this prohibition was lifted for rich and poor alike.

Another remarkable aspect of this mummy is that x-rays revealed the presence of Harris lines in the tibia,[54] indicative of periods of malnutrition. It therefore can be assumed that even the affluent suffered nutritionally when the Nile overflowed, destroying crops. Whether early death resulted from disease or malnutrition, the life expectancy in ancient Egypt was a mere 36 years.

The Erman papyrus, as mentioned, is the only extant text that mentions children and is a psalter of incantations invoking healing gods and exhorting demons to depart. An example follows, and the entire text of the Erman appears in appendix B.

Depart you demon who comes in the dark, . . . who has his nose backwards and face turned missing that for which he came.

Depart you demoness who comes in the dark, . . . who has her nose backwards and face turned missing that for which she came.

Came to kiss the child? I will not allow it.

Came to calm him? I will not allow it.

Came to injure him? I will not allow it.

Came to take him away? I will not allow it.

I have prepared protection against you made of *fzt* herb that makes . . ., of garlic that harms you, of honey that is sweet for humans but terrible for the dead, of the zbdw fish, of the jaw of the . . ., of the back of the Nile perch.[55]

HEBREWS

Unlike Mesopotamia and Egypt, which produced tracts on the medical treatment of infants and children, the Hebrews left no medical texts of any kind. A knowledge of ancient Hebraic medicine derives almost exclusively from the Torah and the Talmud. The first five books of the Old Testament, Genesis, Exodus, Leviticus, Numbers, and Deuteronomy, often called the Pentateuch, constitute the Books of Moses—the Torah. The Talmud consists of 63 tractates of rabbinic opinions and interpretations of the Torah.

There are two Talmuds. The first part of the Babylonian Talmud was redacted and written in the second century and was completed by the fifth century after the time of Christ. It is considered the most authoritative. The Jerusalem Talmud was completed earlier but is less extensive. The traditions of the Talmud, the Mishnah, began to accumulate after the Babylonian captivity (536 B.C.), and the interpretations and commentaries or post-Mishnaic teachings, the Gemara, followed. Together they provide the major sources of ancient Jewish pediatrics.

The Sumerians and Egyptians blamed all illness on malevolent beings and produced texts liberally dotted with recipes for cures by exorcism of demons. The Hebrews attributed most misfortune to the wrath of God and at the same time keenly were aware of man's contribution to human misery. Few early civilizations matched the hygienic public health concerns of the land of Israel. Epidemics in communities were announced by a trumpet blast from the *shofar*.[56] Hand washing was repeatedly emphasized (Berakoth 47b, 53b; Sotah 4b; Shabbath 108b), even in solemn prayer:

Blessed art Thou, O Lord our God, King of the Universe, Who hast sanctified us by Thy commandments and commanded us concerning the washing of the hands. (Berakoth 60b)

Environmental cleanliness was considered an essential element for community health:

A permanent threshing-floor may not be erected within fifty cubits of a city. The place for depositing carcasses, a cemetery, and a tannery may not be erected within fifty cubits of a city. (Baba Bathra 2:8f.)

Children were instructed to eat slowly and chew food well (Shabbat 152a). Neither meat nor wine were recommended for them (Hulin 84a), and breakfast was exalted as the most significant meal of the day (Pesachim 112a).

It was forbidden to keep foods uncovered at night for fear vermin would contaminate it.*

Who eats peeled garlic or peeled onion or shelled eggs or drinks diluted liquors, any of which had been exposed overnight, forfeits his life and his blood is on his own head. (Niddah 17a)

The Arabs had a similar proscription: "When night falls, cover your vessels."[57] Since snakes do not drink heated water (Jerushalmi Terumoth 8:45d), uncovered water was permitted if first boiled. The unrecognized sagacity of this dictum was to destroy all manner of infectious organisms by boiling and therefore sterilizing the water. Drinking from rivers was forbidden to prevent "the water filament" (Abodah Zarah 12b).

The health of the child began in utero, since pregnancy was considered a gift of God. Biblical writers remarkably were aware of the negative effects of alcohol consumption during pregnancy and admonished against imbibing it: "Thou shall conceive and bear a son; and now drink no wine nor strong drink" (Judg. 13:7).

The Old Testament describes a method of parturition similar to the Egyptian custom. Women gave birth with the assistance of midwives in a semi-kneeling position on bricks or stools (Exod. 1:16). Recent excavations from a fourth-century A.D. tomb near Jerusalem uncovered skeletal remains of a 14-year-old girl who died during labor. Analysis of carbonized matter from

---

*The admonition finds validity even today. It is most dramatically illustrated by the story of the Machupo virus that causes Bolivian hemorrhagic fever. In the late 1950s the World Health Organization (WHO) mounted a malaria eradication program, spraying all the straw huts of the Beni region with the insecticide DDT. Shortly thereafter, mortal epidemics of hemorrhagic fever began to appear. Epidemiologists from the Middle America Research Unit (MARU) in Panama, Drs. Karl Johnson, Ron MacKenzie, and Merle Kuns, descended on the region, and Merle Kuns noticed an absence of cats in the region. Villagers commented that cats started to die shortly after the spraying program. The team also learned that the cats used hut walls as scratching posts and, given the cat habit of licking paws, epidemiologists concluded they died of DDT poisoning. Logically, it followed that the absence of this predator of vermin allowed the field mouse population to increase. Kuns therefore hypothesized that the mouse was the carrier-vector of this virus, and he began to examine the quotidian habits of the people and the mouse.

He observed that field laborers, arising early in the morning, ate leftover food from the night before. It was concluded that mice contaminated the uncovered food with urine. Mice that had been trapped were examined, confirming they were carriers of the virus. (Johnson, K. M., Halstead, S. B., Cohen, S. N., *Prog Med Vir* 1967; 9:127–58.)

In a controlled experiment, the village of San Joaquin was divided in half. Mousetraps were set in one half only. Within two weeks, the half with mousetraps had no new cases of the disease.

the abdominal area of the skeleton documented the substance delta-THC or cannabis,[58] an early indication that soporifics were used to ease labor.

The normal newborn was expected to be a little less than a cubit[59] in length (Genesis Rabbah 12:6). After birth, an infant was washed, salted with soda ash, and swaddled. The salt acted as a bacteriostatic astringent. The salting of infants was propagated further by the eminent ancient Roman healers, Galen and Soranus, and adopted by Christians in the baptism ritual. The custom persisted into the seventeenth century. In biblical times it may have had some religious significance, but it seems more likely the custom was equated with cultural superiority from lowly barbaric societies as suggested by the following:

Thy birth and thy nativity is of the land of Canaan; thy father was an Amorite, and thy mother a Hittite. And as for thy nativity, in the day thou wast born thy navel was not cut, neither wast thou washed in water to supple thee; thou wast not salted at all, nor swaddled at all. (Ezek. 16:3–4)

There were recipes for the newborn who suffered distress. One employed heat to warm the body. Another, reminiscent of the Santmeyer reflex,[60] was used for resuscitation.[61] Another resuscitation modality incorporated elements similar to an Egyptian survival ritual that had been assimilated by the Hebrews during their captivity, which called for rubbing the infant with its own placenta.

If an infant cannot suck, his lips are cold. What is the remedy? A vessel of burning coals should be brought and held near his nostrils, so as to heat it; then he will suck. . . .

If an infant does not breathe, he should be fanned with a fan, and he will breathe. . . .

If an infant cannot breathe easily, his mother's after-birth should be brought and rubbed over him, he will breathe easily. (Shabbath, 134a)

Epidemics of diphtheria (*askara*) were treated with an apotropaic diet of lentils and salted water:

Askara is a much dreaded epidemic disease which usually attacks children, is located in the throat, and kills the patient by a painful death from suffocation. (Rabbi Ismael ben R. Jose)[62]

The talmudic texts often intermingled animal and human medicine. Many observations of birth anomalies were based on veterinary observations and comparisons. Congenital esophageal atresia and an anomaly suggestive of tracheoesophageal fistula are known:

If a child's gullet is perforated his mother is unclean, but if his gullet is closed up she is clean. (Niddah 23b)

Membranous imperforate anus and its treatment is clearly defined:

An infant whose anus is not visible should be rubbed with oil and stood in the sun, and where it shows transparent it should be torn crosswise with a barley grain, but not with a metal instrument, because that causes inflammation. (Shabbath 134a)

Suturing of membranes employing ant-mandibles appears in Yebamoth:*

A grain of barley is to be procured wherewith the spot is lacerated. Tallow is rubbed in, and a big ant, procured for the purpose, is allowed to bite in, and its head is severed. (Yebamoth 76a)

Umbilical hernia was treated by bandaging a round object to the navel (Shabbath 66b), a procedure still used by some cultures.

Other congenital anomalies were mentioned, such as head malformations (Bekoroth 43b), scoliosis (Sanhedrin 91a), harelip (Baba Kamma 117a), hairy nevi (Niddah 46a), congenital deafness (Hagigah 2a), and supernumerary digits (Bekoroth 45b). Congenital blindness was mentioned with the assertion that the infant locates the mother's breast by smell and taste (Kethuboth 60a), a fact that only recently has been documented in the medical literature.[63]

Scurvy (Abodah Zarah 28a), epistaxis (Gittin 69a), trachoma (Kethuboth 77b), and epilepsy (Bekoroth 44b) were addressed in the Talmud. Common childhood earache was treated by drinking the juice (urine?) of a goat kidney (Abodah Zarah 28b). Newborn ecchymosis and cholestasis were described but with no insights as to possible etiologies or treatment:

If an infant is too red, so that the blood is not yet absorbed in him, we must wait until his blood is absorbed and then circumcise him. If he is green, so that he is deficient in blood. . . . (Shabbath 134a)

---

*This same technique was used in many parts of the world and continues to this day among tribes of the Amazon basin (Moré, Baure, Movima), in Bhutan and the African continent. Some cultures use termites, and others use beetles; the ant is the most commonly employed. The two edges of a wound are dressed, approximated, and the mandibles of ants are used to clamp the wound. Several ants are used, depending on the length of the wound. Greek barbers in Smyrna were known to use up to 10 ants. Once the ant "bites," the body of the ant is broken off at the thorax, leaving behind the head with mandibles clenched in rigor mortis, acting like a suture, nature's surgical clip! This same technique was recommended by the *Susruta Samhita* and even as late as 1546 by Guy de Chauliac for repair of intestinal perforations. (Gudger, 1925, pp. 1861–64.)

Yet hematemesis was cleverly assessed by dipping a straw into the blood. If clots adhered to the straw it was considered pulmonic in origin; if not, hepatic (Gittin 69a). The total blood volume of an infant was determined by a dilutional technique comparing the color of blood in various solutions (Pesahim 19; Oholath 3:2). This technique would not be duplicated until some 1,500 years later by W. H. Welcker in 1855.[64]

To prevent heatstroke, Middash Shocher Tobitha 19 proscribed outdoor activity between 10 and 3 in the afternoon. The first recorded case of resuscitation involved a Shunammite's son who suffered heatstroke and was revived by Elisha (c.849–786 B.C.):

And when the child was grown, it fell on a day, that he went out to his father to the reapers. And he said to his father, My head, my head. And he said to a lad, Carry him to his mother. And when he had taken him, and brought him to his mother, he sat on her knees till noon, and then died. (18–20)

And when Elisha was come into the house, behold, the child was dead and laid upon his bed. He went in therefore, and shunt the door upon them twain, and prayed unto the Lord. And he went up, and lay upon the child, and put his mouth upon his mouth, and his eyes upon his eyes, and his hands upon his hands: and he stretched himself upon the child; and the flesh of the child waxed warm. Then he returned, and walked in the house to and fro; and went up, and stretched himself upon him: and the child sneezed seven times, and the child opened his eyes. (2 Kings 4:32–35)

Aspiration of a foreign body (especially a bone) was considered so serious the Sabbath laws could be set aside to deal with the emergency (Shabbath 67a).

Animal bites, common misfortunes among children, were addressed by the Egyptians in *The Book of Bites*[65], and by the Hebrews. The Bible (Deut. 8:15; Num. 21:4–9) and the Talmud discussed snakebites (Abodah Zarah 31b). Some biblical scholars (Preuss 1913) interpret the *saraph* snake to be *Dracunculus medinensis*, or the female guinea worm, which can grow to nearly a meter long.[66] In fact, it is possible that other worm parasites and snakes were confused. Reference is made to snakes, most likely tapeworms, being excreted in strips (Shabbath 109b).

The bite of the rabid dog caused appropriate terror, and the child would be given liver from the dog to eat (Yoma 83b). Insect and arachnid bites were recorded, particularly those of the scorpion (Deut. 8:15), which were treated with the gall of a white stork in beer (Kethuboth 50a). Bee (Kethuboth 50a) and hornet (Sotah 36b) stings plagued adults as well as children.

Circumcision of the male was performed on the eighth day after birth (Lev. 12:3), which is about the time the body stabilizes the vitamin K levels that are conducive to the normal coagulation of blood. Originally performed by the mother employing a chipped flint (Exod. 4:25), in time the rite fell to the *mohel*. Hemophilia was recognized as a risk.

If she circumcised her first child and he died, and second one who also died, she must not circumcise her third child. (Yebamoth, 64b)

This brief review of ancient Hebraic child care merely highlights the insights into public health as well as keen observations of congenital anomalies and normal newborn behavior. The Talmud provided the underpinnings that were to be used by the great Jewish physicians of the medieval period.

INDIA

In a system of medicine that evolved between 3,000 and 5,000 years ago, the physician in India was called the *vaidya*. The corpus of Hindu literature pertaining to this system, the *Ayurveda* ("knowledge of life") stems from the four Vedas or books of knowledge. The oldest, the *Rigveda*, was composed about 1500 B.C. The *Sama*, *Yajur*, and *Atharva* Vedas followed. Each Veda is divided into two parts: the mantra, or prayers, and the *brahmana*, or rituals.[67] During this Vedic period, medicine was predominantly apotropaic, and the *Atharva* contained the spells and incantations indicated for children. One example requested long life for a newborn:

Giving life-time, O Agni, choosing old age, ghee-fronted, ghee-backed, O Agni, having drunk the sweet pleasant ghee of the cow; do afterward defend this boy as a father his sons.

Another example invoked protection against worms:

O Indra, lord of riches, smite thou the worms of this boy; smitten are all niggards by thy formidable spell. What one creeps about his eyes, what one creeps about his nostrils, what one goes to the midst of his teeth—that worm we grind up.
The worms that are white-sided, that are black with white arms, and whatever ones are of all forms—those worms we grind up. Up in the east the sun, seen of all, slayer of the unseen, slaying both those seen and unseen, and slaughtering all worms.[68]

It was during the Brahministic period (800 B.C. to 700 A.D.), a time when the Brahman caste of Hindu priest dominated, that the major medical contributions were made. Well-trained *vaidyas* introduced hyoscyamus and cannabis as surgical soporifics. The glycosuria of diabetes was recognized. The associations of mosquito bites with malaria and of plague with rats were understood. The works and redactions of Susruta (second-century B.C.),

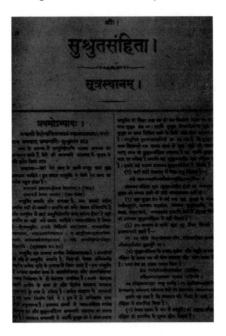

Figure 2.4 First page of the *Susruta Samhita*. Old Sanskrit, dated 576.

Charaka (first century?), and Vagbhata (seventh century) comprised the three basic texts of Brahmanical medicine, which were incorporated into the general corpus of Ayurveda. The collection (*Samhita*) of Susruta contained the significant pediatric focus, and, out of 66 chapters, 11 were devoted to children (figure 2.4). The major part of the text focused on surgical and gynecological medicine, but chapter 1, verse 5, defined the scope of *Kaumara bhrtya*, or pediatrics, as dealing with normal newborn care, breast milk, and treatment of diseases due to vitiated maternal milk or malignant influences.[69] There were physicians called *kumara bhrtya*, or children's doctors,[70] implying a specialized practice already extant in ancient India.

The *Susruta Samhita* described nine evil spirits—the *Bala grahas*, considered responsible for childhood diseases. The legend was that the gods created the *grahas* to punish impious and or unhygienic parents by afflicting their children. Maternal and hygienic neglect, intentional intimidation or frightening of children, and ignorance of incantations deemed proper and appropriate were common behaviors that incited the gods to punish infractions by unleashing one or more of the *grahas*. Each of the supernaturally empowered *grahas* embodied a set of symptoms found in individual ailments, with convulsions of one form or another common to all. As they entered, unseen, into the bodies of children, they induced afflictions that were age-specific, from newborns to adolescents. *Grahas* never worked their evil on adults.[71]

The *Skanda graha*, considered the most evil, caused a complex of symptoms that today would be thought of as edema, melena, facial palsy or rigor, and intestinal dysmotility, signs suggestive of infantile botulism or tetanus:

The child afflicted with *Skanda graha* has swelling of the eyes, bloody odour, an aversion to the breast milk, distorted facial features, fixed eyes, movement of one lid or of one eye only, frightened appearance, half closed eyes, weeps rarely, has clenched fists and passes hard and solid faeces.

The *Skandapasmara graha* inflicted what appears to have been a grand mal seizure:

The child afflicted with Skandapasmara alternately loses and regains consciousness, looks violent with the hands and legs moving as if dancing, passes urine, stool, and flatus, yawns, and foams.

The *Sakuni graha* was marked by a purulent rash of an otherwise undiagnosable syndrome, with smallpox conjoined with sepsis and kidney failure as a possible modern diagnosis:

The child diagnosed as afflicted with Sakuni graha when he is seen to have flaccid limbs, is frightened, has the odour of a bird, is suffering from discharging ulcers all over the body, or from eruption of blisters which are accompanied with burning sensation and suppuration.

Both the *Revati* and *Putana grahas* are enigmatic, with dysentery and cholera as possible diagnoses:

The child afflicted with Revati graha has flushed face, green faeces, and an excessively anaemic or blackish body, has fever, oral sepsis and aches and pains all over the body and always keeps on rubbing the eyes and nose.

The child afflicted with Putana graha has flaccidity of the limbs, sleeps comfortably in the day but not at night, passes loose stools and has an odour like that of a crow; he is distressed by vomiting, has horripilation and remains thirsty.

The symptoms of *Andhaputana graha* resemble the abdominal distress of gastroenteritis or gastroesophageal reflux:

The child dislikes breast milk, has diarrhea, cough, hiccough, vomiting and fever, becomes discolored, always sleeps prone, and emits sour odor.

The diagnosis of the *Sitaputana graha* may have been a choleric malabsorption:

This child is anxious, shivers, weeps too much, has flatulence and severe diarrhea, a bad odor, and has coma.

Mukhamandika graha probably was chronic hepatic failure (cirrhosis) or ascites with renal failure:

The child with Mukhamandika is pale and edematous, is gluttonous, has its abdomen covered over with engorged veins, is restless and smells of urine.

The signs of *Naigamesa graha* resemble those of meningitis with opistotonus:

The child with Naigamesa graha vomits froth, has a bowed trunk, cries out with fear looks upward, has fever, emits a fatty odor, and becomes unconscious.

Some *grahas* were known to be incurable:

The child with rigidity of the limbs, resents breast milk, has recurrent fits of fainting, and possesses all the features of afflictions by the grahas, is incurable and soon dies.

It was believed that most *grahas* could be cured by rubbing the child with *ghrta* (ghee) and sprinkling mustard seeds throughout the house. Additionally, it was prescribed that a lamp of mustard oil be kept burning, and *sarvasugandha* seeds and flowers were to be thrown into the hearth while chanting:

Obeisance to thee, O fire god; obeisance to thee, O goddess Krttika; obeisance to thee, O Skanda; obeisance to thee, O lord of the Grahas. I bow down my head before you. Dost thou accept the offering I have made thee. May my child get rid of the disease and makest it hale and healthy again.

In addition to the above general measures, each *graha* had a specific treatment ritual. The example that follows is for *Sitaputana*:

As it was described by Lord Dhanvantari.

Sprinkling:
The decoction of *kapittha, suvaha, bimbi, bilva, pracibala, nandi,* and *bhallataka* should be sprinkled over the child.

Massage:
Oil duly cooked with the urines of the goat and the cow, *musta, suradaru, kustha,* and with the drugs belonging to the group of *sarvaghandha* should be used.

Medication:
Ghrta duly cooked with the decoction of *rohini*, *sarja*, *khadira*, *palasa*, and with the bark of *kakubha* mixed with milk should be used.

Fumigation:
Fumigation should be done by the fumes of the faeces of vulture, owl, *bastagandha*, cast-off skin of the snake, the leaves of *nimba* and of *madhuka*.

Amulets:
The wood of *lamba*, *guñja*, and *kakadani* should be worn by the child.

Sacrifices:
The goddess *Sitaputana* should be worshipped by the river with food mixed with *mudga* (ground lentils). Offerings of wine and blood should further be made to the goddess. The child should be bathed by a water reservoir.

Chant:
"May goddess *Sitaputana*, who is fond of taking *mudga* and rice, who is habituated to drinking wine and blood and who resides by the side of watery places save thee."

By 200 A.D. a pediatric manuscript existed that made observations about fetal life. "A six months embryo is the last that lives when born and the foetus becomes full-fledged in the tenth month" (Shatapatha Brahmana).[72] The *Navanitaka* of the Bower manuscript was written by a *kumara bhrtya* called Jivaka, a contemporary of Buddha. Newborn observations, among them umbilical hernia (*vttudita*) and the progression of normal dentition were recorded in it.[73]

Childhood ailments and a pediatric pharmacopeia were passed on by oral tradition and through the centuries were redacted into the Ayurveda. Meconium evacuation was encouraged by giving honey. Before first feeding, the wet nurse washed her breasts and chanted the following mantra:

O thou beautiful damsel, may the four oceans of the earth contribute to the secretion of milk in thy breasts for the purpose of improving the bodily strength of the child. O, thou, with a beautiful face, may the child, reared on your milk, attain a long life, like the gods made immortal with drinks of ambrosia.[74]

Directions to the wet nurse to express superfluous milk if the newborn gagged or coughed implies that reflux and aspiration were recognized. Breast milk was tested by adding a few drops to cold water. It was expected to be thin, clear, conch-shell colored, easily miscible with water, neither floating nor sinking, frothing nor curdling. Newborn tetanus that appeared on the ninth day was of an evil spirit, and tears absent after the fourth month was the spirit of serious illness. In point of fact, both of these prescient observations were grounded in acceptable physiological premises. The incubation period of the tetanus spore is usually 7 to 10 days, and a lack of tears bespeaks at least a 5 to 7 percent dehydration.

The *Vagbhata* enlarged on the *grahas*, adding "planetary influences,"[75] and by the seventh century A.D. the major illnesses of children were held to fall into six categories: convulsions, worms, fevers, vomiting, diarrhea, and those of planetary influences (crying, self-mutilation, bloating, swelling, and giving off bad odors).[76] The treatments for those six categories were primarily herbal. Remedies were given in doses to suit the child. The newborn was medicated by adding the drug to milk or ghee or through breast milk absorption. The milk-fed child received a "plum stone-sized" paste dollop, while the child taking rice or other solids was given a "plum-sized" dollop.[77] To obfuscate bitter taste and facilitate administration, licorice and honey were used as base ingredients. (It is of interest that this culture took the trouble to facilitate medicinal administration to children. As late as the nineteenth century the Western world was still medicating children with "bitter-medicine spoons," devices to force consumption.) Some recipes called for fruit, mineral salts, and animal milk. A typical compound read as follows: "For diarrhea mix powdered nutmeg, fruit of palm, cloves, cumin, and borax with goat milk."[78]

The *Vagbhata* expressed both negative and positive attributes for mammalian milks, strongly advocating some while decrying others (table 2.4). (The Hebrews also used mammalian milk for nurslings. Genesis 32:15 makes reference to milch-camels as "mayneket," or wet nurse.)

Surgical procedures also were modified for children, a practice seldom recorded among other cultures. For example, an adult suffering from poisonous snakebite had a tourniquet applied above the wound, an incision of the bite area made for blood letting, and cautery by applying a hot coal. A child was considered too delicate for bloodletting. Instead, a plaster was applied over the cauterized area, and the child was given a decoction of *sarpaganda* of *Rauwolfia serpentina*, the source of reserpine.[79] The major pharmacological effects of reserpine are to lower blood pressure and tranquilize.

The ears of children were pierced to avert the "influence of malignant stars," and this had to be done on the sixth or seventh month under the proper alignment of stars and moon. Little boys had the right ear pierced first, then the left. The opposite procedure was followed for little girls. Oiled lint was threaded through with a needle and then changed every three days, with thicker plugs used to enlarge the opening. The child who needed a surgical procedure underwent incision with a bamboo blade (similar to Egyptian and Roman reeds) because the child's body was deemed too delicate for a metal scalpel.[80]

With the *vaidya*, then, came the first early records of specific attention to children's medical issues, and although not articulated as such, there was a recognition of the physiological differences between children and adults.

TABLE 2.4
USES OF MILK ACCORDING TO THE *VAGBHATA* (5:21–28)

Species	Attribute
Human	Use for eye diseases
Goat	Use for diarrhea/dehydration
Cow	Use for purgative/nutrition
Camel	Can constipate/cause worms
Sheep	Damages stomach
Elephant	Constipates
Buffalo	Use for insomia

CHINA AND JAPAN

The sources of ancient Chinese medicine are to be found in oracle bones, tomb artifacts, and classical texts; most important is the *Huang Ti Nei Ching*. The bones, generally broad, flat scapulae, date from the fifteenth to the eleventh centuries B.C., and the tomb seals of the Chou period from the fifth to the third centuries B.C. The authorship of the *Nei Ching* is attributed to Huang Ti, the Yellow Emperor, and is relegated to the period of 2697 to 2597 B.C. Most scholars consider him legendary and place the composition of the *Nei Ching* somewhere between 1000 and 300 B.C.[81] The text takes the form of a dialogue between the Yellow Emperor and his minister, Ch'i Po. From these collective sources we learn that ancient China, like Egypt, had specialists, among them eye, ear, speech, teeth, abdominal organs, bladder, psychological, and doctors for women and children.[82] Surgical correction of harelip was documented in the Chin dynasty (317–420).[83] During the T'ang dynasty (618–970) the Grand (Imperial) College of Medicine functioned with five branches, one of which was pediatric (Hsiao-fang mi), requiring five years of study to qualify for examination.[84] In the seventh century, Ch'ao Yuan-fang wrote *Chu-ping yuan-hou lun* (On the origins and symptoms of various diseases), which contained six chapters dealing with 255 items that touched on children's diseases. In the eighth century, Sun Ssumiao wrote *Ch'ien-chin fang* (A thousand golden recipes), which contained a chapter titled "Procedures for Children and Infants."[85]

By the eleventh century, practitioners existed with practices devoted exclusively to children, such as Ch'ien Yi (1023–1104), who differentiated measles from scarlet fever and chicken pox from smallpox, and Qian Yi (1032–1113), who wrote a text called *Proven Formulae of Pediatric Medicine*.[86] In 1150, Lui Fang produced *Yu-yu hsin-shu* (A new text for protection of children), and Ch'en Wen-chung wrote *Hsiao-erh tou-chen fang-lun* (On poxes and measles of small children) in 1214.[87]

Newborn tetanus was addressed with close attention during this epoch. In 1156, Sung Imperial College published *Hsiao erh Wei-sheng tsung-wei lun-fang* (A thorough discussion on the hygiene of small children). It described *Ch'i-feng* ("umbilical wind"), which was clearly tetanus marked by cyanosis, muscle spasms, cold, and stiffness, appearing about the seventh to ninth day of life. Most significant was the observation that the clinical picture resembled the symptoms adults developed after receiving an open wound. As a result, a form of moxibustion was devised for infants, utilizing an umbilical branding cake to cauterize the umbilical stump:

As soon as the cord is broken, one should place an umbilical branding cake [fermented soy beans, yellow wax and musk] on the cord stump and burn it three times. The wick of the flames should be of the size of the ears of wheat. If the infant does not cry, use moxa and burn it up to five or seven times.[88]

Procedures and observations in the care of children were made centuries before the Western world even conceived of them. Preventive variolation, for example, was advocated by Wang Tan (957–1017) some 700 years before it was introduced into England, and Hua Shou (c.1360) identified Koplik spots.[89] A major nine-volume text, *Yiu-k'e chun-sheng* (Principles of children's diseases), was published in 1607 by Wang K'eng-t'ang.[90] The earliest special treatise on children's diseases was the *Lu Hsin Ching*, or "The Fontanel." This was an anonymous work in two volumes, written at the end of the T'ang dynasty (c.910 A.D.) or over 500 years before the first pediatric incunabulum appeared in the West.[91]

During the fourteenth century the Wan medical family assumed a prominence in pediatrics that would endure for a hundred years. Wan Ch'uan compiled the collective observations of the family into a text called *Yu-ying chia-mi* (Family secrets on infant-raising).[92] It was a major collection of practical insights and hints on dealing with the common ailments of infants. For example, the text described variations of infant vomiting caused by overfeeding, position, or dribbling—what is now commonly called infantile gastroesophageal reflux:

Vomiting milk occurs because the stomach of a newborn infant, being small and fragile, can not contain too much milk. The nursing mother should thus feed according to degree of hunger, not allowing the infant to be overfed. . . . If nursed until too full and yet placed in a wrong position, he is bound to spill over two or three mouthfuls. . . . Dribbling of milk occurs when a child is seen with milk constantly coming out; it appears often on the corner of his mouth and on his lips.[93]

TABLE 2.5
ISHIMPO TABLE OF CONTENTS[94]

Book	Pages	Contents
1	148	Disease Treatment, Pharmacology, Posology
2	168	Acupuncture and Moxibustion
3	92	Afflictions of the Nervous System
4	68	Whiskers, Hair, Face, Nose, Body Odors
5	120	Eyes, Ears, Mouth, Tongue, Teeth
6	64	Stomach, Heart, Kidneys, Liver, Lungs
7	52	Genitals, Piles, Intestinal Worms
8	72	Nutritional Deficiency, Diseases of Extremities
9	68	Cough, Asthma, Dyspepsia, Nausea
10	88	Hernia, Jaundice, Swelling
11	100	Cholera and Dysentery
12	76	Constipation, Diabetes, Hematuria, Bedwetting
13	68	Consumption, Exhaustion, Insomnia
14	132	Sudden Death, Fevers, Drowning, Freezing
15	92	Boils, Growth in Lungs and Intestines
16	100	Carbuncles, Vicious Swellings, Varicose Veins
17	68	Skin Diseases
18	120	Wounds, Burns, Metal Wounds, Arrow Wounds, Falls from Horses, Dog Bites, Horse Bites
19	112	Various Types of Tonics, Mineral Diet
20	72	Antidotes for Mineral Poisoning
21	60	Women's Diseases
22	76	Women's Diseases, continued
23	96	Obstetrics
24	72	Conception, Sex Prediction, Pregnancy Tests
25	184	Pediatrics
26	80	Geriatrics, Attaining Longevity
27	80	Geriatrics, Mental Hygiene, Breathing Exercises
28	108	Health Principles, Chamber Exercises
29	108	Dietary Adjustments
30	104	Materia Medica: Cereal, Fruit, Meat, Vegetable

Much of the early imperial period wisdom was lost through destruction of texts, but the writing of the *Ishimpo* preserved and provided a window to the ancient medicine of China. The *Ishimpo* was completed by Yasuyori Tamba in 982 and is the oldest medical book extant in Japan. It consists of 30 scrolls (table 2.5), compiled from Chinese medical works—almost verbatim. Of the 110 classic Chinese documents compiled in the *Ishimpo*, only

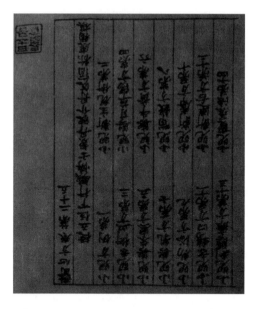

Figure 2.5 First page of scroll 25 of the *Ishimpo* (1849).

two appear to have survived, the rest have disappeared, making the *Ishimpo* an extremely valuable source of ancient Chinese and Japanese medicine—in fact, the major source.[95]

Tamba dedicated his work to the emperor in 984. A second edition was calligraphed in 1145. Thereafter the scrolls were scattered and hidden away by various noble families, preserved as a precious heritage. They were not reassembled until 1859, when woodblock prints of the 30 scrolls were made available to scholars.[96] Scroll 25 of the *Ishimpo* (figure 2.5) focuses on children and is essentially a pediatric textbook of first millennium China.

This text was kindly supplied by Professor Shizu Sakai of Juntendo University and translated by Professor Wai-Yee Chan of Georgetown University. It is discussed in the pages that follow.

The treatment of children in the *Ishimpo* relied on an understanding of Chinese medical principles and pharmacopeia. It was a medical philosophy founded on two opposing forces, the Yang (light, dry, and male) and the Yin (dark, moist, and female), with modifying elements and attributes (table 2.6). A disruption in the balance of forces and elements, resulted in disease, a disharmony of the qi—a plasmic energy and vector of life.

From conception, the Yin-Yang dictated the health of the child and the *Ch'an Ching*, the great obstetric classic, declared:[97]

TABLE 2.6
SINO–JAPANESE CONCORDANCE OF THE FIVE ELEMENTS
AND THEIR ATTRIBUTES[98]

Viscera	Season	Element	Taste	Color	Animal	Grain	Emotion	No.	Planet
Liver	Spring	Wood	Sour	Green	Fowl	Wheat	Anger	8	Jupiter
Heart	Summer	Fire	Bitter	Red	Sheep	Gum	Joy	7	Mars
Spleen	Summer	Earth	Sweet	Yellow	Ox	Millet	Sympathy	5	Saturn
Lungs	Fall	Metal	Pungent	White	Horse	Rice	Grief	9	Venus
Kidney	Winter	Water	Salty	Black	Pig	Bean	Fear	6	Mercury

The child born from combining of Yin and Yang

at midday when the sun is at its zenith will suffer from vomiting and nausea

at midnight when heaven and earth are blocked and not communicating will either be blind, deaf or dumb

during a solar eclipse will be weak in bodily structure as if he had been injured by beating

during thunder and lightning, when the angry heavens display their powers, will easily take on madness

during a lunar eclipse will be unlucky, as will also be his mother

under a rainbow will appear to be committed to do evil and unlucky things

on the days of winter or summer solstice will harm his parents

between the crescent and full moon will side with rebel soldiers or be blinded by the wind

when the parents are intoxicated, or right after a heavy meal, will suffer from fits or convulsions, carbuncles or abscesses

Other elements, such as emotion, the calendar, or the season also conspired to affect newborns. A child born in the last part of the twelfth month would encounter "a hundred devils" and be deaf and dumb. A child conceived of the Yin and Yang of mourning parents was destined to be devoured by "tigers or wolves."[99]

Some are born injured and dead. These are the sons of fire when the combining of Yin and Yang takes place before the lighted candle is extinguished.

Once a baby was born it was too late to affect the predestination aspects of Yin-Yang, but there were auspicious and inauspicious astrological dates that could modify other life forces. Protocols 8, 9, 16, and 17 of the *Ishimpo* address these forces. For example: Protocol 8 suggested dates for the first feeding and dates to avoid. Some were lucky, others ominous. Of interest was the advocated early feeding of rice paste:

One can grind up some grains of rice to make a thick paste like cheese and feed that to the baby in the form of a bean. Feed about 3 beans each time and three times a day. This type of feeding can start on the seventh or tenth day. The amount can be doubled on the twentieth day.

The auspicious date for the first feeding of the baby are: fifth *yin*, fifth *chen*, fifth *chou* and fifth *you*. It also stated that for boys, *jia, yi* are lucky, and for girls, *ren, gui* are auspicious . . . the following days should be avoided for feeding the baby: fifth *xu*, fifth *si* and fifth *mao*.[100] (*Ishimpo*, Protocol 8)

In a similar fashion, Protocol 9 listed dates prescribed and proscribed for the first bath as well as the qualities of the bath water:

[S]oup for bathing newborns should be cooked with roots from plum, pear and peach trees. . . . [I]f porcine gallbladder is put in the bathing soup, it will help the baby to avoid pustules throughout his life.

The auspicious dates to give a bath to the baby are: *chou, yin, mao, shen* and *you*. . . . [T]he ominous dates at which the baby should not be bathed include: *geng xu, ren ji, jia yi, geng xin, ren gui, chen si* and *wu wei*. (*Ishimpo*, Protocol 9)

The code for dressing a child—both the color and weight of the fabric—was dictated by the day on which the child was born, and Protocol 17 addressed these prescriptions in detail:

[C]hildren born on *jia* day and *yi* day should be dressed in black (do not dress them on *geng* day); child born on *bing* day and *ding* day should be dressed in bluish green (do not dress them at midnight). . . . [I]t is not good to use new fabric to make clothes for children because it will hurt the *qi* (vital energy) of children. It is better to use old fabric because cloth that has been in touch with humans is advantageous to the children. (*Ishimpo*, Protocol 17)

Failure to follow any of these protocols resulted in a sick and debilitated infant.

The *Ishimpo* covered topics found in all the *scripturae antiquitatis*,[101] such as wet nurse selection, skin lesions, ear infections, eye mishaps, teething, nosebleeds, hiccups, abdominal pain, genital lesions, parasites, seizures, diarrheas, fevers, scrofula, accidents, and foreign bodies. Some examples follow and the entire table of contents of the pediatric *Ishimpo*, together with the pharmacopeia, definition of units, and sources, appears in appendix D.

Some of the protocols are complex and offer many modalities of treatment such as No. 24, which is called "Protocol for Treating *Bai Tu*" (white balding). This most likely is alopecia secondary to infected seborrhea:

Bing Yuen Lun stated that *Bai Tu* is the conditionl where there are white spots on the scalp. Initially they look like tinea capitis with dandruff on it. Then scab and pustules are formed followed by hair loss. This is called *Bai Tu*. *Ge's Fang* stated that it can be cured by applying sauce with ash from burnt *ji yu*.[102] Another protocol is to use an ointment made with the ash of *li lo*.[103]

Xiao Bin Fang stated that the use of juice from ground *qiu ye*[104] mixed with lard makes an ointment which can be applied to the scalp. *Ji Yiu Fang* said mix ground *yuen hua*[105] and lard until it looks like mud and apply to the scalp. *Lu Yan Fang* suggested to use white fat of bear.

Other protocols prescribed modalities common to many cultures throughout millennia, such as No. 37, "Treating Red and Painful Eyes," or conjunctivitis:

Chan Jing suggested to use 7 pieces of *huang lian*[106] in one cup of human milk to wash the eye. Another protocol uses cotton soaked with a solution containing 3 cups of *zhu li*[107] and 1 cup of human milk to wipe the eye.

Many of the protocols were clearly based on Yin–Yang elements, such as No. 45, which attributed "swallow mouth" (cheilosis, aphthae, thrush?) to organic heat:

Bing Yuen Lun stated that lesions of the lips in children are called *Yan Kou* because they are white like the beak of a swallow. They are caused by the heat rising from the stomach and spleen to the lips. *Qian Jin Fang* stated mix the ash of hair with lard and apply to the lesion. Another protocol stated that wet *qiu bai pi*[108] be put on the lesion 4 to 5 times.

These few examples of the *Ishimpo* serve to inform the format and contents of ancient Sino–Japanese pediatrics. The concepts of etiologies, descriptions, and treatments were and remain strange to the Western medical mind, but what is extraordinarily notable is the existence and recognition of the child as a unique clinical entity very early on in the Oriental culture.

NOTES

1. Robinson, 1995, pp. 12–16.
2. Kramer, 1959, p. 1.
3. These can be found on columns 18 and 19, codes 215 through 227. G.

Contenau, *Le Médecine en Assyrie et en Babylonie* (Paris: Librairie Malonie, 1938).

    4. Saggs, 1962, p. 460.

    5. Ibid.

    6. Saggs, 1984, pp. 226–29.

    7. Jayne, 1979, pp. 92–93.

    8. Kramer, 1959, p. 64.

    9. Abt, 1965, p. 20.

    10. Jayne, 1979, pp. 103–4.

    11. Gordon, 1949, pp. 168–69.

    12. Wilson, 1996, pp. 135–40.

    13. Wilson, 1967, pp. 191–208.

    14. Labat, 1951.

    15. Saggs, 1962, pp. 461–67.

    16. Wilson, 1967, pp. 203–4.

    17. Kramer, 1959, pp. 60–64.

    18. Kramer, 1963, pp. 93–99.

    19. Michie, 1991, pp. 602–5.

    20. Mark 15:23.

    21. Adamson, 1991, pp. 428–35.

    22. Wilson, 1996, pp. 137–38.

    23. Majno, 1975, p. 65.

    24. Oppenheim, 1964, p. 296.

    25. Oppenheim, 1967, p. 118.

    26. Abt, 1965, p. 22.

    27. Kramer, 1959, p. 231.

    28. Herodotus 2:83.

    29. Strouhal, 1992, p. 25.

    30. Erman, 1901, p. 30.

    31. Bryan, 1974, pp. xx–xxi.

    32. Erman, 1901, pp. 9–11.

    33. Leake, 1952, pp. 7–17. A few other fragments are available to scholars, mostly magical in nature and a few prescriptive, written on ostraca. Dawson, 1967, pp. 98–104.

    34. Bryan, 1931, pp. 83–85.

    35. Ghalioungui, 1974, p. 129.

    36. Abt, 1965, p. 13.

    37. Strouhal, 1992, pp. 21–24. The *Vagbhata Samhita* (5:25) also recommends maternal milk for eye infections.

    38. Kuhr, M. D. *Contemp Pediatr* 1991; 8(6):124.

    39. Bryan, 1931, pp. 83–85.

    40. Ibid.

    41. Germer, 1993, p. 77.

    42. Abt, 1965, pp. 13–15.

    43. Strouhal, 1992, p. 245. Three millennia later, in the eighteenth century, worms still were believed to be the cause of irritability, drooling, and even convul-

sions associated with childhood teething (see below).

44. Harris and Weeks, 1973, p. 65.

45. Basset et al., 1980, pp. 1532–34.

46. Germer, 1993, p. 78.

47. Bryan, 1931, pp. 90–94.

48. Abt, 1965, p. 14.

49. Ibid.

50. Steuer and deCusance, 1959.

51. Majno, 1975, pp. 129–30.

52. *Lancet* 1990; 335:724.

53. *Br Med J* 1992; 304:555–56.

54. Wells, 1967, pp. 390–404.

55. Erman, 1901, p. 12.

56. Abt, 1965, p. 27.

57. Rosner, 1978, p. 197.

58. Zias, J., et al., Early medical use of cannabis. *Nature* 1993; 363:215.

59. A cubit is about 50 cm.

60. When air is blown into the face of an infant, an autonomic gasp and swallowing is induced, which is referred to as the Santmeyer reflex.

61. Orenstein, S. R., et al., *Lancet* 1988; 1:345–46.

62. Quoted in Abt, 1965, p. 33.

63. Varendi, H., Porter, R. H., Winberg, J., Does the newborn baby find the nipple by smell? *Lancet* 1994; 344:989–90.

64. Kagan, 1952, p. 39.

65. Manjo, 1975, p. 84.

66. Rosner, 1978, p. 197.

67. Gerson, 1993, pp. 8–12.

68. *Atharva-Veda Samhita*, as cited by Abt, 1965, p. 23.

69. Kutumbiah, 1959, p. 329.

70. Ibid., p. 328.

71. The translation of the Sanskrit *grahas* comes from Kutumbiah, 1962, pp. 200–201, and the translation of the Sitaputana ritual is from Singhal and Mitra, 1980, pp. 79–81.

72. Sena, 1901, vol. 1.

73. Bowers manuscript, pt. 2, chap. 14, verses 1011–99.

74. *Susruta Samhita*, Sarira Sthanam, 10:22.

75. Huard and LaPlane, 1981, 1:18–20.

76. *Susruta Samhita*, Sarira Sthanam, 10:41.

77. *Susruta Samhita*, Sarira Sthanam, 10:29.

78. Sena, 1901, vol. 2.

79. Majno, 1975, p. 280.

80. Ibid., pp. 285–90.

81. Veith, 1972, pp. 4–9.

82. Gwei–Djen and Needham, 1967, pp. 222–37.

83. Vrebos, 1992, pp. 147–49.

84. Huard and Laplane, 1981, 1:9.

85. Ping-Chen, 1996(a), p. 73.

86. Gartner and Stone, 1994, p. 532; Wong and Lien-Teh, 1936, p. 90.

87. Ping-Chen, 1996(a), p. 74.

88. Ping-Chen, 1996(b), pp. 11–13.

89. Huard and Wong, 1968, pp. 40–43.

90. Wong and Lien-Teh, 1936, p. 130.

91. Ibid., p. 87.

92. Ping-Chen, 1996(a), p. 76.

93. Ibid., p. 230.

94. Hsia, 1986, p. xiii.

95. Otori, 1970, pp. viii–ix. Hsia et al., 1986, put the number at 204 documents, 180 (88%) of which have disappeared (p. 11).

96. Sugitatsu, 1984, pp 108–14.

97. Hsia, 1986, pp. 201–2.

98. Veith, 1972, p. 21.

99. Ibid., pp. 203–4.

100. Heavenly Stems [*Tian gan*] and Earthly Branches [*Di Zhi*] are from *Yi Jing*. The Ten Heavenly Stems are *jia, yi, bing, ding, wu, geng, xin, ren, bao*, and *gui*. The Twelve Earthly Branches are *ji, chou, yin, mao, chen, si, wu, wei, shen, you, xu*, and *hai*. Branches and stem equate with years; sole branches, with hours.

101. Berlin papyrus, *Traite akkadien*, *Susruta Shamita*, and the Talmud.

102. *Carassius auratus*, a freshwater fish.

103. The plant *Veratrum nigrum*.

104. Leaves of *Catalpa bungei*.

105. The flower of *Daphne genkwa*.

106. The stalk of *Coptis chinensis*.

107. Sap of bamboo *Phyllostachys nigra*.

108. Bark of *Catalpa bungei*.

Chapter 3

Greco-Roman Pediatrics

Of the three periods of early Greek medicine[1]—the Aesculapian, the Homeric, and the Hippocratic—the Aesculapian is legendary for intermingling human and divine entities in a pantheon of healers. Orpheus, Melampus, Chiron, and Aesculapius coexisted with Apollo, Artemis, Demeter, Pan, and Hades. The transitional Homeric period (c.1000 B.C.)

was marked by theurgical modalities mixed with an innovative focus on anatomy and wounds, as described most prominently in the *Iliad* and the *Odyssey*. The *Iliad* alone detailed nearly 150 different types of wounds.

Children, however, are not mentioned in either the Aesculapian or the Homeric period. Only in the Hippocratic era can reference to early Greek pediatrics be found.

HIPPOCRATES

Hippocrates (460–370 B.C.) was, in today's jargon, a generalist. His teachings, collectively referred to as the Hippocratic Corpus, consist of approximately 60 oral treatises inscribed between 430 and 330 B.C. by a large number of anonymous writers, presumably his students. Hippocrates, according to Aristotle and his pupil Meno, originated from Cos.[2]

Traditionally, the development of case notes and the patient as a teaching model is attributed to Hippocrates. The Corpus reveals to us Hippocrates' mastery of the art of clinical observation.

Hippocrates wrote about medicine, surgery, embryology, nutrition, and even climate.[3] Although he wrote no treatise that properly can be called "pediatrics," there is one specific work on teething, a collection of aphorisms about teeth and pharynx. *On Dentition* describes well-known clinical pictures:

1. Of children, those that be by nature well nourished suck milk not in proportion to their fleshiness.
2. Gross feeders that draw much milk do not gain flesh in proportion.
10. Not all who are convulsed whilst about teeth, die; many come through it safely.
24. With ulcers on the tonsils the presence of a sort of spider-web [membrane] is not favorable.

Maxims 1 and 2 most likely refer to the iron-deficient anemic "milk-baby" known to today's pediatrician, and 24 clearly refers to diphtheria. Number 10 attributes some form of seizure to teething, an unfortunate misconception that persisted into the nineteenth century. The entire text of *On Dentition*, Hippocrates' only treatise on children, is reproduced in appendix C.

Hippocrates' most frequently quoted reference to children appears in section 3:24–29 of his *Aphorisms*. It is often compared with Shakespeare's poetic observations on life cycles in *As You Like It* (Act 2, scene 7) and with the medieval *Le Grand Proprietaire de toutes choses, tres utile et profitable pour tenir le corps en sante.*[4]

24. In the different ages the following complaints occur: to little and newborn children, aphthae, vomit, coughs, sleeplessness, frights, inflammation of the navel, watery discharges from the ears.

25. At the approach of dentition, pruritus of the gums, fevers, convulsions, diarrhea, especially when cutting the canine teeth, and in those who are particularly fat, and have constipated bowels.

26. To persons somewhat older, affections of the tonsils, incurvation of the spine at the vertebra next to the occiput, asthma, calculus, round worms, ascarides, acrochordon, satyriasmus, struma, and other tubercles.

27. To persons of more advanced age, and now on the verge of manhood, the most of these diseases, and, moreover, more chronic fevers, and epistaxis.

28. Young people for the most part have a crisis in their complaints, some in forty days, some in seven months, some in seven years,* some at the approach of puberty; and such complaints of children as remain, and do not pass away about puberty, or in females about the commencement of menstruation, usually become chronic.

29. To persons past boyhood, hemoptysis, phthisis, acute fevers, epilepsy, and other diseases, but especially the aforementioned.[5]

Although Hippocrates was ignorant of helminthic cycles, he demonstrated a fascination with worms—a common trait, it would seem, for millennia.[6] The observation made with respect to worms noted in aphorism 26 is expounded further in *On Diseases*:

Tapeworms, I claim, are produced in the child while yet *in utero*. . . . Roundworms are grown there similarly. The proof is as follows: when children are born women give them with their pap such medicines as cause the feces to pass out of the intestine and not to become dried up, and do at the same time relax the bowel.

On taking this many of the children pass round or tapeworms with the first stool: and if they do not, nevertheless, they are produced in the womb.

Hippocrates recorded other observations regarding children, among them are:

---

*Hebdomadism divided human life spans into seven periods of seven years, *puerulus, puer, adolescens, juvenis, junior, vir*, and *senex*. Tanner (1981) notes that the earliest published hebdomad on human growth was by Solon (c.595 B.C.). Given that seven heavenly bodies were visible to the human eye, each was assigned influence over human growth. Thus, the Moon influenced the infant; Mercury, the child, and Venus, the adolescent. The Sun governed *juvenis*; Mars, the inheritor; Jupiter, the mature man; and Saturn, the old man. Belief in hebdomadism persisted until the medieval period, when assigning humors to the age cycles became popular. *Phlegma* was given over to childhood until 14 years; *cholera*, to youth until 28 years; *sanguis*, to maturity until 60 years; and *melancholia*, to old age (Tanner, 1981, p. 17).

13. Old people bear fasting most easily, then adults, much less youth and least of all children. The more active they are, the less do they bear it.

14. Things which are growing have the greatest natural warmth and, accordingly, need most nourishment.

16. Fluid diets are beneficial to all who suffer from fevers, but this is specially true in the case of children. (*Aphorisms*, sec. 1)

Diphtheria and tuberculosis with Pott's disease also were described:

Difficult deglutition and suffocation in fever without swelling of the fauces is a fatal symptom.

Those who acquire a gibbous spine with cough and asthma, before puberty die. (*Aphorisms*, sec. 2)

The systematic clinical observations Hippocrates made retain their value—and interest. His description of a mumps epidemic in Thasos, for example, remains fresh and fascinating reading:

Many people suffered from swellings near the ears, in some cases on one side only, in others both sides were involved. Usually there was no fever and the patient was not confined to bed. In a few cases there was slight fever. In all cases the swelling subsided without harm and nonsuppurated as do swellings caused by other disorders. The swellings were soft, large and spread widely; they were unaccompanied by inflammation or pain and they disappeared leaving no trace. Boys, young men and male adults in the prime of life were chiefly affected and of these, those given to wrestling and gymnastics were specially liable. Few women took it. Many patients had dry, unproductive coughs and hoarse voices. Soon after the onset of this disease, but sometimes after an interval, one or both testicles became inflamed and painful. Some had fever, but not all. These cases were serious enough to warrant attention, but for the rest, there were no illnesses requiring care. (*Epidemics*, 1.i)

Hippocrates made reference to febrile seizures in several of his treatises, but most thoroughly in *On Prognosis*, 24:

Children are likely to have convulsions if the fever is high and if they are constipated, if they are wakeful, frightened, cry and change color, turning pale, livid or red. This most commonly happens in children under the age of seven. As they grow up and reach adult years, they are no longer likely to be attacked by convulsions in the course of fever, unless one of the most severe and worst signs appears as well, as happens in inflammation of the brain.

In *The Sacred Disease*,[7] Hippocrates elaborated further on a more serious form of convulsion—epilepsy.[8] Several diseases were considered together

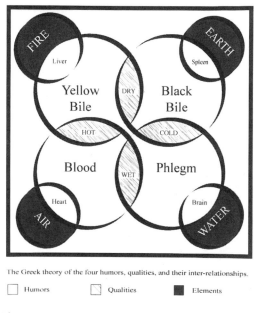

The Greek theory of the four humors, qualities, and their inter-relationships.

☐ Humors ☐ Qualities ◼ Elements

Figure 3.1 The classical humors. DRAWING BY AUTHOR.

under the one common manifestation of motor seizure activity: grand-mal epilepsy, hemiplegia, meningitis, ischemia, and cerebral vascular accidents, for example.

Infants who suffer from this disease usually die if the phlegm is copious an if the weather is southerly. Their little blood-vessels are too narrow to absorb a large quantity of inspissated phlegm and so the blood is at once chilled and frozen, thus causing death. If the amount of phlegm is small and enters both main vessels, or if it enters but one of them, the patient survives but bears the stigmata. Thus the mouth may be distorted, or an eye, a hand or the neck; according to the part of the body in which some blood-vessel became filled and obstructed with phlegm and thus rendered inadequate. As a result of this damage to the blood-vessel, the corresponding part of the body must necessarily be weakened. (*The Sacred Disease*, sec. 2, 5)

In referring to "phlegm," Hippocrates was invoking one of the four "body fluids" or *chymoi* (humors) as the cause of the seizures. The humors and their modifying elements (figure 3.1), like the Yin–Yang, had to be kept in balance in order to maintain a state of health:

Should these routes for the passage of phlegm from the brain be blocked, the discharge enters the blood-vessels which I have described. This causes loss of voice, choking, foaming at the mouth, clenching of the teeth and convulsive movements of the hands; the eyes are fixed, the patient becomes unconscious and, in some cases, passes a stool.[9]

It is possible that Hippocrates was writing about enteroviral poliomyelitis since he places it in a seasonal cycle:

Those who have a very small discharge at a time when the weather is northerly recover without any permanent injury, but there is a danger in such cases that the disease will remain with the child as he grows older.

Such then, is the way in which, more or less, this malady affects children.

Adults neither die from an attack of this disease, nor does it leave them with palsy. (Ibid., 11, 12)

Hippocrates recommended wine for infants:

Infants should be bathed for long periods in warm water and given their wine diluted and not at all cold. (*A Regimen for Health*, 6)

He noted that pica and geophagia contributed to anemia and its physiological consequences:

When children of seven years of age show weakness, a bad color and rapid respiration on walking, together with a desire to eat earth, it denotes destruction of the blood and asthenia. (*Coan Prognosis*, 333)

Finally, in the apocryphal *Epidemics* (bks. 4–7), case histories are recorded of children's thoractomy for empyema (4:4), trephining for head trauma (4:11), tetanus from a wound (5:76), and gangrene from a tooth abscess (6:100). Mastoiditis meningitis (8:5), umbilical hernia with obstruction (7:117), and other conditions requiring surgical interventions also are referred to. Clearly, children in Hippocrates' day were beneficiaries of extant surgical skills.

More than anyone or anything else in his time, Hippocrates and his school of thought divorced medicine from philosophy, religion, and magic. His was a practical medicine that emphasized bedside attention, palpation, auscultation, and the importance of recording observations. His enduring brilliance most significantly recognized the importance of age differences and the variations of disease in growing organisms.

ARISTOTLE

Although Aristotle (384–322 B.C.) was the son of a physician in a family of three generations of physicians, he never practiced medicine. His remarkable genius lent itself to many themes, and he wrote extensively on all of them.[10] Found among his biological treatises are many astute physical and physiological pediatric observations. Some of these he borrowed from midwives, who undoubtedly would have recognized normal newborn appearances and functions. Aristotle's prescience was to record them, with additional comments about prognostic implications. He observed how experienced midwives animated anemic newborns by milking the cord:

Frequently the child appears to be born dead, when it is feeble and when, before the tying of the cord, a flux of blood occurs into the cord and adjacent parts. Some nurses who have already acquired skill, squeeze [blood] back out of the cord [to the baby] and at once the baby, who had previously been as if drained of blood, comes to life again. (*On the History of Animals*, bk. 7)

He described in detail the normal newborn's passage of meconium, transition to normal breast fed stools, and changes in physical appearance:

There is evacuation of excrement sometimes at once, sometimes soon, but always within the day, and this excrement is more than accords with the bulk of the child. Women call it meconium; its color is like blood and it is extremely black and like pitch but after this it already assumes the milk-like character for the infant draws the breast at once.

All children directly they are born have their eyes bluish, but afterwards these change to the sort they are destined to remain. (*On the Generation of Animals*, bk. 5.1)

Modern clinical and chromosomal studies have confirmed in particular the validity of one sagacious observation he made two millennia ago: "In man the male is more often born with deformity than the female" (*On the Generation of Animals*, bk. 6.6).

Aristotle, with careful thought, took issue with some of the prevailing wisdom of his times, such as the practice of giving wine to newborns. This otherwise original thinker, however, did accept some traditional tenets of thinking without challenge:

Generally speaking it is a common thing for convulsions to attack infants especially the better nourished, and those who get milk excessive in quantity or richness. Mischievous as regards this affection is wine, dark more than white, and wine not diluted with water, also most of the windy foods, also if the bowel is constipated. Most [babies] are carried off before the seventh day that is why they give the child its name then, as they have more confidence by that time in its survival. The illness is more severe during the full moon: there is also danger when babies have convulsions beginning in the back as they are getting older.[11] (*On the History of Animals*, bk. 7)

There were other masters of Greek medicine who followed Aristotle, but they gave little if any reference to children. Theophastus (330–225 B.C.) was the most prominent as a medical botanist, with his works *Historiae Plantarium* and *Causis Plantarium*. Praxagoras (c.340 B.C.) emphasized the diagnostic qualities of the pulse. Epicuris (342–270 B.C.) was a naturalist and physiologist.

The last two prominent figures were from Ptolemaic Alexandria. Herophilus (?330–?260 B.C.), horrifically, was given the right to practice vivisection on criminals. He made observations on the normal color, shape, movement, and pulsations of internal organs.* Erasistratus (310–250 B.C.) studied the vascular system, and to him is attributed the application of vessel ligature to facilitate surgical procedures.

With the decline and fall of Alexandria and its museum and library, the masters of Greek medicine had to seek new venues. The sacking of Corinth (146 B.C.), the fall of Ptolemaic Egypt (c.50 B.C.), and the ascent to power of Rome led physicians to Rome. In the new order of Roman world power, five contributors to pediatrics appeared: Celsus, Pliny, Soranus, Galen, and Aretaeus.

CELSUS

Cornelius Celsus (c.30 B.C.–45 A.D.) salvaged some Alexandrian medicine by incorporating it into his major work, the eight-volume *De Medicina* (c.10 A.D.). It was the first complete medical treatise after the Hippocratic Corpus. In the vast interim of centuries between them, in the words of Majno, "there is nothing but debris."[12]

Few pages of the large work specifically addressed children, but one particular line is crucial: "Children require to be treated entirely differently from adults."[13] It is an observation that should be obvious but still manages to elude a vast number of people involved in health management. Celsus, on this point, refused to recommend bloodletting, purgatives, or wine in the treatment of children.

Although most of his thoughts about child care were almost verbatim borrowings from Hippocrates, Celsus did express some unique thoughts—in his description of diphtheria, parasitoses, and tonsillitis, for example. Tonsillectomy was discussed in painful detail:

---

*This was reported by Celsus and confirmed by Galen and Tertullian. Whereas Celsus and Galen reluctantly justified the practice, Tertullian was indisputably disgusted by it: "Herophilus that physician or butcher who dissected six hundred men in order to find out nature, who killed men in order to learn the structure of their frame . . ." (quoted by Gordon, 1949, p. 596).

The tonsils which are indurated after inflammations being covered by a thin capsule should be scratched round and torn out by the finger: but if they are not got rid of thus, then one must seize them with a hook and cut them out with a knife, then wash the raw place with vinegar and smear the wound with some drug by which the bleeding is stopped. (*De Medicina*, 7.12)

He advocated delaying umbilical hernia repair until after the age of seven years (7.4). He recommended trusses for inguinal hernia since he felt herniorrhaphy was not tolerated well by children (7.20).[14] Celsus suggested leaving hydroceles intact, believing that they diminished in size spontaneously and nonsurgically (7.8).

He used infibulation in boys for "preserving their voices" (7.25).[15] This is a curious entry, and its meaning is uncertain. Infibulation was a pinning or stapling used to "seal" foreskins and vulvas against sexual use, but "preserving their voices" seems to suggest keeping testicular function intact and may refer to bringing down the undescended testes into the scrotal sac. Or it may mean the converse: sustaining a "castrati" voice by keeping the testes out of the scrotum.

PLINY

Although not a physician, the historian Pliny the elder (23–79 A.D.) left behind a number of noteworthy pearls of wisdom on pediatric matters. He wrote his 37-volume *Historia Naturalis* over a two-year period in a frenzy of encyclopedic compilation.[16] Among the many tomes with thousands of scattered factual, questionable, and sheer nonsense entries are some gems that, deservedly, have endured.

Pliny advocated smearing rennet on the nursing breast to bind and treat infantile diarrhea (8.173) and the use of the plant *Ephedra* to treat a bloody nose and the cough of asthma (7.365). The ephedrine extracted from *ephedra* still is used for the same purposes.[17]

He described the anatomy of the newborn, appropriately noting that a pulsating fontanel is normal (7.17). He commented on what appears to have been a hypothalamic tumor:

[T]he son of Euthymenes of Salamis had grown to be three cubits [±4.5 ft.] in height at the age of 3 years, that he was slow of gait and dull of comprehension, that at that age he had even attained puberty and his voice had become strong like that of a man. We hear also that he died suddenly of convulsions of the limbs at the completion of his third year. (7)

Pliny was a strong believer in dietetical and botanical medicine as well as homeopathic-strength dosages. For example, to promote the fading of child-

hood freckles he recommended a liniment of garlic, oil, and *garum*.*
Ironically, Pliny, who was distrustful of physicians,[18] bequeathed them a
most memorable aphorism on children, the validity of which has not diminished with time: "At the age of three years, the body of each person is one
half the length that it will ever attain."[19]

SORANUS

Soranus, who lived during the reigns of Trajan and Hadrian (98–138
A.D.), wrote specifically and comprehensively on many pediatric subjects in
his treatise *On Diseases of Women*. (Modern translations title this work,
Gynaecology.)

Before settling in Rome, Soranus of Ephesus (?–129 A.D.) studied in
Alexandria when it was still a great center of learning. Of his pediatric writings most were devoted to neonatal care, nutrition, and rearing: "How to
know what is capable of being reared," "How to divide the cord," "Inunc-
tion," "Swaddling," "Feeding," "Choice of a wet-nurse," "Cord separation,"
"Teething," "Rashes," "Wheezing and cough," "Seiriasis,"[20] and "Flux of
the belly," or diarrhea. The detail with which he wrote regarding initial care
of the newborn is worth noting:[21]

The approved way of salting.† Powdered soda ash either of the fine or coarse sort is
to be taken and sprinkled on the baby, avoiding the eyes and the mouth for any that
falls on these parts produces ulceration and inflammation and choking. And do not
sprinkle with too much salt, for through the excessive acridness, the skin, having a
quality just like seaweed and being very delicate, is eroded; but do not do it with too
little, otherwise the surface is not sufficiently hardened. It is agreed that if the infant
is a weakling the salt should be broken up with honey or oil or with decoction of
barley or fenugrec or mallow. After wiping away the salt the body should be washed
with warm water and all the adhering salt washed off. Then do the same a second
time; sprinkle the salt on, but wash it off with warmer water and with the finger
press out the glairy material which is in the nostril, and clean out the mouth and the
meatus of the ears, and drop some oil into the eyes, for it is good to wipe away with

---

Garum (fermented fish sauce) was a favorite cooking and medicinal ingredient for the
Romans. The fish body was salted to make *salsamentum*, and the head along with the viscera
was used to make *garum*. *Garum*-flavored meat was believed to stir appetite and was used as
part of the *gustatio*. It was incorporated into many medicinal compounds. For example, Galen
used lentils with *garum* for chronic diarrhea, and Dioscorides painted *garum* on infantile
thrush and aphthous ulcers. Curtis, R. I., *Garum and Salsamentum* (Leiden: E. J. Brill, 1991).

†Salting was a long-standing common practice. After birth, an infant was washed, salted with
soda ash or natron, and swaddled. The salt acted as an astringent on the clouts and was bacteriostatic. Salting was adopted by Christians for the baptism ritual. During the medieval

this the very thick moisture which is in them, and if this is not done it happens commonly that the children become blind.

Have the nail of the little finger previously pared, insert the little finger and divide the fine web-like material which has often formed about it [the anus] with a view to the easy passage of excrement; forthwith there is passed what it is customary to call meconium. On the navel put a little pad steeped in oil, or some wool, and one must ask for some cumin as an astringent. The tied-up portion of the cord which is left some bind on to the thigh, but it is better to double it over and roll it in the little bit of wool and then lay it gently against the middle of the navel, for perchance by the pressure of its weight the part will be moulded to a better-shaped depression. (*On Diseases of Women*, 1.13)

His reference to wiping the eyes of "thick moisture" may have been to prevent the eye infection ophthalmia neonatorum of gonococcus or chlamydia. The "pared" little finger nail was a favorite "instrument" of the surgeon, used not only for membranous imperforate anus but also for instant tonsillectomies.

In his comments on the early movements of a child, he once more contributes a remarkably thoughtful, thorough, and useful set of observations and guidelines:[22]

If no one supervises the movements of infants the limbs become distorted in most cases, for the whole weight of the body rests on the legs and the floor is hard and trodden firm and very generally stone paved; when therefore that on which he walks is resistant and the weight carried is heavy and the supporting substance is soft, necessarily the limbs yield as the bones are not yet become firm.

So when he first begins to sit he should be supported by a cloth wound round him, or be propped up by placing beside him something capable of supporting him, and it should not be for long at first. When he progresses as far as crawling and stands a little, stand him beside a wall by himself, but for walking put him up against a wheel-chair. In this way with the gradual development of all his parts he will acquire walking. (*On Diseases of Women*, 1.43)

Soranus gave no indications that he considered the adolescent in the domain of pediatrics. He considered, for example, that, at the age of 14, a girl reached womanhood.[23]

---

period, a child born on a Sunday was called a *sine-sal,* "without salt," because it was the day the salt seller did not work. A *sine-sal* was thought to be unlucky because baptism was not possible on its natal day. Salt sellers sold mined salt or sea salt. Therefore, sometime during the Middle Ages, salting changed from the use of sodium bicarbonate, or natron, to that of sodium chloride, or table salt. At baptisms the priests placed salt on the infants' tongues; this custom persisted into the seventeenth century.

It is good to preserve the state of virginity until menstruation begins by itself. For this will be a definite sign that the uterus is already able to fulfil its proper functions. . . . As a matter of fact in most instances the first appearance of menstruation takes place around the fourteenth year. This age then is really the natural one indicating the time for defloration. (*On Diseases of Women*, 1.33)

Soranus was the first to discuss the "nail-drop" method of testing breast milk consistency to determine its nutritional value. This method was used by physicians and others until the nineteenth century:[24]

Whether the milk will coagulate properly is determined by the fact that if we put a drop on the fingernail or on a laurel leaf or other smooth surface it slowly spreads and when shaken, retains the drop-form; for if it flows at once in all directions, it is watery, but if it coheres like honey and does not change its drop-form, it is too thick. (*On Diseases of Women*, 1.33)

GALEN

Claudius Galen (c.130–200 A.D.) was born in Pergamum, the seat of worship for Aesculapius.* He studied in Smyrna, Corinth, and Alexandria before settling in Rome. In *De Sanitate Tuenda* he focused on infant nutritional needs, astutely recognizing the three soothing modalities infants respond to: food, motion, and sound:[25]

---

*Asclepius (Aesculapius, in Latin) was the Greek god of medicine, associated with serpents and dogs and symbolizing the regenerative powers of earth and medicine. Many votive inscriptions have been uncovered that give healing credit to the lick of a sacred serpent or a puppy. The remains of puppies have been found interred together with newborns, presumably in hope of insinuating the child back to life.

Saliva contains regulatory peptides such as transforming growth factor a^2 and hepatocyte growth factor, as well as antimicrobials, like thiocyanate, and lysozymes (*Lancet* 1997; 349: 1776). Fijian fishermen keep dogs aboard to lick and heal acquired wounds (*Lancet* 1970; 1:615). Experimental animals with salivary glands removed (sialadenectomy) are unable to heal skin ulcers by licking them, as opposed to animals with intact glands (*Lancet* 1970; 350:369).

The saliva of two species of sacred serpents (both benign), *Elaphe longissima* and *quatuorlineata*, have been studied and found to have active polypeptide epidermal growth factor, which may indeed have contributed to the healing of skin lesions (*Lancet* 1992; 340:223). There are no similar data with respect to dogs, but one pediatric record reads:

> A dog cured a boy from Aegina. He had a growth on the neck. When he had come to the god, one of the sacred dogs healed him—while he was awake—with its tongue and made him well. (Cited by Jackson, 1988, p. 146)

Hence children fed on the mother's milk, are not only having the customary food but also the most proper, and nature seems not only to have prepared such nourishment for infants, but at the same time endowed them to use it. For if you place the teat in the mouth of a child just born it sucks and swallows most readily. . . .

If they are distressed and cry, by no means the least of remedies is the teat placed in the mouth. Nurses, taught by experience, have found these three remedies for children: one, that already mentioned, the other two, moderate movement and singing, by the use of which they not only soothe them but also induce sleep. (1.7)

Galen acknowledged the need for exercise to maintain good health, and described its different forms:[26]

Now there are three kinds of exercise, also for corresponding no doubt with differences of movement itself. The movement may be self-produced, it may be produced by some one else, or by medical direction. The third variety is not adapted to the healthy: the other is by boating, horse-riding, riding in a carriage and, as stated already, in cradle, hammock in the arms. The newborn do not require as yet such motion as occurs in a carriage or boat or on horseback, but those who have reached the third of fourth year, may have gentle movement even in carriage or boat. But when children have reached the 7th year, they bear more vigorous exercise, and may now be accustomed to horses. Children begin self-movement when they can crawl and especially when they can walk. But it is not good to compel them lest their legs become bent. Obviously even at this age it is clear how natural exercise is to us; for even though you shut children up you cannot prevent them from running about and jumping like chickens or horses or calves. (1.8)

Finally, Galen made the correlation between an infant's cleanliness and its level of comfort:[27]

I have also noticed that his cot and all his wrappings were too dirty and the infant himself dirty and unwashed, and I have ordered him to be bathed and that she should change his napkins for clean ones, and when these things were done the infant has stopped kicking and has settled off in a long sleep. In this matter there is need not only for forethought but of daily habit. (1.8)

ARETAEUS

Little biographical is known of Aretaeus, other than that he came from Cappedocia. The apex of his career is believed to have been circa 55 to 80 A.D. His major surviving work is *De Causis et Signis Morborum*.

Aretaeus did not specifically write on children's diseases, but in discussing morbid entities he commonly included the child, pointing out where the signs and symptoms differed in contrast to the adult. His clinical descriptions of diphtheria, pneumonia, empyema, cholera infantum, and other infectious diseases are as exacting as are his accounts of diseases of the central nervous system. But his long and detailed account of tetanus is most revealing, expressing the frustration of the physician who despairs in his inability to help:

Opisthotonus bends the patient backwards, like a bow, so that the reflected head is lodged between the shoulder-blades; the throat protrudes; the jaw sometimes gapes, but in some rare cases it is fixed in the upper one; respiration stentorous; the belly and chest prominent. . . .

   An inhuman calamity! an unseemly sight! a spectacle painful even to the beholder! an incurable malady. . . . But neither can the physician, though present and looking on, furnish any assistance, as regards life, relief from pain or from deformity.[28]

Despite the presence of four prominent Roman physicians who could claim expertise in pediatric medicine, Roman mothers looked to both physicians and their gods when their children became ill—and probably not in that order. It is likely, moreover, that they relied on folk medicine and superstitions for healing powers. Prayers to Jupiter for a child's recovery would be followed by dipping the recovered, naked child in the River Tiber on the subsequent feast day of Jupiter. Then, to protect the child from birds of prey that hovered over the Tiber, the mother prayed to Carna. These medical superstitions and curious treatments were commonplace. To strengthen them, Cato the Elder suggested bathing children in the warm urine of a cabbage eater. It was believed that a colicky baby could be calmed by placing goat dung in its diaper.[29] Pliny, in his *Natural History*, admonished nurses to spit on their charges three times at the approach of a stranger. This admonition most likely was an antidote to the evil eye, a malediction and peril considered so common that a special goddess of the cradle, Cunina, always was invoked to protect the infant. Spitting was an anti-*malocchio* remedy promulgated for centuries to protect children. It was practiced by Greeks, Turks, Slavs, Poles, Persians, and Roumanians, with unshakable belief.[30]

   A piece of liver from a slain gladiator was believed to cure epilepsy. Majno relates that children were known to step into the arena after major events and to stroll among the dead combatants, searching out eviscerated corpses in order to find exposed liver. He notes that children must have been inured to the spectacle. A floor mosaic in a Roman Carthage villa suggests as much, with a depiction of eight children playing gladiator and spearing cats and rabbits.[31]

Hippocrates, Aristotle, Celsus, Soranus, and Galen, then, were the major figures of the Greco-Roman period who understood the differences in growing and maturing organisms that necessitated altered and customized treatment modalities: "Ex toto non sic pueri ut viri curari debent."

When Diocletian established Byzantium as the eastern center of the Roman Empire in 285, this conduit between Europe and Asia became Rome's window to medical philosophy and learning from the East. Of the Byzantine groups of physicians, four in particular stand out for their contributions to child care: Oribasius, Aetius, Alexander Trallianus, and Paulus Aegineta.

ORIBASIUS

Like Galen before him, Oribasius (325–403 A.D.) hailed from Pergamum and studied in Alexandria. At the Emperor Julian's request, Oribasius wrote a 70-volume treatise on medicine. Much of this work was not original— rather a collection and compilation of texts from predecessors. Book 5 has similarities to data of Soranus, but Oribasius wrote more completely and with greater detail about children, as is evident in the table of contents:[32]

> On the feeding of an infant
> The qualities of a wet nurse
> On milk
> The correction of milk
> On rashes which occur in an infant
> On cough in an infant, and coryza
> On itching
> On teething
> On aphthae
> On excoriation of the thighs
> On running of the ears
> On seiriasis [meningitis?]
> Regimen from infancy to maturity

Only approximately one third of his encyclopedic magnum opus is extant, but the *Synopsis* he wrote for his son, Eustathios, is complete, and Book 5 contains most of his pediatric observations.

In great detail, Oribasius described Soranus' "nail test" on the quality of breast milk. He also, importantly, suggested a measure, albeit indirect, of milk's protein content:[33]

Pour an eighth part of the milk into a glass vessel, add rennet in proportion and stir with the fingers, then leave it to set and see whether the curd is less than the whey, for such milk is no good, and the reverse is indigestible: the best is that which contains both in equal proportions. (5.3)

His recipe to reduce the discomforts of teething included some curious ingredients to alleviate pain—particularly hare's brain.[34] Still, the prescription endured until the eighteenth century:

If they are in pain, smear [gums] with dog's milk or with hare's brain; this works also if eaten. But if a tooth is coming through with difficulty, smear cyperus with butter and oil-of-lilies over the part where it is erupting. (5.9)

The most salient aspect of Oribasius's work was the keen observations he made in his *Synopsis*[35] on healthy nurturing practices, hygiene, and nutrition. Noting that parents more often gave attention to their horses than to their children, he discussed child rearing from infancy to adolescence:

Infants who have just been weaned should be permitted to live at their ease and enjoy themselves: they should be habituated to repose of the mind and exercise in which little deceptions and gaiety play a part. . . . After the sixth or seventh year, little girls and boys should be confided to humane and gentle teachers: for those who attract children to themselves, who employ persuasion and exportation as a means of instruction and who praise their pupils often, will succeed better with them and will do more to incite their zeal to studies: their instruction will rejoice the children and put them at their ease. Now, relaxation and a joyous spirit contribute much to digestion and favorable nutrition; but those who, on the other hand, are insistent in instruction, who resort to sharp reprimands, will make the children servile and timorous and will inspire them with an aversion for the objects of their instruction: it is by beating them that they expect them to learn and recollect things, even at the very moment when they are beaten, when they lose their courage and presence of mind. It is not necessary either to torment children just beginning to learn by trying to teach them something through the whole length of the day: on the contrary the greater part of the day should be devoted to their games. . . . Children of twelve years should already frequent the grammarians and geometers and exercise their bodies; but it is necessary that they should have preceptors and supervisors who are reasonable and not entirely devoid of experience, so that they may know the amount and proper time for meals, exercise, bathing, sleeping and other details of personal hygiene. Most people will pay a high price for grooms for their horses, choosing for this purpose careful and experienced men, while they will select as teachers for their children, individuals without experience, who have already become useless and incapable of rendering any of the ordinary services of life. (5.14)

The observations on children's needs and behavior made by Oribasius remarkably anticipate by more than a millennium the philosophies of John Locke, John Dewey, and Maria Montesorri, namely, children's need for fantasy and a happy environment ("little deceptions and gaiety"), that they learn through games ("the greater part of their day should be devoted to games"), that a sound psyche facilitates growth ("relaxation and a joyous spirit"), that negative reinforcement impedes learning ("will inspire them with an aversion"), and that their narrow spans of concentration have to be considered ("length of day").

AETIUS

From Mesopotamia, Aetius of Amidis became physician to the Byzantine emperor Justinian I (527–565 A.D.). He wrote extensively on pediatric issues. One of the first medical writers to convert to Christianity, he laced his works with healing invocations such as "May the God of Abraham, the God of Isaac, the God of Jacob deign to give this medicine virtue."[36] Aetius discussed children's health in 26 chapters of volume 4 of his *Tetrabiblon*. Although many observations were not original and were reflections of other writers' works, a debt is owed Aetius for preserving material that otherwise would have been lost. Some of his discussions, however, were indeed original, among them the following chapters:[37]

Chapter 7:   Infants who snore
Chapter 8:   Infants who hiccough
Chapter 10: Inflammation of the eyes
Chapter 11: Childhood opacities
Chapter 14: On consumption of the spine
Chapter 17: Infantile sneezing
Chapter 26: Hairiness in children

He wrote on eye disorders in children, hitherto all but ignored, giving an exact description of trachoma, for example, and dividing the disease into four distinct stages to facilitate prognosis.[38] His chapter on the hirsute is a unique curiosity. Excessive hair is—and presumably was—not a common pediatric complaint,[39] but Aetius nevertheless suggested rubbing the body with the powder of burned dry figs as a cure.

He described childhood encephalitis, and his prognostications about diphtheria were sound:

[C]are should also betaken of the fever, which usually sets in with severity . . . in many cases the uvula is destroyed and, if after a long time the ulceration stops and cicatrization begins, children speak indistinctly and in swallowing, fluid returns through the nose. Thus I have seen a girl die after forty days, who was already in convalescence. Most cases, however, are in danger up till the seventh day.[40]

ALEXANDER TRALLIANUS

The principal work of Alexander Trallianus (525–606 A.D.) is his *Treatise on Pathology and Therapeutics* in 12 volumes. In pediatrics, however, Trallianus is known for a work on parasites. The work is a small manuscript —actually, a letter—sent to his friend Theodore, whose child was afflicted by worms.[41] Trallianus wrote authoritatively on the extant knowledge of worms in children and of vermifuges. (His work was borrowed by Hieronymus Mercuralis and incorporated into a pediatric treatise of 1583 [see below].)

Trallianus treated pinworms with enemas of ether oil; roundworms (*Ascaris*), with common *Artemissa maritima*, thyme, and coriander seeds. To treat *Taenia*, or flatworms, he concocted pomegranate seeds with castor oil. Another major contribution was a description of the various inflammatory lesions of the pharynx.[42]

PAULUS AEGINETA

The last of the pediatric writers from the waning Roman Empire was Paul of Aegina (?625–690 A.D.). Producing few original thoughts, his major contribution to pediatrics was a compilation of seven volumes, the first of which was dedicated to pregnancy and children and followed the known pharmacological wisdom of the day. His advice that mothers give children rhubarb or honey as an aperient remains a safe and time-proven remedy for children. In the event that a stronger laxative was needed, he recommended the use of irritants. Similarly, his suggestion to feed children millet for diarrhea follows basic tenets of ingesting bulk and fiber.[43]

If the child's belly be constipated, a little honey may be put into its food; and if even then it does not obey, turpentine, to the size of a chick-pea, may be added. When the bowels are loose, millet, in particular, ought to be administered. (1.10)

Diarrheas caused by epidemics of dysentery did not respond, of course, to such treatment, and children were the first to die of a choleric dehydration, often within a day of becoming ill. Profuse watery diarrhea, rapidly followed by parched, tenting skin; dry, sandy mouth; and sunken eyes took their toll, with acidosis and labored breathing followed by death. Gregory of Tours (538–594 A.D.) described a wave of dysentery that left many couples childless. Most of the deaths occurred among those under five years old:

[It] attacked young children first of all and to them it was fatal: and so we lost our little ones, who were so dear to us and sweet, whom we had cherished in our bosoms and dandled in our arms, whom we had fed and nurtured with such loving care.[44]

Much of Paulus Aegineta's writing on children was therapeutic in intent, but a few of his lines recommending a method of infantile castration speak volumes to prevailing attitudes regarding children.* Sometimes an abandoned male infant was made a eunuch and forced into prostitution. Castration was performed in infancy when testicles were small and soft:

[C]hildren, still of a tender age, are placed in a vessel of hot water, and then when the parts are softened in the bath, the testicles are to be squeezed with the fingers until they disappear. (6.68)

The hot water accomplished three things: it was a numbing anesthesia; it relaxed the testicles, allowing them to drop into the scrotum; and it softened the tissues.

Hospitals, a major revolutionary concept, appeared in late antiquity. Patristic councils of bishops and church leaders convened periodically to analyze pressing theological, liturgical, moral, and social dilemmas, and they often addressed issues related to the sick and homeless. In 325 A.D., the Nicaea Council ordered that asylums, called *xenodocheion* ("hotel"), be built in all Christian villages. They were to care for the poor, sick, homeless, and abandoned. Undoubtedly motivated by charity and compassion, the necessity for public health measures also informed the decision. The earliest record pertaining to a specific independent institution dedicated to the care of the sick[45] credits Basil of Caesarea in 357 A.D.:[46]

---

*Paulus Aegineta (translation of Francis Adams, 1844). Castration gradually fell into disuse during the medieval period, but reappeared in Spain and Italy in the sixteenth century. Two contributing factors to the resurgence of the mutilation were the prohibition, by Pope Sixtus V in 1589, of women on stage and the need for postpubertal male sopranos for a genre of secular music that was popular at the time. Since only the papal states enforced the proscription of female actors, the Vatican gradually became the capital of *castrati* for both stage and chorus until, in 1903, they were banned by Pius X from the papal chapel. Smith, A. M. Eunuchs and castration. *JAMA* 1991; 266:655–66.

The leaders of the churches founded some of these out of hospitality. They made lepers and other sick people move in there and provided what they needed as much as possible. (Epiphanius, *Panarium*, 75.1)

Basil's own words reveal the generous and egalitarian nature of his concept of the *xenodocheion*:[47]

Are we doing anybody any harm if we build shelters for all passersby who need somebody's attention because of ill health and if we provide them with the necessary relief through male nurses, physicians, and men in charge of transportation—these have to apply the skills needed for saving lives and skills for making life more comfortable. (Basilius Caesariensis, *Epistuale*, 94.1)

It is clear from historical records that these institutions rapidly grew in number throughout the Byzantine Empire. These were predominantly for adults, but a number of *brephotrophia*, or "baby shelters," also appeared. The assumption is that these were "children's hospitals,"[48] since abandoned or orphaned children were looked after in *orphanotropheions*.

There was strong superstition, resulting in extreme ennui, associated with the year 1000. The millennium, it was widely thought, presaged the end of the world, and the attitude suffocated intellectual endeavors of all kind.[49] Certainly, this was the case with Western medicine, and especially as it related to children. Extant Western medical texts were translated, however, into Arabic by Byzantine sectarians and Jewish scholars. During this period only the East produced physicians of renown, whose curiosity about and interest in understanding disease led them to formulate new concepts about and understanding of disease. In the West, medicine came to depend on the monastic scriptorium that translated Arabic into Latin. Monks like Constantinus Africanus (1018–1085) in Carthage and Gerald Cremonius (1114–1187) of Toledo were responsible for continuity of medical thought in Western medicine. The wisdom of Rhazis, Averroe, Haly Abbas, Avicenna, and other Arabic scholars was so widely respected that their works reached the ears even of Geoffrey Chaucer.

NOTES

1. Gordon, 1949, pp. 433–98.
2. Lloyd, 1978, pp. 10–11.
3. All the quotations that follow are from the translation of Chadwick and Mann (1950), Still (1931), or Adams (1849).
4. Aries, 1965, p. 129.

5. Further elaboration on age-cycle diseases appears in *Coan Prognosis*, 502:

The diseases which do not occur before puberty [fourteen] are pneumonia, pleurisy, gout, nephritis, varicose veins of the legs, bloody discharges, cancer unless congenital, white dropsy unless congenital, catarrh of the back, hemorrhoids and ileus of the large bowel unless congenital.

6. The mysterious wiggly creatures living inside the human body always have caused, at the very least, consternation, if not outright revulsion. It is not surprising that in ancient Babylonia, Egypt, Israel, India—and in Hippocrates so much attention to them was devoted to them. They have been blamed for, among other things, teething pain and convulsions. In our day even Hollywood has capitalized on the repulsion they elicit; an example is the larval *Alien* that erupted from the abdomen of actor John Hurt in the film of the same name. A startling fact is that *Dracunculus medinensis* and other parasites do erupt with equally menacing shock.

7. Hippocrates thought the designation nonsense, invented by charlatans. "I do not believe that the 'Sacred Disease' is any more divine or sacred than any other disease but, on the contrary, has specific characteristics and a definite cause."

8. *The Sacred Disease*, 1:2.

9. Ibid., 10.

10. The quotes that follow are from the translations of McKeon (1941).

11. This last entry, regarding "convulsions beginning in the back" may have been in reference to opisthotonos, a physical sign commonly observed in cerebrospinal meningitis.

12. Majno, 1975, p. 328.

13. "Ex toto non sic pueri ut viri curari debent." *De Medicina*, 3.7.

14. Ibid., pp. 20–21.

15. Abt, 1965, p. 43.

16. Pliny's curiosity about all things natural ultimately led to his death as he sailed into the eruption of Mount Vesuvius to study the smoke and gases. The sulfurous emissions suffocated him in 79 A.D.

17. Manjo, 1975, pp. 341–51.

18. "Physicians acquire their knowledge from our dangers, making experiments at the cost of our lives" (8.195).

19. Ibid., 7.16.

20. This is believed to have been meningitis.

21. *Gynaecology*, 2.13.

22. Ibid., 2.43.

23. Ibid., 1.33.

24. Ibid., 2.21–23.

25. *De Sanitate Tuenda*, 1.7.

26. Ibid., 1.8.

27. Ibid.

28. Ruhräh, 1925, pp. 10–11.

29. Rucker, C. W., Folk medicine in the Roman Empire. *Mayo Alumnus* 10(1) (1974): 26–30.

30. Dundes, 1992, pp. 12–38.

31. Majno, 1975, pp. 401–2.

32. Oribasius, *Synopsis* (1876 translation), bk. 5.

33. Ibid., p. 38. In fact, good mature human milk has a casein:whey ratio of 30:70, not 50:50.

34. Ibid.

35. Ruhräh, 1925, p. 13.

36. Ibid., p. 15.

37. Still, 1931, pp. 39–40.

38. Meyerhof, 1984, 2:32–33.

39. Indeed, it is such a curious entry that one is led to speculate whether there might have been an environmental cause or toxin producing hirsutism in children— a botanical agent or fungal contaminant, perhaps. Cyclosporin, for example, is a fungal metabolite known to produce hirsutism.

40. Ruhräh, 1925, p. 16.

41. Walsh, 1911, pp. 49–50.

42. Huard and LaPlane, 1981, p. 36.

43. Paulus Aegineta, 1844 (translation of Francis Adams).

44. Gies, 1987, p. 60.

45. Cited by van Minnen, 1955, p. 157.

46. Ibid., p. 158.

47. Referred to here is not a site of incubation, such as an Aesculapian temple where a patient went transiently for a night's sleep and a theurgical cure, but a free-standing institution specifically dedicated to hospitality for the chronically or ter-minally ill. Besides *xenodocheion*, such an institution also was called a *nosokomeion* (monastery sick ward), a term that would be familiar to today's physician.

48. This, of course, is reasonable hypothesis. To find the origins of a "children's hospital" as we know it today we must refer to the *Krankenhaus* of the eighteenth century. (See below.)

49. Although superstition abounded in the medieval world, most historians con-tend that few people had the knowledge or instruments to know with accuracy when the 1000th year would occur. Nevertheless, there is no doubt that documentation and historical records more than trebled after 1000 A.D., suggesting an intellectual languor related to the millennium.

Chapter 4

Medieval Pediatrics

In the prologue to the *Canterbury Tales*, Geoffrey Chaucer (1340–1400) depicted a doctor of physic who was well versed in all the medical classics—ancient, Eastern, and Western:

> With us ther was a Doctour of Phisyk
> In al this world ne was ther noon him lyk
> To speke of phisik and surgerye, . . .
> Wel knew he the olde Esculapius
> And Deiscorides, and eek Rufus
> Old Ypocras, Haly and Galien
> Serapion, Razis, and Avicen
> Averrois, Damascien, and Constantyn
> Bernard, and Gatesden, and Gilbertyn.

The physik had read the ancient works of Aesculapius, Dioscorides, Rufus of Ephesus, Hippocrates, Galen. Importantly, he also was familiar with a number of medieval Islamic physicians whose manuscripts also had found their way to Europe and were translated into Latin. The writings of these sages filled the void of Europe's barren scientific wasteland of the Dark Ages.

The works of the Islamic writers, Haly Abbas, Serapion, Rhazes, Avicenna, and Averroe, were well known—renowned—throughout Europe, and, with few exceptions, they were the only sources available in the West for topics related to child care. Chaucer kept his doctor mute on the subject of pediatric medicine and gave him a ribald tale to spin for his fellow pilgrims on their way to Canterbury; his list of physicians, however, is remarkable in its implication that the poet could expect his fourteenth-century audience to know the references!*

When Plato's Academy closed in 529, some scholars migrated east to the Jundishahpur University in Persia. There, the medical school flourished as Islamic physicians learned from these new sources about the works of the Greek physicians. Hunayn ibn Ishaq al-Ibadi (809–873) and his collaborators translated the corpus of Greek and Roman medicine, including Hippocrates, Galen, Paulus Aegineta, and Oribasius into Arabic. By the end of the ninth century, Arabic physicians had a core curriculum grounded in Greek, Roman, Byzantine, Chinese, and Indian medicine.[1]

RHAZES

The first of the Islamic writers to have works translated into Latin was Rhazes (865–925), whose full name was Abu Bakr Muhammad ibn Zakariya al-Razi. His *Book on Medicine Dedicated to Mansur* (c.903) was translated into Latin by Gerard of Cremona as *Liber ad Almansoris* in 1187. His major work, the *Kitab al-Hawi fi al-tibb* (Comprehensive Book on Medicine) was published in Latin under the title *Continens* in 1279. Rhazes' major contributions were small treatises on diseases of children, on smallpox and measles. He noted the frequency of smallpox in children and its differentiation from measles, the various presentations of both diseases, and the complications in children. The latter material was appended to *Almansoris*, which totaled 23 chapters detailing major known illnesses of children. It was translated into

---

*Although not named in the Prologue, Chaucer later refers to "Dame Trot"—Trotula de Ruggiero, a twelfth-century practitioner from Salerno known for her treatises on women, *De Passionibus Mulierum Curandarum* and *De Ornatu Mulierum*. The *Passionibus* featured a long and thorough section on parturition and its complications and on *newborn care*. King, 1991, p. 44; Anderson and Zinsser, 1988, p. 525; and Walsh, 1911, pp. 182–86. Karl Sudhoff (1853–1938), one of the great medical historians, argues that "Trotula" probably was collective name for all the Salernian midwives, but this is irrelevant to our purposes. What counts is the existence of an extensive body of Salernian writing on newborn care. Medvei, 1982, p. 92.

Latin under the title *De Aegritudinibus Puerorum et Earum Cura*[2] and was published in Europe multiple times from the tenth to the sixteen centuries. The chapters discussed epilepsy, eye diseases, dental problems, vomiting, dysentery, otitis, cough, constipation, itching, worms, fissures, bladder stones, strabismus, and other ailments. Among them was a curious condition called mater puerorum, which was marked by crying, nocturnal restlessness, insomnia, and fever. It was treated with *Theriaca magna*.*

In chapter 16, Rhazes described infantile diarrhea:[3]

Infants are frequently troubled with flux of the bowels, whether from teething, from catching cold, from spoiling of the milk by choler and phlegm; and the signs of choler are acidity and acridity of the stools, which are rapidly evacuated; and the signs of cold and phlegm are light-colored stools, griping pains in the abdomen on evacuation, which is instantaneous unless the phlegm [mucous] be viscid. (*De Aegritudinibus Puerorum*, chap. 16)

His anecdotal case histories, vividly described with a great deal of warmth and personal involvement, are mainly noted for pathos and a remarkable understanding of pathophysiology. A description of acute glomerulonephritis secondary to measles or streptococcus infection is a case in point:[4]

The little son of Ibn Sawada had a yellow bile fever from his throat. On the fourth day in the morning he began to urinate blood and to pass with the stools green and bloody bile, resembling water in which fresh meat had been washed; his strength decreased suddenly. We were baffled because his malady has been slight and benign and then had changed in one night to this acuteness and severity. . . . When the afternoon came, he had quite black micturition and equally black stools. He died in the early morning of the sixth day. He had had from the beginning a malign form of measles, prone to attack the internal organs. (*Clinical Observations*, case 24)

AVICENNA

The most famous of all the medieval Arab physicians was Abu Ali al Husayn ibn Abd Allah ibn Sina, known in the Latinized world as Avicenna (980–1037). Avicenna's best known works were *Canticum de Medicina*, con-

---

Theriaca magna was considered a "wonder drug." Originally, the compound was formulated by the Greeks to treat the bites of wild animals (Thería). Gradually, the legendary poison antidote, Mithridatium, was added to the compound, rendering it an "all-purpose" drug. Over time, 64 ingredients enhanced the mix, including the flesh of viper and opium. Majno, 1975, pp. 413–16. It was used for all manner of illnesses in all manner of patients, including children. It remained in use until 1884.

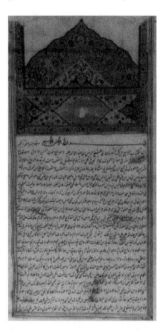

Figure 4.1 Avicenna's *Canonis Medicinae.* COURTESY NATIONAL LIBRARY OF MEDICINE.

sisting of numbered aphorisms in the tradition of Hippocrates, and *Canonis Medicinae* (figure 4.1), an encyclopedic work with four chapters in volume 1 dedicated to pediatrics.[5] The chapters reviewed prior work covered in greater detail by Paulus Aeginata and Rhazes. Nineteen additional chapters on hygiene, exercise, diet, and sleep in the growing child followed in the subsequent volumes.

Avicenna's originality was the attention he gave to preventative measures and to psychic well-being. In the *Canticum* he emphasized the importance of prenatal care for mother and child:

Let care be taken of the infant in his mother's womb, that no harm happen to his body . . . let the mother's blood be kept in good order and let the excess of it, out of which the infant is formed, be kept pure. (*Canticum*, 2.85)

Avicenna's conservative, noninvasive philosophy of care and his recognition of the special needs of infants are two outstanding features of his work: "[B]eware that no opening of a vein be done, and no purging by drug, until he is found to have reached puberty" (*Canticum*, 3.98).

He advocated children's developmental and psychosocial needs 900 years or more before such themes were sounded:

In his waking time put him in the light that he may see the stars and the sky, and show him sometimes various colors that so you may accustom him to the use of his eyes . . . speak to him with a loud voice while you are looking after him so that you may accustom him to speech. (*Canticum*, 3.103)

He eloquently expressed the importance of children's emotional needs, and, perhaps for the first time in history, he made the correlation between the happy mind and the healthy body:

All our study, all our care, should be directed to forming and molding the character of the child. Care must be taken that he does not blaze out with anger, nor be overwhelmed with fear, nor cast down by sadness, nor harassed by wakefulness. So we must always notice what he wants, what he is eager for, and this should be provided for him and given to him, but what he dislikes should be taken out of his way. For hence comes a two-fold advantage, one to the mind, the other to the body: to the mind because he grows up from infancy imbued with good disposition and acquires a fixed habit of this, to the body because just as a bad character is related to some faulty constitutional tendency, so if this bad character is the result of habit, indisposition of like kind is associated with it. (*Canonis*, bk. 1, chap. 4)

Several other Arabian physicians contributed to pediatric thought in the West. Their works have survived in Latin translations. Haly Abbas (?900–994), Albucasis (10th cen.), Averroes (1126–1198), and Avenzoar (?1070–1162) are pertinent to this history.

Haly Abbas's *Liber Regius* contained 20 chapters, many of which were devoted to surgical treatment and invasive procedures such as trocar insertion for ascites (figure 4.2), and methods of cauterization and ligature of arteries.[6] He did, however, make many nonsurgical and pediatric observations. For infants, he recommended digital dilation for anal stenosis, and he annotated differences in the quality of milk in various animal species and their applications in infant nutrition. Haly Abbas's evaluation of human versus cow, sheep, camel, goat, and ass milk suggests that, in his native Persia, there was familiarity with Hindu medicine and the *Vagbhata* Samhita.

Albucasis's major work was the *Altasrif* (Miscellany). Much of his work was taken from Rhazes, but his surgical and procedural opinions were original.[7] Scattered throughout the chapters he noted special methods for children. Among these, Albucasis described inserting thin lead plates between the fingers after separation of syndactyly. Foreign bodies and insects in the ear canal (a common mishap in children) were removed by suction through a copper reed. He described procedures for dealing with infantile hydrocephaly (chap. 1), tooth extractions (chap. 30), imperforate urethra (chap. 55), circumcision corrections (chap. 57), and imperforate anus (chap. 79). The examples that follow refer to hare lip and imperforate meatus and anus.[8]

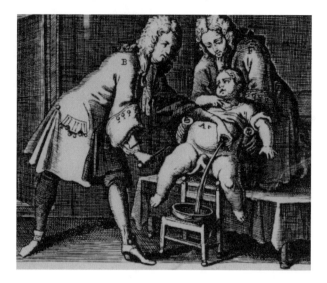

Figure 4.2 Trocar treatment of ascites in a child, from Francisco Suarez de Ribera (?1686–1738), *Clave Medico-Chirurgica Universal* (Madrid: Francisco del Hierro, 1730).

There often occur fissures in the lip to which are given the name of "hares"; they are particularly common in the lips of boys. When you have ineffectually treated these clefts . . . heat a small edged cautery of this shape. The hollow should be as sharp as a knife. Then quickly place it when hot right on to the fissure till the burning has reached the depth of the lip. Then treat with wax plaster till healed. (chap. 18)

Sometimes a boy is born from his mother's womb with the glans penis not perforated. So at the moment of his birth you should be quick and make a perforation with a scalpel figured thus. Then put in the opening a slender leaden sound, tie it and keep it for three or four days. When he wishes to make water, it will be removed and he will do so and then put it back. (chap. 55)

Infants are quite often born with the anus imperforate, closed by a fine membrane; then the midwife should perforate the membrane with her finger or pierce it with a sharp scalpel being careful not to touch the muscle. Then wool dipped in oil and wine should be applied, and treat it with ointment until healed. If you are afraid it may close up, put into the opening a leaden tube for many days, which will be removed when the child wants to evacuate the bowel. (chap. 79)

Averroes was a prolific writer and author of 33 works on philosophy and science, only three of which were medical: a commentary on Avicenna's *Canticum*, a treatise on Theriac, and his *Colliget*, which contained his pediatric thought. Averroes, in consort with this teacher, Avenzoar, disapproved of salting the newborn, advocating instead oil as an emollient. He recommended moderate exercise for children but decried cold bathing, believing that it inhibited growth.[9]

Ibn Qayyim al-Jawziya (1292–1350) from Damascus wrote a child-rearing manual called *Tuhfat al-mawdud*, in which care of the newborn is discussed. Primarily of Hellenistic sources, the focus was secondarily medical. The manuscript observed that first smiles occur at about 40 days of age, which is about the time the infant acquires visual tracking and displays social interaction. Teething irritability was relieved by rubbing the gums with butter.[10]

Arabic medicine preserved ancient wisdom and served as a bridge between the Byzantine and Western worlds. In addition to their interpretations and analyses of the old masters, many original contributions, procedurally and therapeutically, were made (i.e., surgical innovations, botanical treatments from the East, and new physiological concepts).[11] Most significantly, a philosophical outlook best expressed by Rhazes' aphorisms was introduced to Western thought and had important applicability to all, especially to child care. The following examples are cited by Walsh:[12]

Truth in medicine is a goal which cannot be absolutely reached, and the art of healing, as it is described in books, is far beneath the practical experience of a skilful, thoughtful physician.

When you can heal by diet, prescribe no other remedy, and, where simple remedies suffice, do not take complicated ones.

Physicians ought to console their patients even if the signs of impending death seem to be present. For the bodies of men are dependent on their spirits.

Arabic hospitals were indicative of the East's superior medicine and medical care in the Middle Ages. There were teaching hospitals (*bimarestans*) in Baghdad, in Damascus, and in Moorish Cordova, Spain, modeled after the hospital of Jundi Shahpour established by the Nestorians circa 530 A.D.[13] The Mansur hospital of Cairo was completed in 1284, and in many respects it remarkably resembled a modern infirmary. It had separate wards for men and women and specialty wards for wounds, eyes, and fevers. It had a teaching courtyard for lectures, a library, a pharmacy, and the equivalent of the modern psychosocial services in the guise of Koran readers, storytellers, and musicians. There was even a welfare department, which provided convalescence funds to discharged patients.[14]

Although not original, there were two anonymous works that have been cited as important links with the four incunabula of pediatrics that appeared in the early Renaissance.[15] There is evidence that the authors of the incunabula[16] had read both the *Liber de Passionibus Puerorum Galeni* and *Practica puerorum: Passiones puerorum adhuc in cunabulis jacencium*.[17]

The *Liber de Passionibus Puerorum Galeni* was written about the ninth century; it reproduced the aphorisms of Hippocrates and his recommended pharmacopeia of prescriptions. It opens, "As Hippocrates relates in his aphorisms, infants develop many diseases, like cough, vomiting, insomnia, fevers, diarrhea, convulsions, constipation,"[18] and proceeds to present botanical prescriptions for various symptoms, as in the following example:

If it suffers vomiting, make the following plaster and place upon the forking of the breast and on the throat: Rx mastiches, olibani et pulverem rosarum.

Distemper with juice of mint and mallows, if you wish, and if the vomiting has been violent, add a dash of vinegar.[19]

The second anonymous source appeared in the twelfth century. It was a compilation of Greek and Arabic writings on the diseases of children still in the cradle and was called *Practica puerorum: Passiones puerorum adhuc in cunabulis jacencium*. The text addressed some very practical aspects of child care. To assess the quality of milk it employed a variation of Soranus's nail test:[20] "[I]t is put on a mirror or on polished steel, if it keeps its position like a crystal it is good, but if it spreads out like water it is not good."

Each subject, symptom, or affliction was introduced with a conditional aphoristic, "If he suffers . . ."

If a child suffers from fissure of the lips . . . take well combed wool and put it in the juice of plantain and lanceola and a little butter or fresh hen's grease, and smear the lips with a feather either with this liquefied or with the plain juices.

The text favored topical remedies over ingested ones, giving many recipes for plaster and poultice compounds for fever, diaper rash, and parasites. Perhaps ineffective, it was nevertheless innocuous and, in this respect, a safe compendium to follow, adhering in principle to *primum non nocere*:

If he have a fever, take a little barley ground with violet and temper this meal with juice of wormwood, mallows, plantain and navelwort and make a plaster and place it upon the little fork of the breast.

If because of the saltness of the urine and softness of the flesh he suffer excoriation and heat around the legs, sprinkle the place with wheat meal well tritonized or with powder of roses not too fine.

If he has slippery worms in his stomach, take the juice of wormwood and pulp of coloquintida and ox gall and apply to the umbilicus as hot as can be borne.

TABLE 4.1
PHYSICIANS FROM SALERNO WRITING ON CHILDREN

Author	Work	Pediatric Contents
Trotula	*De Passionibus Mulerium*	Normal newborn care
Hildegarde	*Physica*	Normal newborn care
Aldebrandino	*Regime du Corps*	Infant hygiene

In the high Middle Ages, Italian physicians of the so-called School of Salerno touched on pediatrics. Located south of Naples, the school evolved around a Benedictine hospital that had been founded in 820 A.D. The school was independent from the church and was open to all faiths and philosophies and to men and women. It was in its prime during the twelfth to the thirteenth centuries. It organized its curriculum on anatomy and surgery and produced a body of texts that serially covered diseases *a capite ad calcem.* Pediatric data was incorporated into general data and was scattered throughout the text, making the observations on child care difficult to extract. Table 4.1 lists the principal Salernian works that touched on children.[21] For all of that, the issues are minor, meriting acknowledgment only.

Three other European medical works of the early Renaissance are frequently cited by historians, but none mentioned medical care specific to children. John of Gaddesden (1280–1361) wrote and edited the *Rosa Anglica Practica Medicine a Capite ad Pedes*; a monk, Bartholomaeus Anglicus, wrote *De Proprietatibus Rerum* around 1260; and Guy de Chauliac (1300–1368) wrote *Chirugia Magna.*

In sum, medieval Europe produced mostly inconsequential original pediatric thoughts and relied on derivative works, direct translations of works from other eras and cultures. Throughout Europe, simple yet crucial concepts of health, nutrition, and hygiene were yet to be understood and applied. Prevailing ignorance that perpetuated misery and negatively affected longevity persisted for centuries. In the medieval world the sane—and general—attitude was not to expect very much in this life.

NOTES

1. Tschanz, 1997, pp. 23–24.
2. Table of Contents, *De Aegritudinibus Puerorum et Earum Cura* by Rhazes:

De sabasato puerorum	De obliquitate visus
De favositate puerorum	De morbis dentium

De magnitudine capitis puerorum	De pustulis quae accidunt in ore puerorum
De inflatione ventris puerorum	De vomitu in pueris
De sternutatione puerorum	De fluxu ventris puerorum
De vigiliis puerorum	De constipatione puerorum
De epilepsia puerorum	De tussi puerorum
De quadam passione quae dicitus mater puerorum	
De sanie aurium puerorum	De pruritu et vesicis
De veneno fluente de aure	De lumbricis puerorum
De morbis oculorum in pueris	De crepatura puerorum
De lapide in vesicis puerorum	De relaxatione puerorum

The 1513 edition printed in Venice discussed only disease, without mentioning normal newborn care and development.

3. Ruhräh, 1925, p. 21.

4. Meyerhof, 1984, pp. V 343–44.

5. *Kitab al-Qanun fi al-tibb* or *Canon of Medicine*.

6. Walsh, 1911, p. 122.

7. The surgical work was translated into Latin by Gerald of Cremona sometime between 1150 and 1200 as *Liber Alsaharavi de Cirurgia*. Walsh, 1911, pp. 126–27; and Abt, 1965, p. 55.

8. Spink and Lewis, 1973.

9. In these and other points, Avenzoar disagreed with Avicenna, along the way influencing his pupil Averroe to believe the same. Savage-Smith, 1994, p. 10.

10. Gil'adi, 1992, pp. 19–34.

11. Pulmonary circulation was described by al Din ibn al-Nafis (1200–1288), an achievement later attributed to Servetus in 1553. Porter, 1997, p. 103.

12. Walsh, 1911, pp. 115–16.

13. Ziai, 1975, p. 83; Radbill, 1955, p. 412.

14. Hastings, 1974, pp. 28–29

15. A third source from Spain, *Tratatus de fetus generatione ac puerperatum infantium que regimine* by Garibai-Ben-Said (c.975), may have been read by early the incunabulist. It focused on physiological phenomena attending pregnancy, birth, and lactation, progressing to a nurture regimin assuring the health of the child. Vilaplana Satorre, 1934, p. 184.

16. Ruhräh, 1925, pp. 22–26.

17. Latin, of course, was the language of education, religion, and science and served as the *lingua franca* of medicine for over 1000 years. Like the *snwu* who trained in the Egyptian temples or the healers who applied the serpents in the Aesculapian temples, medieval physicians trained in their "temples"—the Church. The most influential of them were churchmen. The cathedral schools that evolved into universities, such as the universities of Montpellier (1181), Paris (1110), Bologna (1113), and Oxford (1167), employed church clerics as professors. Ackerknecht, 1982, pp. 84–86.

18. *Ut testatur Ypocras in afforismus, pueris noviter genitis multae passionibus emergunt, ut tusses, vomitus, vigiline, febres, dyarrie, tremores, ventris constipationes. . . .* Ruhräh, 1925, p. 22.

19. Ibid., p. 23.

20. The examples that follow are from the translations of Karl Sudhoff (1925) as cited by Ruhräh and Still.

21. Walsh, 1911, pp. 141–62.

Chapter 5

The Incunabula and Pediatric Poems

By the end of the fifteenth century, nearly every European city had hospitals and foundling homes (table 5.1). Sick, abandoned, or plague-displaced children found shelter in foundling hospices. They typically were not salubrious institutions but functioned with good intentions. Within this Renaissance of humanistic compassion, pediatric manuscripts first appeared in the West.

Beginning in the late fifteenth century, four great medical treatises on children's physiology and pathology were written. They are collectively referred to as the *Pediatric Incunabula*. Attesting to Europe's increasing

TABLE 5.1

MAJOR EXTANT FOURTEENTH-CENTURY FOUNDLING HOMES

City	Hospital	Date
Florence	Santa Maria de San Gallo	1294
Florence	Santa Maria della Scala	1316
Florence	Loggia del Bigallo	1352
Florence	Santa Maria degl'innocenti	1445
Rome	Santo Spirito de Sassia	1201
Marseille	Saint Esprit de Montpellier	1188
Chartres	L'Aumone de Notre Dame	1349
Embeck	Order of Saint Esprit	1274
Paris	Saint Esprit en Greves	1362
Lyon	Hotel-Dieu de Notre Dame de Pitie	1523
London	Eleemonsynary St. Katherine	?

recognition of and interest in children's growth and development, these seminal texts on child care were widely consulted in their time, and they influenced in a major way the proliferation of pediatric manuscripts of subsequent centuries. The incunabula were written by Paulus Bagellardus a Flumine (?–1492), Bartolomaeus Metlinger (?–1491), Cornelius Roelans (1450–1525), and Heinrich von Louffenburg (1391–1460).

PAULUS BAGELLARDUS

Paulus Bagellardus (?–1492?) studied in Padua and wrote his Latin text, *De Infantium Aegritudinibus et Remediis*, in 1472. It was divided into sections on management of the newborn and on diseases of children. On first reading, it becomes evident that he compiled and somewhat compounded old errors such as treatments using the dung of various animals, burned powders, and even gems hung around the necks of children.

However, his remarks on infant care have endured through the centuries, owing to reasonably accurate advice and, most notably, the elegant expression of Bagellardus's sweet and loving interest in the physical and emotional well-being of infants:[1]

When the infant at the command of God emerges from the womb, then the midwife with eager and gentle hand should wrap it up in a linen cloth . . . noting whether the infant be alive or not or spotted, i.e., whether black or white or of bluish color and whether it is breathing or not. If she find it warm, not black, she should blow into its mouth, if it has no respiration. . . . If the infant is alive and of bluish color, then she should cut the umbilicus. . . . [I]f the umbilicus does not consolidate, then she should cover it with powdered myrrh or aloe, or what is better, powdered myrtle. . . . [F]eed the infant by light and nursing, lest by excessive nursing she should cause coagulation of the milk in its stomach. When the nursing has been finished, let her put the infant in the cradle, placing over it a covering which does not touch its face, push the cradle to and from and thereby with a light motion produce a gentle slumber. Let her chant in a low voice, so that the infant's spirits rejoicing in harmony may become cheerful. Let there be no noise in the room or harsh voice or anything else which might frighten the infant. (*Libellus*, bk. 1)

The section on children's diseases is indexed into 22 parts covering favosity (ringworm), epilepsy, colic, eye diseases, ear discharges, scrofula and mastoiditis, gum problems, the lips, the throat, vomiting and diarrhea, constipation, parasites, swellings, urination problems, bed-wetting, hernias, and sores. The chapters were descriptive and prescriptive. Some had prognostic elements, such as this example that compares a tympanitic abdomen with congenital intestinal obstruction:

Infants are subject to tumor or inflation of the belly so that, by touching or striking, it sounds like the noise of cymbals . . . tumor of the belly from wind, as a condition, is contracted either from birth or from a neglect by the midwife. . . . [If] contracted from birth, it can in no wise be corrected. If from neglect of the nurse who bathes it, let what we are about to say be done [which he treats with].

Rx origani, castorei, cymini—ana partes aequales. Let them be triturated vigorously and mixed and given to the infant in a potion by weight of three grains of barley with milk or aromatic wine. (*Libellus*, 2.17)

Familiar with prevailing medical practice, Bagellardus admonished physicians to treat children with a restraint appropriate to their vulnerable physiology, and he warned about the effects of pharmacopoeia: "The curing must always be begun with the lighter remedies, since all things which provoke sleep are narcotic and in certain measures stupefying" (*Libellus*, 2.4).

Reluctantly and only "upon urgent necessity" did he prescribe an opioid sedative: "Let the infant have some food taken in the form of a biscuit soaked in a decoction of white poppy seed."[2]

Bagellardus advocated the routine use of wet nurses unless the family was poor, in which case the infant was to be nursed by the mother (*si infans pauperculus sit*). Almost a century later, in an edited version of Bagellardus's work, Petrus Toletus rejected wet nursing: "I would have a mother to be the one and only feeder of her child."[3]

Petrus Toletus (1502–?1567), from Lyon, was a graduate of Montpellier. He worked for a time at the Hotel Dieu, where he most likely acquired his interest in children. In 1560 he published an edition of Bagellardus's book with the title *Opusculum recens natum de morbis puerorum*. There was no acknowledgment to Bagellardus on the title page—only grudging mention in the introductory dedication. Although Toletus credits Bagellardus with the thought, Toletus himself, in a succinct poetic couplet, expressed as none had before the essential imperative of pediatric care (emphasis added):[4]

> *Till now the babes oft died with ills unknown,*
> *For none was there with skills to succour them;*
> Of midwife or of mother or of nurse,
> What service each should give, no leech has told;
> Small wonder! hard the task, to sage scarce known;
> This hath Bagaldus of the River writ.
> His book with notes Toletus doth adorn;
> Sure none can write more learnedly than these!
> Sweet reader, buy this book, whoe'er thou art,
> If thou dost care that babes should healthy be.

BARTOLOMAEUS METLINGER

Bartolomaeus Metlinger's first edition of *Ein Regiment der Jungerkinder*[5] in 1473 (figure 5.1) was the first pediatric text printed in the German vernacular. Although there is very little originality in his work, it had a broader readership, presuming that common literate folk knew no Latin. Metlinger's philosophy of child care was largely influenced by Avicenna and Rhazes. It was divided into four parts:

On the care of the newborn up to the age of walking and talking;

On the suckling and feeding of infants and the requirements in a wet nurse if the mother cannot suckle;

On the diseases which most commonly affect children;

On the care and management of children from learning to walk and talk up to the age of seven years.[6]

The subject matter included issues covered by Bagellardus but placed more emphasis on the psychic well-being of the child. Many profferings of *verbum sapienti* on aspects of child care illuminate manifold correlations between sound mind and body:

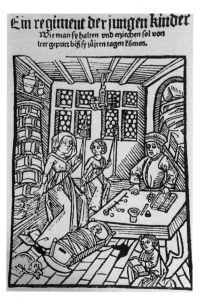

Figure 5.1 Frontispiece of *Ein Regiment der Jungerkinder*. Ruhräh, 1925.

Healthy children have good habits and do not complain. When children whine or cry they are unhealthy, therefore, one should consider their health and care for them in such a manner that they contract no bad habits. One should with great industry see that they do not have unusual movements and if they whine or cry or are angry one should take care to see why they are so and try to prevent it. Children cry either because they have pain, or are troubled, or because they are wet with urine, or wish to stool, or they are too hot or too cold, or have too many clothes on, or have lain too long or they are lying in unclean covering. All these things should be considered and whatever is necessary should be done for the child. Above all things their linen should be kept clean. When one would comfort or quiet a child it can be done in three ways. First, put the mother's breast in its mouth as when one gives the child the breast all its troubles are put to one side; secondly, with song, for a mild voice reaches its heart; and thirdly, that one softly rocks the cradle.

It also should be understood that when children begin to creep around the floor and to reach after things one should make for them a little pen of leather so that they do not hurt them- selves. And finally one should never leave them long and unprotected. (*Ein Regiment*, bk. 1)

Metlinger's third chapter covered 25 diseases, *a capite ad calcem*, that he considered more frequent in children. His medicine was for the most part mainstream. Observations, however, on several uncommon diseases were a singular novelty; these were described with detailed, anecdotal embellishment, as with his comments on hydrocephaly:

It begins generally after the seventh day and, on account of the great changes in the appearance, these children are called changed children. I have seen a child whose head was so large that it could not raise the body and it increased daily in size until the child died. (*Ein Regiment*, 3.2)

Metlinger opined on the causes of bladder stones and elaborated on symptoms:

Urine stones come in children because the mother eats too much cheese, or, according to others, many brown berries, whortleberries or elderberries. The signs of urine stones are that the child urinates frequently and little and may desire to pass urine without being able to do so. Or perhaps there may be erections of the penis or the child catches hold of the genitals and scratches. (*Ein Regiment*, 3.21)

He prescribed a potion of onion juice, walnuts, and thistle for the ailment, adding, "If this does not help, it is advised not to try medicine further but one should let it be cut by masters as undertake such things."[7] It appears that Metlinger did not complete the clinical process of follow-up with his patients, suggesting, for example, that stones or sediment be retrieved by parents and given to him or that surgeons report back to him. In such cases, he would not have been able to confirm his diagnoses.[8]

He was on safer ground when he prescribed mercury and sulfur for seborrhea and dandruff:

Scurf is a sort of roughness that affects children on the head and face and numerous places. It is of two kinds. One is accompanied with itching and biting and the other with itching and biting and scales. . . . The children should have their hair cut and the irritated place covered with a malt poultice to draw out the bad moisture and when the scurf is off, one should use a white and yellow salve of each a half ounce, the whites of two eggs and one ounce of ash lye. If the scurf is accompanied with itching and scaling and horny like crusts the child's head should be washed in the morning with two parts steaming water and one part maserva water and then anoint it with white and cold salve of which a half ounce, quicksilver and sulphur and vinegar, of each one quintel. (*Ein Regiment*, 3.1)

Metlinger's compassionate exposition in the final pages of his book of the general principles of child rearing endearingly emphasized the importance of kindness and tenderness in raising children. In noting libidinal instincts at puberty, Metlinger tacitly acknowledged the compelling factors in children's psyches that inform all of the stages of their development:

It should be known that children should not be too severely punished. . . . In modesty and goodness should parents bring up their children. . . . Punishment is to be praised when it is just and not too severe and a small fault in a child may be over-looked to prevent some greater one. . . . It should be marked that children who have reached six years should be sent to a teacher to be taught. They should not be kept at it continually but have recesses. . . . Of whether or not to give to children, it should be understood that they are to have no wine until they arrive at the age in which nature begins to assert itself, that is twelve in women and fourteen for men. (*Ein Regiment*, bk. 4)

CORNELIUS ROELANS

Cornelius Roelans published his pediatric writings in a *Buchlein*, or Latin compendium, in 1483 in Louvain. The text has no title page and begins simply with a preface. He refers to himself as "aggregator," or compiler, and gives frequent credit to the work of others:

That the order of procedure in this compilation of diseases of children and infants may be grasped, I shall as compiler explain it in a few words. Firstly the name of the disease will be stated, secondly the causes, thirdly the symptoms, fourthly the prognosis, fifthly the treatment in accordance with the opinions of the most experienced.[9]

His index, however, was far more extensive than in the prior two mentioned incunabula, covering, as it did, topics such as nightmares, cataracts, hiccuping, palsy, and "wasting" (failure to thrive). Roelans read widely, and his major service was in the extraction and collection of pediatric information from a huge database (table 5.2).

Intermingled with medically sound annotations on child care were non-sensical, quasi-magical explanations of the origins of diseases and dubiously

TABLE 5.2
AUTHORITIES CITED BY ROELANS IN HIS TREATISE ON CHILDREN

Ancient	Arabic	Medieval	
Hippocrates	Avicenna	Johannes Matthews	Jacques Despars
Galen	Rhazes	Nicholas Florentinus	Gerald of Cremona
Dioscorides	Avenzoar	Solanus	Peter of Albano
Rufus	Serapion	Jacob of Forli	Bernhard von Gordon
Sextus Placidus	Mesue	Gentile de Fulgineo	John of Gadesden
	Haly Abbas	Franz von Piemont	Gilbert Anglicus
		William Placentinus	Arnold of Villanova
		Marsilius de Sancta Sophia	

effective recommendations for treatment. Roelans's prescription for hydrocephaly is but one example: nasal drops concocted from a potion of bile from cranes and vultures, aromatic oils, wild bitters, crocus, and sugar to induce sneezing. His instructions were exact:

Let them be ground very fine and made into a paste with the juice of psyllium viridis and grains be molded from these lentils and dried in the shade and one grain dissolved in rose water every day and dropped for three days in the nostrils in the morning.[10]

HEINRICH VON LOUFFENBURG

The final incunabulum of child care was not a proper medical treatise or compendium. Written by neither a physician nor a midwife, it was a narrative rhyme on the "Care of the Body" (*Versehung des Leibs*) written in 1429 by the monk Heinrich von Louffenburg but not published until 1491. It was one of a genre of medical writing in poetic form and the first of its kind to mention children (table 5.3).

TABLE 5.3
THE PEDIATRIC POEMS

Poem	Date	Author	Language
Versehung des Liebs	1491	H. von Louffenburg	German (Swabian)
L'Esperon	1532	Anton du Saix	French
Puerile ad Pueros	1536	Nicholas Bourbon	Latin
La Balia	1550	Luigi Tansillo	Italian
Hebammen Buch	1554	Jacob Rueff	German
Paedotrophia	1559	Giulio Alessandrini	Latin?
Paedotrophia	1584	Scaevola de Sainte Marthe	Latin
De Custodienda	1593	Jacob Truncon	Latin
Callipaedia	1655	Claude Quillet	Latin
Infancy	1774	Hugh Downman	English

Executed in a doggerel rhyme, it evidently was popular. It was reissued as *Ein Regiment der Gesundtheit für die jungen Kinder* in 1532, 1544, and 1549. The text was illustrated with woodcuts (figure 5.2), furthering its appeal to the lay audience for whom it most likely was intended. The vernacular German, simplicity of expression, and illustrations all suggest a handbook or guide for mothers, rather than doctors.

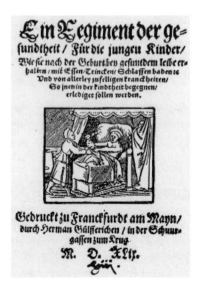

Figure 5.2 *Ein Regiment der Gesundtheit für die jungen Kinder,* 1549 ed. Ruhräh, 1925.

The poem had seven chapters. The first was a form of astrological calendar auguring predictions for each month and delineating preventive or protective measures. The second talked about the planets and their influences. Chapter 3 explained the zodiac. The fourth chapter described the four humors and the four elements. Chapter 5 concerned safeguarding health; chapter 6 dealt with pregnancy, and chapter 7 was about the plague (*die Pestilenz*).[11]

Proper Care of the Body

This little book conveys information
on the different months of the year, as to
natural conditions and the influences of the stars.
It further gives instruction
on food, drinking and purging,
on bathing and the guidance
of pregnant women,
on the bringing up of children,
and on the way to avoid pestilence.
Accordingly it is a book of medicine.[12]

The verses postulated traditional precepts on prenatal care and postnatal management of the newborn, such as anointing with oils, salting the neonate, and applying myrrh to the umbilical stump. Advice on toiletry and feeding and practical instructions on what to do when weaning, for teething, and so on were given in rhymed couplets. Each part began with a question from the mother, followed by a descriptive and prescriptive answer.

A baby frail is born to me,
My mead, I ween, good care should be.

Now will we hearken while is told
What care a young child should enfold,
With all that appertains thereto,
Its food and drink, and all that's due
At night, at morn, asleep, awake,
What care moreover we must take
When, born by nature weak and frail,
Great care the babe must needs entail:
And first when from its mother's womb
The tiny babe newborn doth come,
Then shalt thou mix with all good speed
Rose-oil and salt and these shalt knead
And sprinkle him therewith apace,
His trunk, his arms, his legs, his face;
Or salve him well with oil of oak,
For this no evil can provoke
And strengthens well his every limb
And hardens too his skin for him.
Then cut the cord with care in twain,
Four fingers breadth there should remain.
Thereafter take yet further care
And where the cord is cut prepare
To spread some powder, it is good
Of bolus made and dragon's blood,
Of sarcocol and myrrh combined
And cumin of the Roman kind;
Then wood that's soaked with oil all through
Lay on the part and bind it true
With linen soft applied with skill
And bathing him be careful still
No jar upon the cord to make
Until itself away doth break.[13]

Louffenburg's description of gum care during teething remains both colorful and perplexing. The ever-popular hare brain was considered a major ingredient for alleviating a baby's irritability and the travails of teething:

Now when your baby's teeth appear
You must for these take prudent care
For teething comes with grievous pain,
So to my word take heed again.
When now the teeth are pushing through,
To rub the gums thou thus shalt do,
Take fat from chicken, brain from hare,
And these full oft on gums shalt smear.[14]

Attesting to the popularity of the verse form in the fifteenth and sixteenth centuries, other pediatric poems were written in that period, and are mentioned here. Luigi Tansillo (c.1510–c.1569) wrote *La Balia* (The Wet Nurse) sometime around the middle of the sixteenth century. Tansillo was a soldier with a bent for poetry who dabbled in medical advice. He strongly advocated maternal breast-feeding and was scandalized by mothers who "dried" their breasts with drugs and alcohol:

Oh how grievously you sin Madam
When with alcohol and herbs and powders
You dry those sacred fountains![15]

He warned mothers of all kinds of dire misfortunes that infants, deprived of mother's milk, were prey to, from spoiling and illness to even substitution (the changeling):

Once exil'd from your breast, and doom'd to bring
His daily nurture from a stranger spring,
Ah who can tell the dangers that await
Your infant, thus abandoned to his fate?
Say, is there one with human feelings fraught
Can bear to think, nor sicken at the thought,
That whilst her babe, with unpolluted lips,
As nature asks, the vital fountain sips;
While yet its pure and sainted shrine within
Rests the young mind, unconscious of a sin,
He with his daily nutriment should drain,
That dread disease which fires the wantons' vein;
Sent as the fiercest messenger of God,
O'er lawless love to wave his scorpion rod?

Strange is the tale, but not more strange than true
And many a parent may the treachery rue,
Who for their child, neglected and unknown,

Receive a changeling, vainly deem'd their own.
For witness, Ariosto's scenes peruse;
—Who shall a poet's evidence refuse?
But say what end the impious fraud secures?
—Another's child thus takes the place of yours.
Meanwhile, secure the crafty dame can wait
Her ripening project, and enjoy the cheat;
Reap for her son the fruit of all your toils,
And bid him riot in your children's spoils.
Then, hopeful of reward, no more she hides
Her guilt, but to his secret ear confides;
Delighted thus a double boon to give,
First life itself, and next the means to live.

What ceaseless dread a mother's breast alarms
Whilst her lov'd offspring fills another's arms!
Fearful of ill, she starts at every noise,
And hears, or thinks she hears, her children's cries
Whilst more imperious grown from day to day,
The greedy nurse demands increase of pay.
Vex'd to the heart with anger and expense,
You hear, nor murmur at her proud pretense;
Compell'd to bear the wrong with semblance mild,
And sooth the hireling as she sooths your child.
—But not the dainties of Lucullus' feast
Can gratify the nurse's pamper'd taste;
Nor, though your babe in infant beauty bright
Spring to its mother's arms with fond delight,
Can all its gentle blandishments suffice
To compensate the torments that arise
From her to whom its early years you trust,
—Intent on spoil, ungrateful, and unjust.[16]

JACOB RUEFF

The rhymed couplets of Jacob Rueff's (1500–1558) obstetric text, *Hebammen Buch* (1554), devoted a section to newborn care. A regimen of massage and exercise for the newborn (a current, modern vogue among mothers) was the only original material about children:

Bathe only so long until his skin
Is reddened from the foot to chin,
When from the bath the babe you take,
This admonition must I make

The water, lukewarm, with honey fine
Anoint the child, then cleanse he ey'n
But here you must not be severe
And likewise wash each little ear.
With a white cloth the child you dry
And olive oil you then apply.
Then must you exercise each limb
Bending them up and down and in
The leg, the neck, the hands, the back,
The arm, the sides, the hip—no lack
The body's uses manifold.
By this process you help unfold.[17]

SCAEVOLA DE SAINTE MARTHE

A French lawyer, Scaevola de Sainte Marthe (1536–1623), also called Sammarthanus,[18] wrote a pediatric book in Latin hexameter, the *Paedotrophia*. It consisted of three books, totaling 1,726 lines, dedicated to King Henry III.

Sainte Marthe was mayor and comptroller of the town of Loudun when his son became ill. Frustrated by physicians' failure to cure the boy, Sainte Marthe consulted texts on the healing arts in order to help his child. In the process he became quite knowledgeable, and, in his book he covered a broad range of subjects—prenatal care, labor, postnatal care, feeding and weaning, and, in the final section, diseases of children. Although there was nothing original in its contents and the Latin was ponderous (some translations into English were not much more readable), the *Paedotrophia* became a very popular textbook; between 1584 and 1742, twenty editions of the work were published.[19] Historian Tallmadge describes the work as "a mélange of fable, history, philosophy, and medicine, done in the neoclassical manner, and nevertheless it contains many precepts which have not been altered but only confirmed by four hundred years of medical experience."[20] The following exemplifies Sainte Marthe's writing style:

The bristly bear on the cold mountain's head
The spotted tigress in low valleys bred
And all the monsters of the savage throng
With their rude nipples feed their infant young.
And wilt thou, woman, grac'd with gentlest mind
Become more fierce than this terrific kind?
Say, does thy infant likeness touch thee not
When with complaints he strains his little throat?

Will you not pity and his wants relieve
When still he begs what none but you can give?
Is not his being thine, his blood thy own
And stand'st thou deaf and stupid at his moan?
Unhappy boy! whose pleasing burden seems
Too hard for thee, bewitch'd with other dreams
Delight'st thou not his beauteous head to lay
On thy soft breast, to see him smile and play?
Who else should cherish thy neglected young
Hear their first voice and calm their lisping tongue?[21]

Sainte Marthe tackled some weighty material in verse, such as describing anal prolapse:

Why shou'd I name how the Posterior Pipe
Is apt the Bounds in weakly Babes slip?
The Muscles, moistn'd when the Belly's loose,
Their nat'ral Duty to discharge, refuse;
And out the Anus hangs, a grievous Pain;
Nor is it easily got in again.
The Body bind, foment it when 'tis out,
And gently with thy Hand replace the Gut.[22]

Sainte Marthe recommended that fever and earache be treated with warm violet oil and poultices of milk and barley. Hare brain, honey, and coral were advocated for teething:

For Teeth the Stomach serve, and Life maintain,
And none can have the Tooth, without the Pain.
The suff'ring Infant tells it by his Cries,
His driv'ling Mouth he with his Fingers plies,
He strives to help himself, but strives in vain,
The Nurse's Help must ease him of his Pain.
In a Hare's brain his little Fingers dip,
Or what Sicilian Bees from Roses sip.
The raging Gum, the Sweets and Softness sooth,
And white amidst the Red appears the Tooth:
As the white Iv'ry in red Coral shines,
Which wrought with curious Art, the Workman joins.[23]

Sainte Marthe was influenced by the works of Oribasius and insisted on exposing children to calm voices, gentle touch, and kind discipline. Infants, he advocated, should be placated by gentle rocking and lullabies.[24]

The work concluded with reasonable advice to parents:

Call the Physician to your Aid; advise
With him, and do not think yourself too wise;
Do not to ev'ry idle Tale attend,
Nor on old Womens Recipe's depend.
Too much the learn'd into this Error give,
Are thus deceiv'd themselves, and thus deceive.[25]

JACOB TRUNCON

The didactic poem *De Custodienda Puerorum Sanitate*, written by Jacob Truncon in 1593, is remarkable for the author's self-congratulatory verse and the absence of scientific merit:

The thousand wondrous ills that may befall
Frail childhood, these thy monumental scroll,
Destined to last as long as years shall roll,
Has safely banished. For this book of thine,
Trunconius, on thee shall glory shine
For ever and for ever, and its bounds shall be
Unchecked by bounds of earth or sky or sea.[26]

Some curious examples of the genre appeared at the turn of the sixteenth century as broadsides. These illustrated poems focused on the conjoined twin, considered to be a favorable birth omen.[27] Several were written, some describing conjoined heads and others conjoined chests or viscera (figure 5.3).

CLAUDE QUILLET

Medical verse written in Latin hexameter endured as a genre until as late as 1655, when its popularity faded. A didactic poem of major importance, *Callipaedia seu de Pulchrae Prolis Habendae Ratione* (The Way to Have Beautiful Children), was published by Claude Quillet (1602–1661) in Leyden in 1655. Quillet moralized about and warned against premarital sex: "Twelve Springs compleat, before she thinks to wed, / Their Vernal Bloom must in the Virgin shed."[28] Accurate astrological timing was essential to produce a healthy and beautiful child. According to Quillet, food and wine affected gender:

Sufficient for the Nuptial Joy's the Vine,
And lusty Boys are got by gen'rous Wine.
But most, Oh Burgundy! thy Nectar warms
Their Hearts, and burnishes their Bridal Arms.[29]

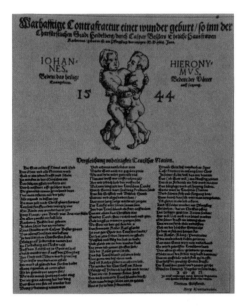

Figure 5.3 Poem broadside by Heinrich Vogtherrn (1544) on the Heidelberg twins. Hollander, 1921.

Like Shakespeare,[30] he warned about the consequences of excess:

> Let reason in your Cups direct your Draught
> The Ship is often sunk when over fraught.[31]

Quillet believed in eugenics and maternal transference. Transference was a concept from primitive times, when congenital malformations were ascribed to mysterious forces beyond human control. Primitive cultures believed that some transmutations occurred during intercourse. In Gen. 30:32–42, Jacob produced spotted cattle by having them view spotted stakes while conceiving. Empedokles (490–430 B.C.) posited the theory that maternal sensory input (*phantasiai*) determined an infant's phenotype. He asserted that "women who have fallen in love with statues and pictures frequently give birth to children who resemble them."[32] Soranus cited examples of women who gave birth to monkeys after having seen monkeys during coitus.[33] As late as 1820, Edwin James recorded the stories of American Plains natives who described instances of anomalous births of newborns who had animal features as a result of their mothers having seen just such animals during coitus.[34] The more general belief was that mutations occurred by sensory transmissions catalyzed by a mother's chance experience—casual or dreadful. For example, Daniel Turner's *Treatise of Diseases Incident to the Skin*, published in 1714, ascribed a child resembling a cat caused by a cat's getting into the mother's bed and a hairy child born to a mother who saw a drawing of a bear:[35]

> Since by foul Objects filthy Births are made,
> And the vile Picture's to the Womb convey'd,
> A pregnant Wife will ne'er behold a Whale,
> Nor Porpus, nor the Dolphin's Azure Scale.
> Nor thee, Oh Proteus, will she see, nor you
> Tritonian Monsters, while she's Teeming, view;
> But let her on the lovely Nereids gaze,
> And fix her Eyes on ev'ry charming Face.[36]

> As well as sound, the Lover shou'd be strong,
> And never to the Wrinkled wed the Young.
> A Youth ne'er couple to a Wife decay'd,
> Nor to a Cripple match a blooming Maid.[37]

HUGH DOWNMAN

From 1774 to 1776, Hugh Downman (1740–1809) wrote his *Infancy, or the Management of Children: A Didactic Poem in Six Books*. The obsolete format and lack of originality contributed to its having been long forgotten, but one passage deserves quoting because it describes the essence of the art of pediatrics—of studying the patient who cannot speak but who reveals his illness only to the close and keen and interested observer.:

> Because the child, with reason unendow'd
> And power of speech, by words to express his grief
> Nature permits not; some believe the source
> Of anguish and affections is conceal'd
> From every eye, and deem assistance vain.
> Or to the nurse, or vaunting midwife trust,
> Who cases manifold and similar
> Have oft beheld, and never fail'd to cure:
> For each her nostrum boasts; if harmless this,
> And trifling, it were well, did not the wing
> Of time speed fast the irrevocable hour
> Of wish'd redress. But frequently the drug
> They praise, the cordial drops are fraught with death,
> Hurrying convulsions on of direst kind;
> Or with narcotic venom strong imbued,

Plunging the patient in eternal sleep.
Yet nature, in thy child, tho' not in words,
Speaks plain to those who in her language vers'd
Justly interpret. Are the different tones
Of woe unfaithful sounds? can he, whose sight
Hath traced the various muscles in their course,
When irritated in the different limbs,
Retracted, or extended, or supine,
Fix no conclusion on the seat of pain?
Is it of no avail to mark the breath,
How drawn? the face? the motions of the eye?
The salient pulse? the eruptions on the skin?
The skin itself, constructed or relaxed?
The mode of sleep? or waking? heat? or thirst?
From which, and numerous traits beside arranged,
Combined, abstracted, and maturely sigh'd,
Judgment its practice forms? Are characters
Like these which ask the nice decyphering soul,
Intelligible to beldames old,
Who wrapped in darkness, utter prophesies
And lying oracles, which cheat the ear,
Or followed, to destruction lead the way?
Oh! may good angels, kindling in thy breast
The lap of reason, guard thee from their snares!
Blind guides assiduous to deceive the blind.[38]

NOTES

1. The translation of Bagellardus that follows is by H. F. Wright. The entire text of Bagellardus appears in Ruhräh, 1925.

2. *Libellus*, 2.4.

3. Still, 1931, pp. 64–66.

4. Translation of Still, 1931, p. 68.

5. The quotations that follow are from the translation of Ludwig Unger, *Das Kinderbuch des Bartolomäus Metlinger* (Leipzig & Wien, 1904).

6. 1. Das erste Capitel sagt wie man erst geborne kind halten sol biss sy gon und reden lernent in eynes gemein; 2. Das ander Capital sagt wie man kind saugen und speisen sol und wan sy ir eigen mutren nit saugen kunnendt wie die saugam gestalt sein wol. Auch wan man sy abmutren sol unnd wie; 3. Dras drit Capitel sagt vom den kranckheiten die kinden zum merem teil zu stond; 4. Das vierde sagt wie man die kind halten und ziehen sol so sy gon und reden lernent biss das sy ergreiffent das alter siben iare. (Still, 1931, pp. 69–70)

7. Ruhräh, 1925, p. 92.

8. Metlinger, in fact, most likely was describing uncomplicated urinary tract infections, since children rarely get bladder stones. Even with today's technology for detection—urolithiasis—stones are uncommonly found in children. *Mayo Clin Proc* 1993; 68:241–48.

9. Conelius Roelas aggregator ut ordo processus aggregationis egritudinum puerorum seu infantium capiatur brevibus eum explicabo. Primo egritudinis nomen declarabitus secundo causae, tertio signa, quarto prognostica, quinto cura secundum expertissimorum sentencias. (Roelans, 1483; Latin text in Sudhoff, 1925)

10. Ibid. Rx fellis gruis, fellis vulturis, castorei, fustium rutae silvestris, macis et croci, sacchari alba.

11. Some authorities believe the work to be a translation of *Regimen Sanitatis Salernitanum*, a Latin poem, published in 1484, expounding rules of hygiene and medical treatment established by the School of Salerno. Clendening, 1960, p. 76; Ruhräh, 1938, p. 3; Ruhräh, 1925, pp. 465–66.

12. Dis buchlein ist also gemacht / wie dz jar nach de monat wirt geacht / Nach natur vn inflüss d' stern / auch thut es weiter lern / Uon speiss tranck vn purgieren / baden lassen und regieren / Schwager frawe die fruchtber sind / wie man ziehen soll die kind / Uor d' pestilencz sich machen frey / darub ist es ein buch d' arczney. (Translation of Hermann Collitz as cited by Ruhräh, 1925)

13. Translation of Still, 1931, pp. 86–90:
Ich hab geborn ein Kindlein zart, / Verdient hab das man mein wol wart. / Nu woln wir hören wie man sol / Die jungen kind regieren wol, / Mit allem das in höret zu, / Mit essen trincken, spat und fru, / Darzu mit wartung sonderleich / Wenn ir natur ist schwach und zart / Drumbs notig ist das man ir wart. / Zum ersten, so die kleinen kind / Von mutter leib geboren sind, / So solut bald zusammen stossen / Salz und Rosen wol zu massen, / Und es damit besprengen rein / Den Leib, das Antlitz, Arm und Bein, / Oder salb es wol mith Eichel öl / Denn solches thut dem Kindlein wol, / Und Stercket sein glieder all, / Sein haut ims auch hart machen sol. / Denn schneit im ab dden Nabel fein / Vier finger breit vom Leiblin sein, / Darnach soltu sein weiter pflegen / Und auff den schnid des Nabels legen. / Ein pulverin, das machts im gut, / Von bolus un von Trachenblut, / Sarcocollo und Myrrehn rein, / Romisch Kümel darbey sol sein / Leg Baumwol drauff die da genetzt / In Baumwol, und verbinds denn fest / Mit weichen tuchlin fleissiglich, / Wenn du das badst thu seuberlich / Das im am Nabel kein gewalt / Geschehe, bis das er selbst abalt.

14. Ibid., p. 90.

15. O quanto, Donne, gravemente pecca
Colei, che con liquori, od erba, o polve
Quelle fonti santissime dissecca! (Roscoe, 1798, p. 52)

Tansillo borrowed many of his ideas from *Noctes Atticae* by Aulus Gellius, and some passages are cited almost verbatim. Foote, 1919, pp. 217–19.

16. Translation of William Roscoe, 1798.

17. So lang baden, bis dass sein leib / Ganz rotlicht wirdt, dan ist es zeit, / Dass due es nimmest aus dem bad, / Jedoch so merck auch diesen rath. / Das Wasser sol nur lawlecht seyn, / Darnach salb es mit honig fein. / Nach dem so wasch ihm one laugen, / Die öhrlein sauber und die augen. / Trückne es dann mit tüchlein weiss, / Zuletzt soltu es auch es auch mitfleiss, / Mit Baumöl gar wol ersalben / An seinem Leibe allenthalben. / Dann soltu auch all seine glieder / Biegen, hin her, auff und nieder, / Die Bein, den Halz den Rück die Hendt, Die Arm die Seiten und die Lend, / Nach dem sie sollen sein gestalt, / Solches bringt in nutzen manigtalt. Ruhräh, J., *Am J Dis Child* 1932; 44:181–84.

18. Aries and Duby, 1989, 2:314.

19. Still, 1931, p. 176.

20. Tallmadge, 1939, p. 292.

21. *Paedotrophia*, 1.175–92.
   Ipsae etiam Alpinis villosae in cautibus ursae,
   Ipsae etiam tigres et quidquid ubique ferarum est
   Debita servandis concedunt ubera natis:
   Tu, quam miti animo Natura benigna creavit
   Expsuperes feritate feras? nec te tua tangant
   Pignora nec querulos puerili e gutture planctus
   Nec lacrymas misereris opemque iniusta recuses
   Quam praestare tuum est et quae te pendet ab una?
   Cuius onus teneris haerebit dulce lacertis
   Infelix puer et molli se pectore sternet?
   Dulcia quis primi captabit gaudia risus
   Et primas blaesae voces et murmura linguae?

22. Ibid., 3.423–34.

23. Ibid., 3.271–93.

24. "Placidumque soporem, Concilia motis ad blandula carmina cunia." Ibid., 2.385.

25. Ibid., 3.513.

26. Portenta heu nimium teneris infesta puellis, / Quae tua, Trunconi, haec cunctos monumenta per annos / Victura ostendunt tuto removere, parata / Unde tibi aeternum tanta est jam gloria, nullis / Terrarum trifidive coercita finibus orbis. Ruhräh, J., *Am J Dis Child* 1932; 44:1074–76.

27. Ruhräh, 1938, pp. 52–56.

28. Ruhräh, 1925, p. 496.

29. Ibid., 1925, p. 497.

30. "[I]t provokes the desire, but it takes away the performance" (*Macbeth*, act 2, scene 3).

31. Ruhräh, p. 497.

32. Garland, 1990, p. 34.

33. Ibid.

34. Bremner, 1970, p. 393.

35. Turner, 1736, chap. 12, pp. 60–61.
36. Ruhräh, 1925, p. 498.
37. Ibid., 1925, p. 496.
38. Downman, 1802, pp. 160–64.

Chapter 6

Renaissance and Reformation

The intellectual fervor of the sixteenth-century Renaissance in Europe encompassed the humanities, arts and sciences, and medicine. In medicine the outstanding works were those of Valerus Cordus (1515–1544), Girolamo Fracastoro (1484–1553), and Andreas Versalius (1514–1564). Cordus wrote an extensive botanical pharmacopeia. Fracastoro formulated the concept of contagious diseases. The Galenic theory of humors (see figure 3.1) was disputed by Paracelsus (1493–1541). Versalius, considered the father of modern anatomy, challenged, with direct observations of anatomy, long perpetuated errors of Galen. Ambroise Pare (1510–1590) revolutionized the treatment of wounds and revivified the arterial procedure of ligature. Michael Servetus (1509–1553) described pulmonary circulation. The origins of conceptual epidemiology, chemical pharmacology and operative intervention began with these achievements.

Extraordinary advances during the seventeenth century followed: the elucidation of cardiocentric circulation by William Harvey (1578–1657), microanatomy descriptions by Marcello Malpighi (1628–1694), the microscopy of Anton van Leeuwenhoek (1632–1723), the physiological concepts of Jean Baptiste van Helmut (1577–1644), the collective elaborations of Aselli, Pecquet, Bartholin, and Rudbech on the lymphatic system, and the systematic detailed bedside observations of Thomas Sydenham (1624–1689). Jan Swammerdam (1637–1680) elucidated the composition of red blood cells and demonstrated that the newborn lung floats only after breathing,[1] an observation that was used in a medicolegal dispute regarding an alleged stillborn.[2]

Beginning early in the sixteenth century, a significant number of physicians appeared whose works focused on the diagnosis and treatment of children's diseases.

EUCHARIUS ROESSLIN

The first pediatric work of the sixteenth century was the *Rosegarten*, a manual of midwifery written by Eucharius Roesslin (?–1526) and published in 1512 in Strassburg as *Der Swangern Frawen und hebammen Rosegarten*. It

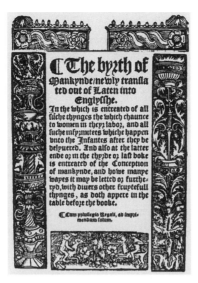

Figure 6.1 *Byrth of Mankynde* by Richard Jonas (1540). COURTESY NATIONAL LIBRARY OF MEDICINE.

was popular with the public for two centuries. Between its initial publication and 1730 the book was translated into several languages and reissued 40 times. The first English version, by Richard Jonas in 1540, was entitled *The Byrth of Mankynde* (figure 6.1) and was dedicated to "Lady Queen Catherine [Howard] wife and most derely beloved spouse unto the most myghty sapient Christen prynce Kyng Henry the viii."[3]

Roesslin's observations on midwifery were based on the writings of Soranus, as well as on firsthand knowledge gleaned from having witnessed and assisted at a number of parturitions—an exceptional achievement for the times given the traditional taboo of male attendance at births. His descriptions of accouchement, devoid of idealized or romantic notions, warned in graphic language about the potential dangers for mother and infant in the birth process:

[The mother] . . . will undergo much pain and suffer many grave infirmities, injuries, and accidents. The poor vulnerable infant may be rendered defective and die in the process, perhaps before it receives holy baptism, and thereby be robbed of eternal life; such are the hazards of pregnancy and childbirth.[4]

Roesslin's study was remarkable and systematic for the time. He recorded 18 predictors of difficult birth, 3 types of miscarriage, proper positioning in a birthing chair to check cervical dilatation, fetal repositioning (podalic version), actual delivery techniques, and immediate postnatal care. One detailed section described an embryotomy (dissection) in utero of the dead child.

The pediatric parts of his book were influenced by the Arabic School. Chapter 10 was devoted to the care of the newborn; 11 covered nursing, weaning and nutrition; and 12 reviewed diseases focusing on the 35 most commonly recognized ailments of children. Although the information in this section of the book was similar to that found in the pediatric incunabula, the overall tone of Roesslin's writing was warmer and more compassionate than that of others, most probably contributing to the book's popularity.

With the exception of recommending the use of the opioid poppy, Roesslin suggested children's remedies in homeopathic strengths safe for children's use. A sampling of his remedies appears in table 6.1.

The following illustrates his concern for even commonplace disturbances experienced by children:

Children may have terrifying dreams which come generally from overfilling so to help it do not allow it to go to sleep with a full stomach. And give it a little honey to lick so that it may digest in its stomach and pass out in the stool.

Give everyday the seventh part of an electuary named dyamuscum dyapliris and more healthy is theriac given with milk as Rhazes says.[5]

After the *Rosegarten*, several minor manuscripts on children's conditions were written by others. Leonello Vittori (Leonelli Faventide Victorius) (?–1520) published *De aegritudinibus infantiu tractatus* in 1544. Neither novel nor inspired, it consisted of 33 chapters detailing common ailments and their treatments. In 1537, Gabriel de Zerbis published *Anatomia Infantis*, describing the anatomy of aborted fetuses. In 1539 appeared Michael Angelo Biondo's (1497–1565) *De Affectibus Infantium and Puerorum*, which modeled diagnosis and treatment after Rhazes. Johannes Lange (1485–1565) wrote a chapter on chlorosis, or iron deficiency anemia, of pubertal girls, titled "De Morbo Virgineo." It appeared in *Medicinalium epistolarum miscellanea, varia et rara* (1554):

[W]ith what kind of disease is she afflicted: since the qualities of her face, which in the past year was distinguished by rosiness of cheeks and redness of lips, is somehow as if exsanguinated, sadly paled, the heart trembles with every movement of her body, and the arteries of her temples pulsate, & she is seized with dyspnoea in dancing or climbing the stairs, her stomach loathes food and particularly meat, & the legs, especially at the ankles, become edematous at night. From these accidents indeed, & from the pathognomonic signs of the disease, which betray the cause and nature of the disease . . . as it is peculiar to virgins, might indeed be called "virgineus." (*Epistola*, 21)[6]

TABLE 6.1
EXAMPLES OF ROESSLIN'S THERAPEUTICS[7]

Canker sore	Chicken fat, aromatics, honey
Diarrhea	Plasters of roseseed, caraway, and anise to stomach, goat milk, soft egg yolk, boiled bread orally
Constipation	Suppositories of honey and oil
Convulsions	Bathing in mullein (figwort) water
Cough	Honey, crushed almonds boiled with fennel oil, quince with sugar
Asthma	Maple seed mashed with honey or cottonseed cooked in egg yolk
Oral blisters	Crushed violets applied directly
Chapped lips	Salve of plantain, butter, chicken fat
Otitis (ear infection)	Ear plug soaked with honey, wine, alum
Swelling	Wrap the body part with cloth soaked in elderberry juices and wine
Sneezing	Inhale crushed basil
Sleeplessness	Poppy products
Hiccups	Crushed indian nut and sugar
Nausea and vomiting	Ground cloves, barley corns
Tenesmus (rectal urgency)	Ground cress and caraway seeds in butter
Diaper rash	Salve of myrtle, roses, mandrake, and camphor

In the same year in which Lange's manuscript was published, Jean Fernel (?1497–1558) described fatal appendicitis in a seven-year-old girl:[8]

On opening the body the caecum intestinum was narrowed and constricted; also the quince was found adherent to the inside and stopping up the lumen, so that it absolutely could not pass through any other way: whence it happened that this acrid and corrupt material prevented from passing; the obstacle overflowing opened up itself an unusual route into the abdominal cavity, by a necrosis and perforation a little above the obstructed place; from whence the gut just as by the outlet & the passage escaping it filled up the abdomen to its entire capacity. (*Universa medicina*, vol. 6, chap. 10)

One other minor pediatric manuscript appeared, written by Otto Brunfels (1488–1534), a Carthusian monk who in 1521 had become a reformist. In 1537 he published *Weiber und Kinder Apothek*, a wholesale adaptation of Metlinger's work. G. F. Still labeled him an "unblushing plagiarist."[9] He did produce original works: a botany book entitled *Historia Plantarum* (1530) and a book of urbanity, *On Disciplining and Instructing Children* (1525).

Brunfels's training as a monk colored his attitude regarding children. He believed their day should be controlled from awakening until retirement:

Sleep neither too little nor too much. Begin each day by blessing it in God's name and saying the Lord's Prayer. Thank God for keeping you through the night and ask his help for the new day. Greet your parents. Comb your hair and wash your face and hands. Before departing for school, ask Christ to send his spirit, without whom there is no true understanding, remembering also, however, that the Spirit only helps those who help themselves. . . . At school be happily obedient; do everything wholeheartedly. When called on, answer quickly and modestly. Expect disgusting behavior not only to be rebuked with sarcasm, but punished firmly. Above all, do not let the teacher strike you with cause. Harm neither your teachers nor your peers in either word or deed. Try to learn from those who criticize you rather than simply turn them aside. . . .

Read something specific from Scripture every day; do not go to sleep until you have memorized a few new verses. Punish yourself when you have neglected your readings. . . .

After school go directly home; do not tarry in the streets. If your parents need help when you arrive, obey their requests without question. If you have time after your chores, use it to review and reflect on what you have read at school, remembering that nothing in this life is more precious than time, for once time is lost, it is lost forever.[10]

SEBASTIAN OESTEREICHER

In 1540, Sebastian Oestereicher (Sebastianus Austrius) (?–1550) of Alsace published a collection of pediatric aphorisms called *De puerorum morbis* (figure 6.2). Oestereicher extolled the benefits of maternal breast milk and advised: "Up to dentition, feed the child on milk alone."[11] Secure in the knowledge that maternal feeding provided superior nutritional and emotional superiority for infants, he exhorted natural mothers to accept responsibility for their nursing infants instead of delegating them to the arms and breasts of surrogates. Oestereicher bowed, however, to the power of the entrenched age-old custom of employing wet nurses and offered maxims providing guidance to parents as they considered possible candidates:[12]

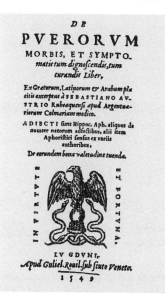

DE
PVERORVM
MORBIS, ET SYMPTO_
matis tum dignoscendis, tum
curandis Liber,

Ex Graecorum, Latinorum & Arabum pla
citis excerptus à SEBASTIANO AV_
STRIO Rubeaquensi apud Argentua-
riorum Colmariam medico.

ADIECTI sunt Hippoc. Aph. aliquot de
nouiter natorum adfectibus, alii item
Aphoristici sensus ex variis
authoribus,
De eorundem bona valetudine tuenda,

IN VIRTVTE
ET FORTVNA.

LVGDVNI,
Apud Guliel. Rouil. sub scuto Veneto.
1549

Figure 6.2 Sebastian Oestereicher's *De puerorum morbis.* COURTESY NATIONAL LIBRARY OF MEDICINE.

A wet-nurse of good morals, good constitution and in the prime of life is always to be chosen.

If nurses keep a good diet, they will produce milk of good composition, supplying rich juices to the growing child.

He remained resolute in his attempts to persuade readers that the best candidate to nourish an infant was the biological mother:

Since we are made of it and nourished by it, the mother's milk, generated from accustomed and known blood, is more suitable to the infant's welfare than other natural milks.

Intent on arousing strong reactions in his readers, he used arguments against wet nursing that employed distasteful animal analogies and warnings of alienation of affection:

As young goats fed by sheep produce finer hair and lambs fed by goat's milk produce coarser wool, so too, children brought up by strange mothers differ markedly, in essential characteristics, from their own mothers.

Those who abandon their infants, who thrust them from themselves and give them to others to bring up, cut and destroy the spiritual bond and the affection by which nature binds parents to their children.

You can tell that an infant has been sent away from home to nurse by its eyes: for the strong affection for the mother is slowly and gradually extinguished and is centered alone upon her who nurses the child, which has no further inclination or love for the one who gave it birth.

Despite three editions, Oestereicher's book was not particularly popular. He modeled the materia medica after Roelans, but his use of a quasi-aphoristic format was original.

THOMAS PHAER

Thomas Phaer (1510–1560), called by some the "Father of English Pediatrics,"[13] published in 1544 a true text of pediatrics—a manuscript, in English, exclusively devoted to diseases of children. It was named the *Boke of Children* (figure 6.3).

Phaer and other medical writers of the time exhibited unusual—unique—perspicacity in recognizing the special requirements of clinical thought and application in the treatment of children. The table of contents is an indicator of the thorough scope of Phaer's book:

Aposteme of the brayne [meningitis]

Swellyng of the heed.

Scalles of the heed.

Watchyng out of measure.

Terrible dreames.

The fallyng evill.

The palseye.

Crampe.

Styfnesse of lymmes.

Bloodshoten eyes.

Watryng eyes.

Scabbynesse and ytche.

Diseases in the eares.

Pesyng out of measure.

Bredyng of teeth.

Canker in the mouth.

Quynsye, or swellyng of throte.

Coughe.

Sreaytnesse of wynde.

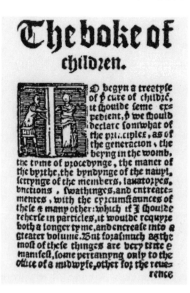

Figure 6.3 *Boke of Children* by Thomas Phaer. "To begyn a treatyse of ye cure of children, it shoulde seme expedient, that we should declare somewhat of the principles, as of the generacion, the beyng in the womb, the tyme of procedynge, the maner of the byrthe, the byndynge of the navyl, settynge of the members, lavatoryes, unctions, swathinges, and entreatementes, with the cyrcumstaunces of these & many other: which if I shoulde reherse in particles, it woulde requyre both a longer tyme, and encrease into a greater volume. But foreasmuch as the most of these things are very rite & manifest, some pertainyng only to the office of a midwyfe, other for the reverence" (Ruhräh, 1925).

Feblenesse of the stomacke & vomiting.

Yeaxyng or hycket [hiccups].

Colyke and rumblyng in the guttes.

Fluxe of the belly.

Stoppyng of the bellye.

Wormes.

Swellyng of the navill.

The stone.

Pyssyng in bedde.

Brustynge [hernia].

Fallyng of the skynne.

Chafyng of the skynne.

Small pockes and measels.

Fevers.

Swellyng of the coddes.

Sacer ignis or chingles.

Burnyng and scaldyng.

Kybbes [chilblains].

Consumpcion.

Leanenesse.

Gogle eyes.[14]

Using phraseology reminiscent of Sebastian Oestereicher, Phaer also encouraged the biological mother to nurse her own infant. His variation to this argument is based on the adage "You are what you eat":[15]

[I]f ye lambes be nourysed with ye milke of goates, they shall have course wolle, like the heare of goates: and yf kiddes in lyke maner sucke upon shepe, ye heare of them shalbe soft lyke wolle. . . . wherefore as it is agreing to nature, so it is also necessary & comly for the own mother to nourse the own child.

His recommended treatment for severe, scabbing seborrhea of the infant scalp resembled the current home-remedy method of softening the flakes with baby oil, followed by a washing. Phaer, however, used a wine base for the shampoo:

If ye se the scalles lyke the shelles of oysters, blacke and drye, cleavinge upon the skynne . . . apply a soft plaistre of the same herbs, with gose grese or butter, usynge thys styll, tul ye se the scabbe removed, and then washe it with thy iuce of hore-hound, smallach, and betony, sodden togither in wyne.

If the seborrhea became secondarily infected and sore, he used a lead oxide plaster as an antiseptic—effective but for the potential lead toxicity, about which all were ignorant:

Take white leade and lytarge, of every one, v drammes, lye made of the asshes of a vyne iii drammes, oyle of roses, an ounce, waxe, an ounce, melte the waxe fyrste, than putte to the oyle and lye with the reste, and in the ende ii yolkes of egges, make an oyntmet, and laye it to the head. Thys is the composicion of Rasis.

Phaer restored the elements of common sense to medical advice, which had disappeared after the great Avicenna. For example, Phaer understood that adequate rest was a fundamental as well as a vital adjunct to sound and proper nourishment for infants:

Slepe is the nouryshement and foode of a suckyng chylde, and as much requisite as the very tete, wherfore wha it is deprived of the naturall reste, all the hole body falleth in distemper, cruditie and weakenes.

His comments on two problems common to latent children—night terrors and bed-wetting—indicate he was a sensitive observer and interpreter of childhood experiences. In appreciating the involuntary nature of bed-wetting and advocating therapy rather than punishment, Phaer anticipated, if not modern treatment, certainly modern opinion:

On pyssyng in the bedde. Many times for debility of vertue retentive of the reines or blader, as wel olde men as children are often times annoyed, whan their urine issueth out either in theyr slepe or waking against theyr wylles, having no power to reteine it whan it cometh, therfore yf they will be holpe, fyrst they must avoid al fat meates, til ye vertue retentive be restored againe, and to use this pouder in their meates and drynkes.

The "pouder" Phaer prescribed was made from the ground trachea of chickens. He suggested it be taken three times a day. Most likely, Phaer had observed that chickens did not produce urine and therefore believed that a remedy made from chickens would act as an urine inhibitor.[16]

With regard to night terrors, his judgment that they were caused by indigestion was the same as Roesslin's:

Often tymes it happeneth that the child is afraid in the slepe, and sometimes waketh soodainly, and sterteth, sometime shriketh and trembleth, which effect commeth of the arysyng of stynking vapours, out of the stomake into the fantasye, and sences of the brayne, as you maye perceyve by the breath of the chylde: wherfor it is good to geve him a litle hony to swallow, and a lytle pouder of the seedes of peonye, and sometymes treacle, in a litle quantity with milke, and to take hede that the chylde sleepe not with a full stomake, but to beare it about wakying, tyl part bee dygested, and whan that it is laide, not to rocke it much, for overmuch shaking letteth digestion, and maketh the chylde many tymes to vomyte.

Phaer, like his contemporaries, believed in the efficacy of charms and amulets. He especially credited coral with much healing power, advocating that children wear it as an amulet and as a teething aid (figure 6.4). Further, he suggested that coral, ground into powder, be given to children in treating episodes of epilepsy and bleeding:

To cause an easie breedyng of teethe . . . red coralle in lyke maner hanged about the necke, wherupon the chylde shuld oftentimes labour his gummes . . . to declare this of coral that by consent of al authours, it resisteth the force of lyghtening helpeth

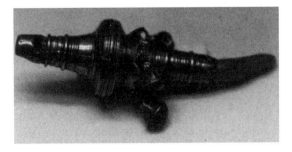

Figure 6.4 Teething coral rattle-cum-whistle. MUSEUM OF THE ROYAL COLLEGE OF SURGEONS, EDINBURGH.

the chyldren of the fallynge evyll and is very good to be made in pouder & dronken agaynst al maner of bleeding of the nose or fundament.

Despite these lapses into what now is recognized as medical nonsense, Phaer's understanding of children's physical and psychic development and his sense of mission to serve the pediatric community commend him to the front ranks of pioneers among pediatric medical writers. The book's final declaration, in which Phaer reemphasized his dedication to study, diagnose, and offer treatments specifically for children's diseases, served as a model for future writers. Clearly, he had no doubt that children's diseases required distinct, special study and treatment by physicians tutored in and sensitive to children's unique medical needs. In that analysis he was indeed an insightful pioneer:

These shall be suffycient to declare at this time in this litle treatise of the cure of children, which yf I may know to be thankefully received I will by gods grace, supplye more hereafter, ney ther desyre I any lenger to live than I will employ my studyes to the honour of god and profit of the weale publike

Thus endeth ye boke of
childrene composed by
Thomas Phayer
Studiouse in Phi-
-losophie and
Phisike.[17]

The discussion of diseases of children as a distinct medical subject was beginning to be validated throughout Europe. In France, Gabriel Miron, physician to King Louis XII, published *De Regimine Infantium* in Lyon in 1544. Although the book merely recited the opinions of Galen and Avicenna, it introduced the term *pedenemice*, meaning "management of children and treatment of diseases in children"[18]—a linguistic antecedent to modern-day *pediatrics*.

De Infantium Febribus was written in 1558 by Jerome de Monteux (Hieronymus Montus, 1495–1560). Although the title would lead one to think it dealt with fevers of childhood, it was in fact an uninspired catalog of treatments for known ailments.

Despite the appearance of several manuscripts in vernacular languages, Latin remained the common and universal academic medium for scholars, enabling physicians in England, France, Spain, Italy, Germany, and elsewhere to share the same texts as well as prevailing common wisdom. Writers like Phaer, however, had begun to write books in their own languages on general health and disease as these pertained to children. These books contributed to a broader understanding of illness and health, as they enabled a wider dissemination of medical information to both doctors and the general populace.

In Spain, Ludovico Lobera de Avila published a vernacular text in 1551 entitled *Libro del Regimiento de la Salud y de la Esterilidad de los hombres and mugeres y de las Enfermedades de los niños*. It was the first Spanish text on diseases of children and contained a puericulture chapter.

The Mallorcan, Damian Carbon (?–1554) wrote a newborn-care text for nurses entitled *Libro del Arte de las Comadres* (1541). Luis Mercado (1525–1611) wrote several volumes on children, the most significant of which was *Curare docet puerorum morbos* (1611), encompassing treatment and education.[19]

In France, *Cinq livres: De la maniere de nourir et gouverner les enfans de leur naissance* was published in 1565 by Simon de Vallambert (1537–1565). Vallambert decried premasticated weaning (i.e., having food chewed by the mother or nurse then inserted into the mouth of the infant). He believed "foreign" saliva caused parasites and was in general harmful. Many cultures throughout the world, however, still engage in "food-kissing" as a weaning process, with no evidence of detrimental effects. Vallambert was all the same an original observer. He described epidemic *du pourpre*, or fever associated with petechiae resembling flea bites.[20] He described congenital syphilis for the first time:

I saw at Tours a goldsmith who for 14 or 15 years since he had the Great Pox had felt no ill and seemed quite well, nevertheless all his children that he has had since then had the Pox soon after they were born, at seven or eight days old.[21]

Georg Maler (Georgius Pictorius, 1500–1569) published *Frawenzimmer* in 1569, written in the vernacular German expressly as a home health guide for

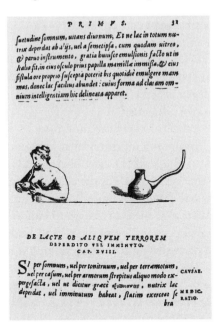

Figure 6.5 Breast milk suction glass from Ferrarius. COURTESY NATIONAL LIBRARY OF MEDICINE.

women. There are sections on midwifery and personal feminine hygiene followed by, in a handbook format, advice on dealing with childhood illnesses.

Another German text, by Walther Hermann Ryff (?–1548), was published in 1580. Historian Still dismissed Ryff as "the most shameless plagiarist"[22] for his book, *Von allen Kranck-heiten bösen Zufällen und Gebrechen der jungen Kinder . . .*, which was based entirely on unacknowledged translations of other authors' treatises on the diagnosis and treatment of children's diseases.

During the Ming dynasty in China, Hsueh Chi and his father, Hsueh K'ai, published *The Complete Writings on Infant Protection* in 1556. Importantly, the text was published by the government, reflecting official professionalization and recognition of pediatric medicine.[23]

OMNIBONUS FERRARIUS

In 1577 in Verona, Italy, Ognibene Ferrari, better known by his Latinized name, Omnibonus Ferrarius, published an illustrated book, *De arte medica infantium*. A popular text, it had many printings, the last one in Leipzig in 1605. It was written in three parts on the topics of breast-feeding, newborn care, and childhood disease. Aphoristic as well as descriptive, the book was

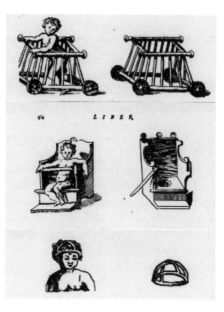

Figure 6.6 Walker, potty chair, and helmet from Ferrarius. COURTESY NATIONAL LIBRARY OF MEDICINE.

liberally illustrated by Ferrarius. His section on breastfeeding included a drawing of a nursing suction glass, or breast pump (figure 6.5), that could be used to relieve engorged breasts and supply breast milk as a mixing medium for pap. The extracted milk also could be used in a feeding horn for infants who were unable to suck milk.

Ferrarius was an original proponent of "baby-proofing" homes to minimize the danger of accidents.[24] He strongly supported developmental apparatus for children, including walkers, potty chairs, and a "helmet" to prevent head injury (figure 6.6):

And as the power of reasoning is not yet awakened in them we should keep out of the way of the child stones, pieces of wood, sticks, knives, glass and all steel instruments of any kind whatever which are capable of hurting, pricking, cutting, fracturing or injuring, and it is equally important that the child should be kept away from fire, from water, from wells, from heights, and from places where animals congregate or pass which are prone and liable to injure by bite or horns or hoof. (bk. 2, chap. 13)

In contrast to Vallambert, Ferrarius advocated premasticated food:

When the child is seven months old and the first central and lateral incisors have appeared and are fully cut, then it is good for the infant to accustom himself to more solid food but without giving up the milk. And first chewed bread is to be put in the baby's little mouth, and later vegetables previously cooked, and chewed by the nurse and then meat and the like. (bk. 2, chap. 2)

Ferrarius's sensitive insight regarding the impressionable minds of children is his most enduring legacy to the pediatric literature:

The greatest care must be taken that he does not see terrifying pictures, nor should the one who has charge of him shew himself to him with a stern look on his face, lest he cause him fright, and so through depression and overmuch grieving he be ill affected and fall into bad ways and infirmities. For many have escaped illness simply through cheerfulness, and many through depression have become ill. Let the nurse always cheer the child with a bright and loving countenance when the child comes to her. For spirit transmitted through the glance of the eye can bewitch and make or mar, so that it is no wonder that in a similar way diseases of mind and body can be given or taken away.

Some of the aphorisms Ferrarius appended to his text proselytized about the issue of using wet nurses:

Infants savour of the nature of the person by whom they are suckled.

It seems an inhuman and monstrous thing to have conceived a child and without legitimate reason to feed him on the milk of some entire stranger. (Aphorisms, 1:5, 6)

Some reflected sensitivity to and appreciation of sound common wisdom:

Infants never cry without legitimate cause: having as yet no speech they show their trouble by crying, screaming, anger and restlessness. (Aphorisms, 2:43)

Many of the aphorisms, however, repeated age-old absurdities that do little more than illustrate the tenacious hold superstitions have on the imagination:

It is the general opinion . . . that certain old women, witches . . . suck the blood of infants that they may thereby regain their youth as far as they are capable. (Aphorisms, 2:30)

A dead man's tooth . . . when hung on the neck of an infant soothes and disperses the pain of teething. (Aphorisms, 3:76)

FELIX WURTZ

The Childrens Book, was written in 1563 by Felix Wurtz (1518–1574) and published in Basel under the title *Practica der Wundartzney, darin aller-*

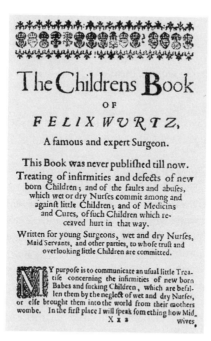

The Childrens Book
OF
FELIX WURTZ,
A famous and expert Surgeon.

This Book was never published till now.
Treating of infirmities and defects of new
born Children; and of the faults and abuses,
which wet or dry Nurses commit among and
against little Children; and of Medicins
and Cures, of such Children which re-
ceaved hurt in that way.

Written for young Surgeons, wet and dry Nurses,
Maid Servants, and other parties, to whose trust and
overlooking little Children are committed.

MY purpose is to communicate an usual little Treatise concerning the infirmities of new born
Babes and sucking Children, which are befal-
len them by the neglect of wet and dry Nurses,
or else brought them into the world from their mothers
wombe. In the first place I will speak something how Midwives.

Figure 6.7 Felix Wurtz's *The Childrens Book.* COURTESY NATIONAL LIBRARY OF MEDICINE.

lei schädliche Missbräuche des Wundartes. It proved very popular and was translated into French and English. The excepts that follow are taken from the English text published in 1656. *Surgerie in Four Parts* (figure 6.7) was a traditional manuscript with marginal annotations as a form of table of contents. Wurtz expressed a particular sensitivity regarding the manner in which, in his view, children should be cared for:[25]

[I]f the hands are kept clean, because their work in hand is about Silk, fine Linnen, Lace of Gold or Silver, is Man not more precious and worthier to be kept clean than all these? especially when that young tender Children are not able to speak or complain against those, which deal roughly with them, more than their nature and body is able to brook withall, by hard pressing, thrusting, pinching, burning, &c. and thus such unhappy girds, Children are put unto.

He reminded his readers of the sensitive and frail nature of newborns:

A Vein broken Child is like to flesh wrapped in a naked skin, as everyone may observe also, who had a swelling or wound on his body which is but newly healed how tender and soft that new skin feeleth; even so is it with a new born Child. If a man doth but scratch his finger, or is pinched, if a heat comes to it, how soon he complaineth of it; or if he be hurt any other way, thrust, &c. whereby some danger he falls into, and that place is more painfull unto him than others, which are not hurt. These things any one may be sensible of; much more will be new born Babes, if roughly or rudely handled, or are hurt in the least manner either with hard hands, rough woolen clothes.

His text is replete with reminders to handle infants with care and delicacy, warning against, for example, the common mishap of hot water scalding:

Touching Baths of Children, it is known that they are bathed sometimes so hot, that the heat thereof is scarcely sufferable to an old bodies hand, whose skin is strong: we must note here, that if a water bath be made for any one, which seemeth to him to be not very hot, at that time when he was scabby, and went in the first time; so the skin of a Child is so thin and tender, as his, who is full of scabs. . . .

The bodies of such little Children may be compared to a young and tender root or twigg of a Tree, which in the such is not so grosse as an old root or branch of a Tree; take heed you cause no paines unto little Children.

Wurtz discussed the orthopedics of children more than any extant text. Two sections of his book were dedicated to "Crooked and Lame Children" and "Dislocated Leggs." Rendered in verse, he offered some very appropriate and reasonable advice on the treatment of fractured or deformed extremities, placing great import on patience and tincture of time:

Have a care you bind the Joint not too hard,
then surely is done neither hurt nor smart.
Do not begrudge your time at all,
a timely cure on the party will fall.
Be exact with your tying and setting,
then the crooked joint will right come in.
Give not over, be willing, not timorous,
the Joint grow'th right as a wick must curious.

In his book, Wurtz departed from the traditional, abstract references to "patients, subjects, invalids, the injured" and to diseases. Employing a simple semantic device, Wurtz, in referring to the "child" and "children" in his manuscript, kept in focus the image of the human child under consideration, whether afflicted with disease or for whom model care was being discussed. Moreover, Wurtz's prose was richly imbued with concern and compassion for children and set the standard for future texts. The closing supplication exemplifies this: "This much of childrens infirmities. Let all be to Gods Glory, and the good of Children: Amen."

HIERONYMUS MERCURIALIS

Hieronymus Mercurialis (1530–1606) was a prolific writer in all medical disciplines. He wrote two pediatric works, *Nomothelasmus seu ratio lactandi infantes*, which appeared in Padua in 1552, and *De Morbis Puerorum*, printed in Venice in 1583. The latter was written by one of his students as the title page informs us: "From the mouth of the Most Honorable Geronimo Mercuriali of Forli, the famous Doctor, and digested into three books: with permission and approval by John Chroscieynosky."[26]

Diseases, fevers, and worms were discussed in three separate parts of the book, all culled from the writings of Hippocrates, Aristotle, Galen, Avicenna, Trallianus, and Celsus. Nonetheless, Mercurialis was court physician to Emperor Maximilian and chair of medicine at the University of Padua, and his fame and reputation ensured a favorable reception and wide distribution of his book. He did, however, achieve a unique contribution for the pediatric literature in a collated, extensive, section devoted to childhood stammering, which he ascribed to either Galenic humors and qualities or to a tongue tie:

The cure of faulty speech is applied in children only when they have already been weaned; for this reason, because before that time it cannot be known whether their speech is faulty or not; and all the more so because often it also happens that children up to the sixth and seventh years stammer and yet are cured of their own accord. Therefore when it is certain that the disease is not to be ended of its own accord, the following cure should be promptly attempted.

Mutes, who are at the same time deaf, should be dismissed altogether. . . .[27] If the child is impeded in speech because of excessive binding of the bridle, all cure lies in manual operation alone. Galen indeed writes that obstetricians were accustomed with their nails to cut away that membrane which is called the bridle; but whether it be because of the inexperience of our obstetricians or whether it be that sometimes this operation alone does not suffice, it is necessary to use another operation. Celsus [proposes] an operation of such a kind that the tongue is elevated toward the palate, so that it touches it, then with a very smooth hook that membrane is stretched, afterwards it is entirely cut off with a very sharp knife, yet so that the veins are in no wise broken. When this has been done, the mouth should be washed out with posca [vinegar and water], then sprinkled with powder of manna, of incense.[28]

AMBROISE PARE

Although remembered primarily for his writing on wounds, Ambroise Pare (1510–1590) did address some childhood problems, particularly, inguinal hernia, taking note along the way of the persistence of the eunuch:[29]

Because children are very subject to Ruptures, but those truely not fleshy or varicous, but watry, windy, and especially of the Guts, by reason of continuall and painefull crying and coughing: Therefore in the first place we will treate of their cure. Wherefore the Surgeon, called to restore the Gut which is fallen downe, shall place the child, either on a table, or in a bed, so that his head shall be low, but his buttocks, and thighes higher; then shall he force with his hands by little and little, and gently, the Gut into its proper place; and shall foment the Groine with the astringent formentation . . . but the chiefe of the cure consists in folded clothes, and Trusses, and ligatures artificially made, that the restored gut may be contained in its place, for which purpose he shall keepe the child seated in his cradle for 30. or 40. dayes . . . and keepe him from crying, shouting, and coughing. . . . Truely I have healed many by the helpe of such remedies, and have delivered them from the hands of Gelders, which are greedy of childrens testicles, by reason the great gaine they receive from thence.[30]

A few minor contributions of the late sixteenth century deserve mention. Guillaume de Baillou (1538–1616) described the pertussis epidemic of 1578: "The summer was glowing and burning hot. Boys four months old, ten months old and a little older were attacked by fever, which carried countless off. Especially that common cough, which is formally called *quinta*."[31]

In 1578, Giovanni Ingrassias (1510–1580) distinguished scarlet fever from measles and severe chicken pox from mild smallpox.[32] Oswald Gabelkhover (?–1616) in 1596 wrote a short treatise on therapeutics for children, and, writing in Spanish, Geronimo Soriano (1536–1618) advocated starvation to diminish the fecal output of diarrhea.[33] In *Metodo y Orden de Curar las Enfermedades de los Niños*, published posthumously in 1690, Soriano, according to Vilaplana Satorre,[34] first described athrepsia (marasmus).

By the end of the sixteenth century, the number of books written in the vernacular on pediatric topics had encouraged physicians and parents to greater sensibility regarding the care of children and to adopt more realistic expectations of child behavior and developmental milestones. Writers like Metlinger, Phaer, Vallambert, Wurtz, and de Avila, by explaining the nature of children's diseases, advanced the development of improved medical treatment available to children.

Most important, these writers established the matrix for a series of truly original pediatric texts published in the seventeenth century that contributed to the formulation of the evolving concept of pediatrics as a distinct discipline.

During the seventeenth century, European textbooks on childhood diseases continued to be published predominantly in Latin (table 6.2); in China the vernacular was used to set down medical wisdom in a traditional and familiar conversational format. Europe's publications in general reaffirmed time-

TABLE 6.2
SEVENTEENTH-CENTURY PEDIATRIC TEXTS

Author	Place	Title (Date)
Johannes Ceckius	Bologna	*De puerorum tuenda valentudine* (1604)
Marius Zuccharius	Naples	*Tractus de Morbius Puerorum* (1604)
Jacques Guillemeau	Paris	*De la nouriture et governement des enfans* (1609)
Wang K'eng-t'ang	Northwest China	*Principles of Children's Diseases* (1607)
Johannes Hucherus	Montpellier	*De Diaeta et therapeia puerorum* (1610)
Hsu Tsan	Northwest China	*One Hundred Questions on Infants and Children* (1610)
F. Perez Cascales	Madrid	*Liber de affectionibus puerorum* (1611)
Johann Strobelberger	Leipzig	*Brevissima Manuductio ad curando pueriles affectus* (1625)
David Herlitz	Stettin	*De curationibus . . . et infantium* (1628)
Daniel Sennert	Wittenberg	*De Mulierum et Infantium morbis* (1632)
Amthor	Schleussing	*Nasocomium infantile et puerile* (1638)
Guillaume de Baillou	Paris	*Epidemiorum* (1640)
Ezekiel DiCastro	Verona	*Il Colostro* (1642)
Melchior Sebisch	Strassburg	*Problemata medica de infantium et puerorum morbis* (1649)
P. Gerhard Grüling	Nordhausen	*Tractat von Kinder Kranckheiten* (1660)
Michael Ettmüller	Leipzig	*De Infantum morbis* (1709)

honored valid and classical precepts and reemphasized for the scientific and scholarly communities the importance of recognizing the unique aspects and treatment of diseases of children.

Moreover, texts began to question old, ineffective tenets and reflected the profound influence of revolutionary scientific postulates that had been made and that continued to evolve. In Europe, clinical-pathological correlates (autopsy observations and analyses) in children began to be examined, and a renascent scientific approach to studying and treating the ills of children emerged.

The progress, however, was very slow and is best exemplified by tracing the publication of several books on rickets, the debilitating and disfiguring disease that was common throughout Europe and especially in England, Switzerland, and Holland.

The first mention of this disease in the English *Bills of Mortality* did not appear until 1634.[35] In 1582, Jerome Reusner (1558–?) perfunctorily described a disease, most likely rickets, that occurred only in children and was marked by "weakness, distortion of the chest, and bandy legs"[36] (see figure 1.5). The Danes also referred to the condition as *varum*, a term closer to the medical designation for the bowing deformity of the lower extremities called *genu varum*. In 1609, Jacques Guillemeau (1550–1613) described the chest beading of rickets. Thirty-six years later, Daniel Whistler (1619–1684), in a doctoral thesis published in 1643, *De morbo puerli Anglorum quem patrio idiomate indigenae vocant the Rickets*, presented a catalog of the symptom complex of rickets. Whistler described the enlarged liver, deformed, swollen joints and ribs, fevers, vomiting, diarrhea, and irritability. He also speculated on the etymology of rickets, which, he said, came from the surname of a "quack" who treated these children or from one of the symptoms: shortness of breath, or "rucket."[37] Modern scholars believe it comes from the old English *wrikken* meaning "to twist." Whistler listed what he considered the seven prognostic signs:[38]

1. Those who have the disease from birth or before all die.
2. More of the female sex suffer but these more quickly and certainly convalesce.
3. Those with hydrocephalus which separates the suture die.
4. Those who bear movement of the body best recover most easily.
5. Those whose feet are affected are cured most easily, and those who are older.
6. Where the head can scarely be held on the neck cure is rare; also those with great difficulty in breathing. With suppuration of the lungs never.
7. A small unequal and rapid pulse, especial a weak one [is a bad sign].

In London, Arnold Boot (1606–1650) published *De Tabe Pectorea* (1649), in which he described the chest and rib deformities of rickets—*nodi in costis*—known to today's clinician as a "rachitic rosary."[39] It was not, however, until the Englishman Francis Glisson published *De rachitide sive morbo puerli qui vulgo "the rickets" dicitus, tractus* in 1650 (figure 6.8), that notable progress in scientific writing on the subject of rickets was made.

FRANCIS GLISSON

Francis Glisson (1597–1677), Regius Professor of Physic at Cambridge, advanced pathophysiological correlations and an enlightened scientific approach in his book. He performed postmortems on rachitic children,[40] and for the first time conjoined valid pathological observations with clinical symptoms of a disease of children:

The Signs which belong to the disproportioned nourishment of the parts.

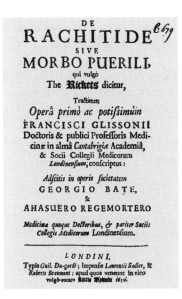

Figure 6.8 Francis Glisson's *Treatise of the Rickets.* COURTESY NATIONAL LIBRARY OF MEDICINE.

First, there is an unusual Bigness of the Head.

Second, the fleshy parts are daily more and more worn away.

Third, certain swellings and knotty excrescences, are observed about some of the joynts.

These are chiefly conspicuous in the wrists, and somewhat less in the ankles. The like tumors also are in the tops of the Ribs, where they are enjoyned in the gristles in the Breast.

Fourthly, some bones wax crooked, especially the bone called the shank bone, and the Fibula or small bone of the leg.

Fifthly, the Teeth come forth both slowly and with trouble.

Sixthly, the Breast in the higher progression of the disease becomes narrow on the sides.[41]

Astutely, Glisson observed that these children often suffered from coexisting scurvy:

[T]he Scurvy is sometimes conjoyned with this Affect. It is either hereditary, or perhaps in so tender a Constitution contracted by infection, or lastly, it is produced from the indiscreet and erroneous Regiment of the Infant, and chiefly from the inclemency of the Ayr and Climate where the Child is educated.[42]

While Glisson was unable to define the etiology of rickets and scurvy, he importantly ascertained that it was neither contagious nor congenital. He therefore established that rickets was not related to the bone disease caused by congenital syphilis, as was thought in some medical circles:

If the French Pox chance to be complicated with this Diseas it is either derived from the Nurse's infection or from the Parents by Inheritance. For it is a Diseas altogether distinct from this and hath scarce any affinity with it.[43]

Sensing the debility and weakness of rachitic children, Glisson advocated the use of rhubarb as a mild and safe aperient:

But in this [rickets] as well as in other Diseases of Children, where Catharticks take Place, Rhubarb is to be preferred to all other Purgatives, upon several Accounts. It is both efficacious and gentle in its Operation . . . never brings on Superpurgation, unless it be given in too large a Dose.[44]

For all of his insights, Glisson remained ignorant of the nutritional deficiency of vitamin D that caused the common form of rickets. He and his colleagues treated rickets in the conventional manner of the time: swaddling was employed to straighten bones and suspension to decrease the scoliosis, gibbus, and other deformities of the spine.

The same year in which Whistler's book was published, John Mayow (1643–1679) was born. In 1674, Mayow wrote *Tractatus Secundus*.[45] It acknowledged Glisson's work and enlarged on it, departing from Glisson only with respect to pathology. Whereas Glisson believed the rachitic bone abnormalities were due to unequal circulation, Mayow felt they were due to muscle weaknesses induced by poor nerve impulses.

It took nearly another 100 years for this common, disfiguring, and painful disease to be clinically and carefully described and an additional 300 years before the cause of the disorder was established.

ROBERT PEMELL

Robert Pemell's (?–1653) *A Treatise of Diseases of Children* was published in England in 1653. Pemell introduced the small volume "for the benefit of such as do not understand the Latine tongue" and predicted it would be "very useful for all such as are House-keepers and have Children." As can be seen in its table of contents, the 58-page book was able to describe a full range of pediatric complaints:

Of ulcers and sores in childrens heads.
Of lice.
Of the Falling sicknesse and Convulsion.

Of Feavers.

Of the scab and Itch.

Of pain the ears and inflammation.

Of breeding and coming of teeth.

Of small Pox and Measels.

Of inflammation of the mouth and throat with ulcers and sores thereof.

Of watching out of measure and want of rest.

Of worms.

Of fear, starting and terrible Dreams.

Of the Hicket.

Of Rheums, the Cough and shortnesse of breath.

Of Vomiting and weaknesse of the stomach.

Of the consumption or leannesse and the Rickets.

Of Gripings and fretings in the belly.

Of looseness and flux of the belly.

Of costivenesse and stopping of the belly.

Of Ruptures and Burstings.

Of pissing in bed.

Of swelling or coming forth of the Navel.

Of inflammation of the Navel.

Of falling of the Fundament.

Of the Stone and difficulty of making water.

Of the disease called Saint Anthonie's fire, or wilde fire, as also of burning and scalding.

Of fretting, chafing or galling of the skin in the groines.

Except for his advice about teething, Pemell's thinking paralleled that of his colleagues. For the irritable baby awaiting the eruption of teeth, Pemell recommended the traditional unction of honey, butter, hare's brain, and hen's grease. He went a step further, advising the lancing of the gum. It was the first reference to gum lancing in the English vernacular:[46]

If these medicines prevail not, as many times comes to passe, then the best way is to cut the gums, for this is very safe and were it more used fewer Children would die; for I am confident the want hereof doth occasion the death of many a child.[47]

Pemell astutely attributed many illnesses to the lack of cleanliness and advised that sick parts of the body be bathed. For persisting wounds he advocated adding to lotions either wine, with its antiseptic property of alcohol; silver and gold, for their bacteriostatic properties; or sulfur (brimstone), for its bactericidal nature. He additionally prescribed covering or sealing lesions with balsam lotion to curtail further infection:

First, let the child's head be bathed with a decoction of Mallows, and Barly, or with a decoction of Dock roots, mallows, Celendine the greater, Wormwood, Fenegreek, Cicers, Lupines, Beans, &c. If there be need of greater cleansing, you may boyl the foregoing herbs in wine; or make a Lotion with decoction of Marshmallow roots, made with Urine of the infant alone, or mixt with barley water. Then anoint the head with oyl of Roses and oul of bitter Almonds mixed with a little litharge of gold or silver in fine powder; or take of the juyce of Beets and Celedine the greater of each one ounce, Hogsgrease two ounces, boyl them together a while, then being almost cold put in of Brimstone in powder a drachme, make an ointment, with which anoint the parts affected morning and evening. Or wash the head with soap-suds made strong. If these ulcers eat to the skul, then use hony of Roses mixed with a little spirit of Wine, and afterwards the powder Birthwort and natural Balsam.[48]

The frequency with which wounds and ulcers became infected was a well-known problem for adult patients, especially for soldiers with battlefield wounds, and Pemell's recommendations reflect his knowledge of contemporaneous medical prescriptions for battlefield injuries. His prescriptions, however, were specifically and appropriately modified for use in treating children. For example, Ambroise Pare advocated applying scalding hot oil to gunshot wounds. Pemell, understanding the principle of the healing balm of oil, modified Pare's procedure and suggested using warm oil mixed with binary metal salts on children.[49]

Pemell's approach to treatment was cautious and observant. He noticed and recorded the many safe cures he effected. He presented fundamentally sound advice, as in the treatment of common and often dangerous infantile diarrhea, for example: keep the child hydrated and temporarily suspend milk from the diet:[50]

If the Infant suck or not, and the flux be of some continuance, means must be used to stay it, and such means as first cleanse and then bind the body, as sirup of Roses solutive, or hony of Roses solutive. Clysters may be used.

Some commend the maw of a Kid, or Hare, if ten grains thereof be given, and the child to take no milk that day, least it curdle in the stomach; but give it bread boyled in water with Rosewater and Sugar.

Pemell was an able clinician who wrote clearly and concisely. He was well liked and respected by his contemporaries as the closing quartet of an introductory poem by his friend John Elmeston attests:[51]

Who then, to skilful Pemell can repay
His due reward? whose care has been so great, . . .
Let this good friend by thy Physitian,
Whose skilfull Counsell, and Direction,
Shall either keep thy head in healthfull case;
Or by his Art, away the Evill chase.

One of two lesser pediatric works published was *Partes Duae De Morbis Puerorum* by James Primerose (c.1598–1659), appearing in 1659. This work reiterated the work of Galen and Soranus. Primerose advanced the notion that tears healthily cleansed the brain: "Tears are serous Humours discharged by the brain through the eyes." His source, most likely, was Sainte Marthe, who wrote in his *Paedotrophia* (1584):

And moderate cryings come oft not in vain
They stir a dull and cleanse a watery brain.[52]

The other text, published in London in 1664, was *Childrens [sic] Diseases Both Outward and Inward* by J. Starsmare. The table of contents replicated Pemell's work. The book did feature an interesting frontispiece. It had an illustration depicting various aspects of children's health care: nutrition, bedside attention, pharmacopeia, and development, including a visual reference to "walking-ribbons" that were sewn on children's clothing as a restrainer to prevent toddlers from falling down (figure 6.9).

Starsmare's book contained one new entry: chapter 3, "The King's Evil," known to us as scrofula:*

The Kings Evill is a hard or Schirrous Tumour contrary to nature, growing for the most about the Neck and chiefly of Children. . . . [T]he Children of poor persons are more troubled with this Disease than the Children of rich men, because they eat grosse and ill Diet which makes and foments the humour. . . . [T]he Cure is . . . A Convenient Diet, let the Air be hot and dry, the sleep little, exercise moderate.[53]

---

*The term refers to a tradition in which a king touched a patient with scrofula, effecting a cure. Edward the Confessor was the first monarch reported to have done so, in 1058. The origin of the superstition probably is rooted in classical times. The historian Tacitus claimed Emperor Despasian cured many diseases by touch.

Whatever the origin, the royal hand as a treatment and cure was universally accepted, reaching its peak of popularity during the reign of Charles II (1660–1685). This king was said to have touched over 100,000 loyal and believing subjects. In his childhood, Samuel Johnson (1709–1784), however, was unsuccessfully touched by Queen Anne. Camp, 1973, pp. 11, 126.

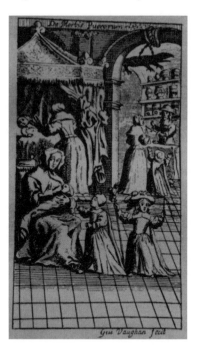

Figure 6.9 Frontispiece of Starsmare's book showing a child with walking ribbons, another playing with a horse and quirt. One visits an apothecary and another is sick in bed. COURTESY NATIONAL LIBRARY OF MEDICINE.

Paracelsus had started the movement to discredit the concept of humors as disease causative elements, but as can be seen in the works of both Primerose and Starsmare, a millennium of Galenic influence was difficult to eradicate overnight. Starsmare, however, was correct in his observations that cervical lymph node tuberculosis appeared most commonly in children susceptible to poor hygiene and overcrowded living.

A military surgeon, Richard Wiseman (1622–1676), wrote a short piece on scrofula.[54] In extending beyond examining tubercular nodes in his descriptions, Wiseman anticipated what would come be recognized as Pott's disease:

The King's-Evil is a Tumour arising from a peculiar Acidity of the Serum of the Blood, which whenever it lights upon a Gland, Muscle, or Membrane, coagulates and hardens; when it mixes with Marrow always dissolves it, and renders the Bone carious. . . . Children that are born of strumous Parents, or who have sucked strumous Nurses, are usually troubled with this Disease. They whose Blood inclines to Acidity, and the Serum apt to coagulate, as also Children that are Rickety, are very obnoxious to it. . . .

In a Child of six Years old, I saw them spreading all over the Body, some superficial in the Skin, others deep. The Viscera are often found with great Strumae growing in them, out from them. Thus we find the Liver, Lungs and Spleen, frequently strumous, and sometimes weighed down with scrophulous Appendages. ("King's Evil" [1676])

An important epidemiological and demographic study was issued by a highly improbable source. London haberdasher John Graunt[55] (1620–1674) had observed the common interest—and gossip—generated by the *Bills of Mortality*, the weekly publication that recorded deaths, causes of death, and the number of burials that had occurred. He envisioned a more fruitful use of the *Bills* as a tool for epidemiology and demography, and over the years he studied them, gathering and analyzing the data. Finally, in 1663, he published *Natural and Political Observations Mentioned in a Following Index and Made upon the Bills of Mortality*. Regarding children, Graunt's figures indicated that more males were born than females and that infants more commonly died of infections and accidents—rarely of suffocation, or "overlaying," as commonly held. In analyzing 229,250, or nearly a quarter-million deaths, he could find only 529 infants—0.23 percent of deaths—reported to have died of overlaying and suffocation.

FRANCIS DE LE BOE SYLVIUS

A posthumous book by Francis Sylvius (1614–1672) from Amsterdam originally was published in 1674. Entitled *De morbis infantium et aliis quibusdam memorater dignis affectibus*,[56] it is notable because of its careful clinical observations, a fact not surprising, coming from a man who described the brain structures, Sylvian fissure, the aqueduct of Sylvius, the ventricle of Sylvius, and the Sylvian artery.

Sylvius's book was a small, 11-chapter work. It surveyed the most common childhood ailments: jaundice, diarrhea, vomiting, hiccups, lethargy, seizures, teething, rashes, worms, measles, smallpox, and rickets. Sylvius had a propensity to prescribe opium for nearly all ailments,[57] earning him the cognomen, "Doctor Opiate":[58]

Take Fennel and Parsley waters of each an ounce, Mint water half an ounce. Spirit of Nitre six drops, Syrup of white Poppies half an ounce, Laudanum one grain, Spirit of Salt eight drops; Mix them . . . [give until] his pain and crying abate and he take rest.[59] (chap. 2, p. 17)

Opium undeniably can be quite dangerous, yet paradoxically, Sylvius's reliance on the potentially dangerous opium deviated from his otherwise cautious use of therapeutics:

For it may happen to Infants as to people of years, that all are not alike easily, speedily or largely purged by any Medicine: for which cause, lest they should get harm by a strong Medicine, it is better to give a gentle Purge at several times, and but a little at a time, rather than together and at once. *For a Physician cannot be too cautious, seeing children are tender, and may die upon a small occasion.*[60] (chap. 3, p. 24)

It would appear that Sylvius feared dehydration from a purge more than the risk of opiate sedation and anoxia. The emphasis is added to the quotation to highlight European society's growing consciousness of infant and child vulnerability.

Sylvius used his 12-bed infirmary in Leyden to teach medicine:[61]

I led them by the very hand into the practice of medicine, i.e. I took them daily into the public hospital for the purpose of seeing the sick to whose complaints and other notable symptoms I directed attention, asking immediately afterwards what they had observed in the disorders of the patient; their views as to the causes and proper treatment and the reasons for the same. (Epistola Apologetica [1664])

NICHOLAS CULPEPER

Several vernacular texts on childhood diseases written by the English herbalist Nicholas Culpeper (1616–1654) contain material largely gleaned from ancient sources.[62] One of the books, *A Directory for Midwives*, made several shrewd and practical observations. There were sections related to pediatric diets and diseases, consisting of 39 pages entitled "A Tractate of the Cure of Infants," which appeared toward the end of the book.

Of weaning, he advised: "It is best to wean in the Spring and Fall in the increase of the Moon and give but very little Wine."[63] In a chapter entitled "Of Great Watching" he observed:[64]

A Child newborn sleeps more than he wakes, because his brain is very moist and he used to sleep in the Womb. If you cannot make them sleep by singing or rocking nor the like, it is a Disease. (chap. 9)

Despite whimsical notions of moist brains, Culpeper correctly recognized the disturbed sleep of a sick infant. His overall descriptions of childhood ailments were not original, and he readily admits that his fund of knowledge derives from the ancients. However, he applied his herbalist training beneficially, with the use of botanical remedies that were both time-proven and safe. Culpeper's prescriptions of frankincense to treat stomach ailments and myrrh to treat thrush, for example, continue to this day to be the preferred therapy in many parts of the world.

Culpeper's *The English Physician* was published in the colonies in 1708 with ten "secret" remedies to cure children's ailments, which were, in fact, no different from Culpeper's known herbal formulas. Despite the title, the 94-page manual was published for the lay colonial reader. The book warrants mention because it was the first medical handbook published in the new America.[65]

FRANCOIS MAURICEAU

Eighteen chapters in the third section of Francois Mauriceau's (?1650–1709) text, *Traite de maladies des femme grosses* (published in Paris in 1668) dealt with newborns.[66] The care of normal newborns was thoroughly discussed, and Mauriceau additionally described both normal physical variations and newborn abnormalities, such as wide skull sutures or imperforate anus. Of especial interest is a chapter on congenital syphilis, one of the earliest to focus on newborn lues. Otherwise, Mauriceau's book was not particularly illuminating. His recommendations on infant care followed prevailing practices with regard to swaddling, choice of wet nurse, nourishment, and the like, but he dismissed common wisdom on the issue of teething:

There are many Remedies which divers persons assert have a peculiar property to help the cutting of the Teeth, as rubbing them with Bitches milk, Hares or Pigs brains, and hanging a Vipers tooth about the neck of the Child and such like trifles: but since they are founded more on superstition, than any reason, I will not trouble myself to enlarge upon what is so useless.[67]

Mauriceau is an important figure in the timeline of pediatric history as a respected obstetrician and gynecologist in a world without pediatricians. Sick children routinely were referred to him and to others of his specialty. Much respected in his community, anything Mauriceau wrote about the newborn, being verisimilar, was accepted without question.

THOMAS SYDENHAM

Thomas Sydenham (1624–1689) wrote no work specifically about child care, but his vibrant and compelling clinical descriptions of diseases that afflicted children in particular merit special mention.

Measles, one infective ailment of childhood, caused by a paramyxovirus, was presented in *Processus integri* (1692). The book became a vade mecum of the English physician, remaining so for more than a century. Scarlet fever, an infection due to a β-hemolytic streptococcus, was discussed in *Observationes medicae circa Morborum actorum historiam et curationem*, published in 1676.[68]

Although failing to mention the intraoral lesions of Koplik, Sydenham's narrative on the measles prodrome—the intensification of the rash with its caudal march and ultimate desquamation—was the most accurate of the day:[69]

The measles generally attack children. On the first day they have chills and shivers, and are hot and cold in turns. On the second they have the fever in full—disquietude, thirst, want of appetite, a white (but not a dry) tongue, slight cough, heaviness of the head and eyes, and somnolence. The nose and eyes run continually; and this is the surest sign of measles. To this may be added sneezing, a swelling of the eyelids a little before the eruption, vomiting and diarrhoea with green stools. These appear more especially during teething time. The symptoms increase till the fourth day. Then—or sometimes on the fifth day there appear on the face and forehead small red spots, very like the bites of fleas. These increase in number, and cluster together, so as to mark the face with large red blotches. They are formed by small papulae, so slightly elevated above the skin, that their prominence can hardly be detected by the eye, but can just be felt by passing the fingers lightly along the skin.

The spots take hold of the face first; from which they spread to the chest and belly, and afterwards to the legs and ankles. On these parts may be seen broad, red maculae, on, but above, the level of the skin. In measles the eruption does not so thoroughly allay the other symptoms as in small-pox. There is, however, no vomiting after its appearance; nevertheless there is slight cough instead, which, with the fever and the difficulty of breathing, increases. There is also a running from the eyes, somnolence, and want of appetite. On the sixth day, or thereabouts, the forehead and face begin to grow rough, as the pustules die off, and as the skin breaks. Over the rest of the body the blotches are both very broad and very red.

About the eighth day they disappear from the face, and scarcely show on the rest of the body. On the ninth there are none anywhere. On the face, however, and on the extremities—sometimes over the trunk—they peel off in thin, mealy squamulae; at which time the fever, the difficulty of breathing, and the cough are aggravated. (*Processus integri*, chap. 14, part 1)

Similarly, without mention of the pharyngitis, Sydenham vividly described scarlet fever:

Scarlet Fever (Scarlatina) may appear at any season. Nevertheless, it oftenest breaks out towards the end of summer, when it attacks whole families at once, and more especially the infant part of them. The patients feel rigors and shiverings, just as they do in other fevers. The symptoms, however, are moderate. Afterwards, however, the whole skin becomes covered with small red maculae, thicker than those of measles, as well as broader, redder, and less uniform. These last for two or three days, and then disappear. The cuticle peels off; and branny scales, remain lying upon the surface like meal. They appear and disappear two or three times. (*Observationes medicae*)

Unaware of the association of chorea as a late sequela of scarlet fever and the β-hemolytic streptococcus that caused it, Sydenham nevertheless vividly described the neurological abnormalities and motor contortions of chorea:

This is a kind of convulsion, which attacks boys and girls from the tenth year to the time of puberty. It first shows itself by limping or unsteadiness in one of the legs, which the patient drags. *The hand cannot be steady for a moment.* It passes from one position to another by a convulsive movement, however much the patient may strive to the contrary. Before he can raise a cup to his lips, he makes as many gesticulations as a mountebank; since he does not move it in a straight line, but has his hand drawn aside by the spasms, until by some good fortune he brings it at last to his mouth. He then gulps it off at once, so suddenly and so greedily as to look as if he were trying to amuse the lookers-on. (*Processus integri*, chap. 16, part 1)

Sydenham repopularized the use of cinchona,* which had fallen out of favor in Europe:

The Peruvian bark, commonly called Jesuit's bark, has, if I rightly remember, been famous in London for the cure of intermittent fevers for upwards of five and twenty years, and that rightly. The disease in question was seldom or never cured by any remedy before it. Hence agues were justly called *opprobira medicorum*. (*Epidemic Diseases*, Epistle 1, p. 17)

Sydenham's clinical skill in caring for children evolved with long practice and insightful observations. His legacy to child care resided in the careful annotations he made of the progression of signs and symptoms of diseases in childhood. He also serves as an example for pediatricians of a practiced clinician whose diagnostic skills derive from thoughtful clinical examination and observation, eschewing invasive procedures whenever possible.[70]

THOMAS WILLIS

Like Sydenham, Thomas Willis (1621–1675) left no treatise specifically about children, and, like Sylvius, he is best remembered for his study of brain anatomy. The confluence of vessels seated deep in the brain still is called the "circle of Willis."

---

*Cinchona comes from Lady Anna di Osoria, the countess of Cinchona, wife of the Viceroy of Peru, who, in 1638, after receiving an elution of the bark, recovered from an intermittent febrile disease. When she returned to Spain in 1640, she took back a supply of quinabark; thus, in Europe the powder was called *pulvis Comitissae*. When the Jesuits sent samples back to Rome, it became known as the "Jesuit's bark" and thus fell into disuse because of Protestant disapproval of the eponym, with its papist connection. Osler, 1921, pp. 183–84.

Willis focused on children in his discussion of epilepsy. His description of the seizure and the postictal phase of this neurological disorder was clear and distinct. Most remarkable was his persistent effort to determine the etiology of the disease by studying autopsy data:

Children and Young People are more subject to this Disease than Adults, or those who are advanced in Years; but in Infants for the most Part it goes under the name of Convulsions.

The Epilepsy is either hereditary or acquired. . . .

But that I might more certainly discover the morbifick Matter in Convulsions I have opened the Bodies of a great many who died of this Disease. I could never discover the Cause of it, in the Stomach or Intestines: but the Heads of many of them I have observed a Collection of a serous Liquor contained within the Cavity below the Cerebellum and distending that Membrane which covers the Medulla Oblongata, compressed the Origin of the Nerves. In others, not one apparent Cause of this Disease was to be found.

Sometime ago a Woman in this City had several Children who died of this Disease: at length we dissected the Head of the fourth Child, which died within the first Month like the rest.[71]

Although Willis did not determine the cause of epilepsy, he established that epilepsy was an organic disease, not devil possession requiring exorcism, as was widely believed. His example encouraged further study of postmortem examinations for clues of its etiology.

STEPHEN BLANKAART

Ziekten der Kinderen by Stephen Blankaart (1650–?) was published in the Netherlands in 1684. It was the first book on childhood diseases published in Dutch. Like that of Glisson and Willis, Blankaart's work reflects extensive reliance on the autopsy. Understanding the value of anatomical–pathological correlations, he performed and wrote about more than 200 autopsies. The frontispiece of his book features a disquieting depiction of an autopsy scene and an urinoscopy, juxtaposed with portraits of a rachitic child and a sick infant (figure 6.10).

Two common topics in cold, canal-laced Holland were discussed thoroughly by Blankaart in chapters entitled "Of Children Fallen into Water and Half-Drowned," and "How to Deal with Children Who Have Fallen into the Fire." Throughout Europe, childhood accidents continued to cause significant morbidity and mortality.[72] Drownings and falls were the most common causes.

Blankaart's opinion on child rearing deviated from the prevailing stern, puritanical philosophy. He proposed a moderate and gentler course of dis-

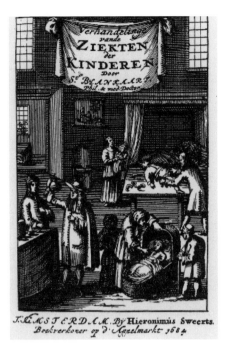

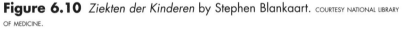

Figure 6.10 *Ziekten der Kinderen* by Stephen Blankaart. COURTESY NATIONAL LIBRARY OF MEDICINE.

cipline that, in his view, would produce stable, industrious and productive citizens:

Children should not be brought up in too niggardly a style, nor too strictly, and they should not be deprived of things which other children have: on the other hand, they should not be brought up extravagantly, for then their choice will more often be the tavern than the church. Some check is to be put upon their will but not with the thump of a blacksmith but rather with gentle admonition, leading up their ideas to something higher and better, studies, trades, professions; they are to be trained to be in earnest.[73]

WALTER HARRIS

In 1689, Englishman Walter Harris (1647–1732) wrote a Latin text entitled *De morbis acutis infantum* (figure 6.11). In it, Harris articulated for the first time in modern medical literature the challenge that pediatric care presents to physicians. He informed his readers of the magnitude of and practice in the skills required to determine from the *infans* ("the voiceless") pertinent signs and symptoms leading to diagnosis and treatment.[74]

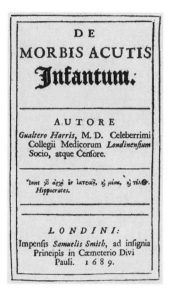

Figure 6.11 Harris's book, *De morbis acutis infantum* (1689). Ruhräh, 1925.

[F]or sick Children, and especially Infants, give no other Light into the Knowledge of their Diseases, than what we are able to discover from their uneasy Cries, and the uncertain Tokens of their Crossness; for which Reason, several Physicians of the first Rank have openly declared to me, that they go very unwillingly to take care of the Diseases of Children, especially such as are newly born, as if they were to unravel some strange Mystery, or cure some incurable Disease.

By his own admission, Harris's book offered no new medical information. His contribution to pediatric history is in having established a pediatric age group—infancy to 14 years of age—and insightfully noting that, once treatment was begun, the prognoses of illnesses generally were more favorable for children—and the younger, the better:

There can be no Doubt but that a perfect Cure of the Disease of Children is as much to be desired by all, as any Thing else whatsoever in the whole Art of Physick. Nor is it of consequence only to the noble, the powerful, and the wealthy, who are desirous of having Heirs, and preserving them, but to all Parents of any Rank whatsoever; for Nature has instilled into all Men an almost invincible Love and Care of their own Offspring. Wherefore I shall think myself happy, if I can strike out a few Hints, which others of greater Abilities may improve, and bring to Perfection. . . .

Under the Name of a Child I comprehend all from that Age to the fourteenth Year. And the younger the Patient is, the more easy will be the Cure of any severe

Disease, as I have found from the best Reasoning, confirmed by manifold Experience.

Harris decried the use of opiates in children, "except in violent Vomiting," and deplored the euphemism "cordial" to describe opiates:

The Name of Cordial has been very artfully contrived, to impose upon female Pretenders to Physick and Country People, who lying at a considerable Distance from Physicians, are supported by my Lady's Cordials out of Charity, which her Ladyship exhibits promiscuously in every Disease with very great Applause; for be the Event what it will the Cordial, to be sure, must never be blamed. In short, it has been invented to amuse all the ignorant Dablers in Physick, who think here they have a Medicine that can cure Death itself. For who can suspect any Mischief from a Cordial? And yet some of the wisest of Physicians are so ill-bred as to suspect whether a greater Number of Children who have escaped violent Deaths, have perished by Diseases or those favourite Cordials.

He scolded about the abusive use of wines and spirits:

Wine of all Sorts taken too freely, as well as all Sorts of Spirituous Liquors, destroys the natural Ferment of all Stomachs, especially those of Children: they impair the Appetite, burn up the Coats of the Stomach.

Harris acknowledged the hereditary nature of some diseases and volunteered some eugenic advice:

There is no one who will deny, that there are hereditary Diseases, proceeding either from one or other of the Parents; or question but that the Gout, Epilepsy, Stone, Consumption, etc. sometimes flow from the Parents to the Children. Whole families proceeding from the same Stock, often end their Lives by the same Kind of Disease. For the prolific Seed often so rivets the morbid Disposition into the Foetus, that it can never afterwards be removed by any Art or Industry whatsoever. But let those who prefer a strong, vigorous and healthy Offspring before Money, take care to avoid epileptic, scrophulous, and leprous Mothers.

Unequipped with the concepts of microbes, Norwalk agent, or rotavirus, he did perceive the nature of seasonal diarrhea:

From the Middle of July to about the Middle of September, the Epidemical Gripes of Children are so rife every Year, that more of them usually die in one Month, that in three or four at any other Time.

He also recognized that infancy was a fragile state requiring mild aperient therapies:

Of all the purging Medicines, I know none more suitable to the puerile Age, or more innocent in itself, than Rhubarb,* which is so well known, and so much in Use.

Interestingly, long before the role of low calcium in tetany was known, Harris treated the spasms with calcium in the form of oyster shells.[75]

Harris's most profound insight was his understanding that the value of clinical observation is significantly enhanced by a parental or nurse's medical history of a child, and he considered this an indispensable diagnostic tool:

The Diagnostick of the Disorders of Children is not to be formed from their own Account, or from the Consideration of their Pulse, or from a curious Examination of their Urine, so much as from the Answers of their Nurses, and of those who are about them.

The last of 18 editions of Harris's widely popular book appeared in 1742. German, English, and Dutch translations attest to the book's far-reaching influence. A pediatric vade mecum of English physicians, it was not replaced as such until 1784, when Michael Underwood's *A Treatise on Diseases of Children* appeared.

Harris's book and *Phthisiologia, seu exercitationes de phthisi* by Richard Morton (1637–1698) both were first published in 1689. Ruhräh (1938) admiringly credits Richard Morton with a first diagnosis of chylous ascites in a living child. Morton described a two-year-old male with cough, fever, and dyspnea:

[At] the very beginning of the Fever his Belly began to be distended with a Dropsical swelling, which increased strangely every day; his Cough and shortness of Breath at the same time growing worse: All which Symptoms were at length accompanied with an Atrophy of the Parts, even to the degrees of a Marasmus. But yet when his Body was a perfect Skeleton, and the Dropsie at a high Tide (which was very remarkable) he had a brisk and healthful look, and a lovely Countenance, without the least Tincture of a Yellowness, and a good, or rather greedy Appetite, and that to the very day he dyed. From whence I did rightly conjecture, and always told his Friends, as my Opinion, that his Dropsie was truly Chylous, caused by the Chyle flowing into the cavity of the Belly by the Lacteal Vessels, upon some rupture that had been made in them; which appeared very plainly from the Event. For in Tapping of the Child's Belly, whilst he was yet alive, we took out several Pints of Milky Chyle.[76]

---

*Rhubarb originated in Korea via China. Transported along the continental trade routes, it was very expensive—three times that of opium and saffron. Attempts to grow it in the West repeatedly failed until seeds were smuggled out of China via St. Petersburg. Some seeds taken to England by one of the tsar's physicians were successfully planted. By 1797 abundant harvests assured ready supplies available to all (Camp, 1973, pp. 79–81).

JOHN PECHEY

The last pediatric treatise of seventeenth-century Europe was a generally lackluster work by John Pechey (1655–1716) entitled *A General Treatise of the Diseases of Infants and Children*, published in 1697. Since, however, it was a compilation of the writings of others, most notably Glisson, the book sustained diagnostic and treatment modalities for children that reflected the progress that had been made throughout the century. The preface to the book merits attention since, in it, Pechey reinforced concepts of parental duty, obligation and responsibility tempered with parental understanding and good example:

Children if they are virtuous are great Blessings and a publick good. It is therefore the duty of Parents to inure them betimes to a Regular course of Life; nor ought Persons of the best Quality to think the guidance of their Children beneath them. . . . And certainly it is best and safest for Parents to have their Children under their own Eye and inspection. But above all, the Fathers Example is of greatest force to instruct the Son, and his Actions Authorise the same in the Child, nor can the Father chastize him for what himself is guilty.[77]

One last aspect of seventeenth-century medicine was significant—the evolution of the concept of infectious diseases. As noted, the idea of contagious diseases was promulgated principally by Girolamo Fracastoro (1484–1553). His manuscripts *Syphilis, sive morbus Gallicus* and *De Contagione* warned of infection "at a distance, or by fomites or by contact."[78] He contributed to the understanding of a body of diseases that was predictable in epidemiology, progression, and prognosis. The vague descriptions of epidemics of "fever" or "flux" or "ague" were being replaced by more sophisticated diagnoses of specific infective syndromes and the age groups each disease afflicted. Even the Tudor historian Holinshed, writing in his *Chronicles* about the "sweating sickness" epidemics of sixteenth-century England, commented: "It is to be noted, that this mortalitie fell chieflie or rather upon men . . . few women, nor children, nor old men died thereof" (*Chronicles*, vol. 3).[79]

The evolving understanding of single disease entities is best illustrated by reference to the number of publications (table 6.3) on the infective syndrome now called diphtheria.

Meissner, in *Grundlage der Literatur der Pädiatrik* (1850), collated several groups of pediatric manuscripts (table 6.4) that indicate that other diseases and various areas of specialization also had been studied in the seventeenth century.

Finally, lest it be thought the totality of the medical literature about children of seventeenth-century Europe was a prelude to works in the Age of

TABLE 6.3
SEVENTEENTH-CENTURY WORKS ON DIPHTHERIA

Date	Author	Work
1611	Jo. Alfonzo de Fonteca	[de affictionem] vocatam Garrotillo
1611	Perez Cascales	Liber de affectionibus puerorum puerorum . . . vulgariter Garrotillo appellato
1636	Aetius Cletus	De Morbo Strangulatorio
1646	Tho. Bartholin	De Angina Puerorum
1646	Renat Moreau	De Laryngotomia [Tracheostomy]
1652	M. A. Severinus	De paedanchone maligna seu de theriomate faucium pestis vi pueros praefocante [On malignant child-choking or ulcer plague of the fauces which suffocates]

Enlightenment, the book *De Infantum Morbis*, written by Michael Ettmüller (1644–1683) and published in 1680, dispels such a notion. Nonsense and superstition prevailed among physics like Ettmüller, as well as among townspeople; the peasantry especially clung to fears of bewitched infants:

One puts a vessel full of springwater under the cradle, and throws an egg into it. If this swims on the surface the child is bewitched, but if it falls to the bottom there is nothing of the sort.[80]

Belief in faith healing remained strong and was reinforced by writers like Tobias Katz (1652–1729). His encyclopedic *Masehtuviah*, containing 16 chapters on the ailments of children, accepted illness due to witchcraft, the *malocchio*, or the breath of a menstruating woman. Katz routed these malevolent auras and spells by reading specific passages from the Bible,[81] or by the use of tissues believed to be imbued with magic, such as the placenta:

The placenta of a first child dispels all witchcraft, thus doing away with emaciation due to magic. The placenta is pulverized and given to the baby to drink either in some liquid or together with its mother's milk.[82]

In North America the colonists, recovered from the tragic disappointments of failed settlements in Jamestown and Plymouth, established settlements in scattered sitesup and down the eastern shores. Exhaustion, starvation, and disease had taken their toll on the populace, but dogged persistence and obstinate endurance ultimately were rewarded with self-sufficient confidence

TABLE 6.4

NUMBER OF PEDIATRIC MANUSCRIPTS APPEARING DURING THE SEVENTEENTH CENTURY ON SELECTED TOPICS

Subject	No. of Manuscripts
Infant nutrition	18
Congenital anomalies	69
Teething	5
Worms	29
Hydrocephaly	8
Scrofula	7
Smallpox	114

and economically autonomous colonies. The journals of Puritans John Robinson and William Brewster best expressed the attitude: "We are well weaned from the delicate milke of our mother countrie."[83]

Matters of education and medical care were handled by individual families, but Europe's influence, information, and supplies remained heavily relied on until such time as these aspects of culture and civilization could take root in the colonies.

The colonies had a small tax base and were slow to establish schools, so children were taught at home. Attention to children's health care still was an admixture of folklore, grandmotherly advice, and herbal recipes from commonplace books. An example is a seventeenth-century family handbook, *The Fletcher Family Medical Book*, filled with ineffective prescriptions based on nonsensical and superstitious lore that throughout history captured the imaginations of people desperate for cures for common scourges. The prescribed treatments for rickets, for example, reflect the ignorance that passed for medical advice:

In the morning when the child arises, anoint the region of his liver and spleen with the liniment made of liverwort and fresh butter. . . . [T]he rest of the day he must drink only of the ale following, and in the night also; take a gallon of wort, boil among it of polypody roots, of sarsaparilla roots, of each an ounce. Of hindstongue, maidenhair and liverwort, of each an handful . . . [plus tamarisk, ash-tree, maces, lentils, raisins] they must be boiled until the third part of the wort be spent, then strain it, and work it with barm. . . . Every night, or (if the child be weak) every other night bathe him softly with this water, rubbing his legs and thighs with the herbs softly. . . . These things may be done until his breath or vital spirits begin to fail.[84]

Advice did not emanate only from books, as the following letter received by the Reverend Joseph Perry of Windsor, Connecticut, illustrates:

Rev'd Sir:

In ye Rickets the best Corrective I have even found is a syrup made of Black Cherrys. Thus, take of Cherrys . . . put them in a vessel with water. Set ye vessel near ye fire and let ye water be Scalding hot. Then take ye Cherrys into a thin Cloth and squeeze them into ye Vessell, & sweeten ye Liquor with Melosses. Give 2 Spoonfuls of this 2 or 3 times a day. If you Dip your Child, Do it . . . in ye morning, head foremost in Cold water, don't dress it Immediately, but let it be made warm in ye Cradle & sweat at least half an Hour moderately....Let a little blood be take out of ye feet ye 2nd Morning . . . before you dips of ye Child give it some Snakeroot and Saffern steep'd in Rum & Water . . . syrup made of Comfry, Hartshorn, Red Roses, Hog-brake roots, knot-grass. . . . Physicians are generally fearful about diping when ye Fever is hard, but oftentimes all attempts to lower it without diping are vain. . . . I have found in a multitude of Instances of diping is most effectual means to break a Rickety Fever.[85]

The first American medical publication was narrow in scope but practical. It was written by a clergyman, not a physician.

THOMAS THACHER

A Brief Rule to guide the Common People of New England how to Order themselves and theirs in the Small Pox and Measles (figure 6.12), incorporating advice on pediatric care, was written by Reverend Thomas Thacher (1620–1678) and published in 1677 in response to the ongoing wave of smallpox epidemics afflicting both the child and adult populations. Endemic in England during the entire seventeenth century, viral agents of smallpox were carried to the colonies on ships from England. The Massachusetts Indians in 1633 and Connecticut tribes in 1634 were the first to be struck with the disease. Ongoing epidemics raging in England from 1667 to 1676 continued to spread to the colonies.[86]

Thacher's broadside, measuring about 12 by 17 inches, listed 13 descriptive and therapeutic elements regarding smallpox. These were essentially expectant and supportive since preventive inoculation had not as yet been popularized. Thacher's approach to therapy was based on his notion that smallpox was due to an impure element attempting to leave the body through the skin lesions. First, he thought, the body produced an "ebullition"—a high fever—followed by the "flox" of spreading pocks. He theorized that this process should be therapeutically facilitated, and, as in the following, deplored treatment then popular that intruded on this process:

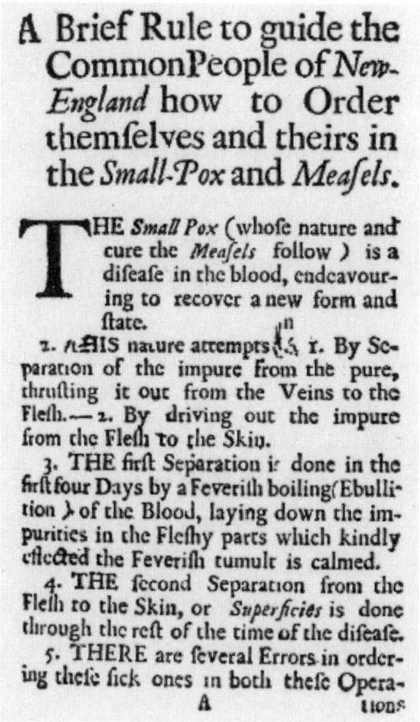

> ## A Brief Rule to guide the CommonPeople of New-England how to Order themſelves and theirs in the *Small-Pox* and *Meaſels*.
>
> THE *Small Pox* (whoſe nature and cure the *Meaſels* follow) is a diſeaſe in the blood, endeavouring to recover a new form and ſtate.
>
> 2. THIS nature attempts in 1. By Separation of the impure from the pure, thruſting it out from the Veins to the Fleſh.—2. By driving out the impure from the Fleſh to the Skin.
>
> 3. THE firſt Separation is done in the firſtfour Days by a Feveriſh boiling(Ebullition)of the Blood, laying down the impurities in the Fleſhy parts which kindly effected the Feveriſh tumult is calmed.
>
> 4. THE ſecond Separation from the Fleſh to the Skin, or *Superficies* is done through the reſt of the time of the diſeaſe.
>
> 5. THERE are ſeveral Errors in ordering theſe ſick ones in both theſe Opera-
>
> A tions

Figure 6.12 Thomas Thacher's broadside on smallpox. COURTESY NATIONAL LIBRARY OF MEDICINE.

The same separation is overmuch hindered by preposterous cooling that Feaverish boyling heat, by blood letting, Clysters, Vomits, purges, or cooling medicines. For though these many times hastens the coming forth of the Pox, yet they take away that supply which should keep them out till they are ripe, wherefore they sink in again to the deadly danger of the sick.[87]

One other written piece of medical advice in seventeenth-century colonial America was a letter written to Governor John Winthrop (1588–1649) of Massachusetts by his physician friend Edward Stafford. Cone (1979) relates that Winthrop had written Stafford asking for therapeutic guidelines and recipes. Using John Gerard's *Herball* (1597) as a source, Stafford's response was a four-page letter dated 6 May 1643, comprising "the first written pediatric prescriptions" in the colonies.[88] There were formulas for epilepsy, dysentery, fractures, and the like, as well as one for jaundice, which apparently subscribes to the belief that "like cures like":[89]

For the yellow Jaundise or Jaunders—Boyle a quart sweet milke, dissolve therein as much bay-salt, or fine Salpeter, as shall make it brackish in taste and putting Saffron in a fine linen clout, rubb it into the Milke, until the Milke be very yellow; and give it the patient to drink.

The common epidemics of smallpox, measles, diphtheria, whooping cough, and dysentery that afflicted children in the mother country were experienced as well in the colonies by both Native American and colonial children. Sadly, the same ineffective treatments also were used in efforts to combat the diseases.

Puerperal fevers and perinatal deaths remained common, and the superstitious and religious prejudices of the period often led to charges against the mothers.

For example, when Mary Dyer gave birth to an anencephalic infant girl in Boston, October 1637, she was accused of being a heretic and giving birth to a monster—an Antichrist. After more than two decades in jail, she was condemned to death on 11 June 1660.[90]

Mortality records in the colonies reveal up to 30 percent of children did not survive to celebrate their first year of life.[91] Initially, eighteenth-century America experienced little change in child morbidity and mortality. A persistent stagnation in the progress against childhood diseases was to prevail for some time.

NOTES

1. Ackerknecht, 1982, pp. 94–127.

2. Schoepffer, J., *Dissertatio Juridica de Pulmone Infantis Natante vel Submergente.* (1747).

3. Still, 1931, p. 98.

4. Roesslin, 1654, p. 32; Ozment, 1983, p. 102.

5. Ibid., pp. 149–82.

6. Translation of R. H. Major (1932) in Ruhräh, J., *Am J Dis Child* 1934; 48: 393–96.

7. Reynald translation, 1654, p. 173.

8. Ruhräh, J., *Am J Dis Child* 1934; 48: 630–32.

9. Still, 1931, p. 102.

10. Ozment, 1983, p. 139.

11. Ruhräh, 1925, p. 137.

12. All the quotes of Oestereicher are from the translation of Albert Allemann as cited by Ruhräh, 1925, pp. 135–38.

13. Ruhräh, 1925, p. 147.

14. All the citations that follow are from a 1547 edition of the *Boke of Children* held by the Royal Society of Medicine and reprinted in entirety by Ruhräh, 1925, pp. 157–95.

15. Ibid., p. 158.

16. He would not have known that birds excrete uric acid and renal detoxification products mixed in feces.

17. Ruhräh, 1925, p. 158.

18. Vilaplana Satorre, 1934, p. 185.

19. Ibid., pp. 184–86.

20. "comme de petites piquerures de puces" (Still, 1931, p. 138).

21. Still, 1931, p. 139.

22. "der unverschamste plagiarius" (Ibid., p. 146).

23. Ping-chen, 1996(a), p. 78.

24. All the quotations of Ferrarius are from Still's (1931) translation, pp. 147–56.

25. Wurtz, 1563, (1656 ed.), pp. 342–58.

26. "Ex ore Excellentissimi Hieronymi Mercurialis Forliniensis Medici clarissimi diligenter excepti, atque in Libros tres digesti: Opera Johannis Chroscieyoioskii cum licentia, et privilegio" (Ruhräh, 1925, p. 222).

27. Fellow countryman Cardanus (1501–1576), from Pavia, disagreed and actually proposed a speech-teaching modality for the deaf. He also suggested a tactile writing for the blind, anticipating braille.

28. Translation of H. F. Wright, Ruhräh, 1925, pp. 225–36.

29. "For the Gelders whilst they feare least when the cure is finished, the relaxation may remaine, pull with violence the process of the peritonaeum . . . by which things ensue great paine, convulsion, effluxe of bloud, inflammation, putrefaction, and lastly death, as I have observed in many whom I have dissected, having died a few days after their gelding. Although some escape these dangers, yet they are deprived of the faculty of generation for all their life after." (Pare, 1585, pp. 110–11)

30. Pare, 1585, pp. 101–2.

31. Ruhräh, 1925, p. 242.

32. Ruhräh, 1938, pp. 57–58.

33. Bloch, 1993, p. 86.

34. Vilaplana Satorre, 1934, p. 186.

35. Ruhräh, 1925, p. 256.

36. Still, 1931, pp. 156–58, 199–211.

37. Ibid.

38. Ruhräh, J., *Am J Dis Child* 1934; 48:858–63.

39. Ibid., pp. 212–14.

40. In 1565, Elizabeth I had granted permission for anatomical dissections if performed within the college walls.

41. *De Rachitide*, 1650, chap. 21.

42. Ibid., chap. 20.

43. Ibid.

44. Anon., 1742, p. 212.

45. Ruhräh, 1925, pp. 341–49.

46. Dally, 1996, p. 1710.

47. Ruhräh, 1925, p. 293.

48. Ibid., p. 292.

49. Clendening, 1960, pp. 192–93.

50. Ruhräh, 1925, p. 295.

51. Ibid., p. 287.

52. Foote, 1919, p. 226.

53. Starsmare, 1664, pp. 15–22.

54. Ruhräh, 1925, pp. 313–20.

55. Rothman, 1996.

56. One of his ward pupils, Richard Gower, published the English translation of Sylvius's book in 1682.

57. Still, 1931, p. 272.

58. "[H]is extravagant Fondness for certain Chymical Preparations . . . nay almost constant use of opiates, even in the youngest Infants (whence he had deservedly gotten the name of the Opiate Doctor)" (Walter Harris in *De Morbis Acutis Infantum* [1689]; cited by Still, 1931, p. 270). Thomas Sydenham also was given a nickname— "opiophilus"—because of his common use of laudanum. Ruhräh, 1925, p. 327.

59. Gower, 1682, p. 35.

60. Ibid., p. 37.

61. Ruhräh, 1925, p. 300.

62. Culpeper also studied contemporary authors and is credited with editing the English translation of Glisson's *de Rachitide*.

63. Culpeper, 1700, p. 338.

64. Ibid., p. 350.

65. Cone, 1979, p. 31.

66. The Latin version appeared in 1681 under the title *De mulierum praegnantium, parturientium, et puerperarum morbis tractatus*.

67. *Gynaecology*, 1668, 3:28.

68. Clendening, 1960, p. 194.

69. All the Sydenham excerpts are from the 1848 translation by the Sydenham Society, London.

70. Sydenham considered a pediatric text written by his student, Walter Harris, far superior to any of his own works. He wrote Harris: "I never flatter any one, and I say it without any compliment, you are the first I ever envied. It is my sincere opinion that this little book may be of greater service to mankind than all I every wrote." Cheyne, 1801, p. 1.

71. This citation is from Anon., *A Full View of All the Diseases Incident to Children*, 1742, p. 173.

72. Late-medieval hagiographical catalogs of healings (miraculous cures attributed to saints) detailed accounts of 135 childhood injuries. Near-drowning accounted for 76; concussion, for 17; and near-asphyxia, for 16. Gordon, 1991, p. 150.

73. Still, 1931, pp. 288–89.

74. The English translation of Harris's book is by John Martyn (1742) and is cited in Ruhräh, 1925, pp. 350–64.

75. Abt, 1940, p. 486.

76. Ruhräh, J., *Am J Dis Child* 1934; 47:629–31.

77. Ruhräh, J., *Am J Dis Child* 1930; 39:179–84.

78. Clendening, 1960, pp. 106–22.

79. Thwaites et al., 1997, p. 581.

80. Colón, 1987, p. 35.

81. Abt, 1945, p. 12.

82. Ruhräh, J., *Am J Dis Child* 1934; 47:399–401. Katz may have based his precept on the passage in Shabbath 134a, which advocates placenta rubbing for infant distress.

83. Illick, 1988, p. 346.

84. Pollock, 1987, p. 101.

85. Earle, 1930, pp. 8–9.

86. Viets, 1977, p. xxvii.

87. *A Brief Rule . . .*, pt. 7.

88. Cone, 1979, p. 13.

89. Ibid., p. 14.

90. Jacobi, 1902, p. 460.

91. Cone, 1979, p. 27.

Chapter 7

The Eighteenth Century

Initially, eighteenth-century America experienced little change in child morbidity and mortality. The persistent stagnation in scientific progress prevailed for some time and left communities helpless in the struggle against cyclical eruptions of epidemics—smallpox, measles, whooping cough, diphtheria, scarlet fever, mumps, and cholera—that decimated a multitude of their children.

Of all the plagues, smallpox was feared the most because of its immediately evident bullous disfigurement, soaring fevers, crushing debilitation, and terrifying mortality rates. During the epidemic of 1721, inoculation, untried in the West though long extant in the East, finally was introduced in America.

As far back as the eleventh century, Chinese doctors granted some degree of immunity against small-pox by prescribing that patients sniff, as from a snuff box, powdered crust from smallpox pustules. Turkish physicians of the fifteenth century lanced open a vein and inserted pustule material into it. It was in Constantinople, while living there in 1718, that Lady Mary Montague (1689–1762), daughter of the Duke of Kingston,[1] observed the Turkish procedure and had her six-year-old son inoculated.[2] Upon her return to London, she instructed a surgeon to inoculate her five-year-old daughter. The surgeon used an equally successful variation of the Turkish method—a thread soaked in pustule secretion drawn through the skin. In time the process was refined into the scarification method employed until the eradication of smallpox in this century. Scarification produced a large eschar, leaving a plaque-like scar that often required protection.

The experiment in America was encouraged by clergyman and author Cotton Mather (1663–1728) and executed by Boston physician Zabdiel Boylston (1679–1766). Boylston inoculated his six-year-old son by lancing the skin and applying 9- to 14-day-old pustule detritus from a smallpox patient. He covered the site with a piece of cabbage leaf and awaited the reaction. He inoculated an additional 280 individuals, of whom 65 were children under 15 years of age. He kept a careful log of the study and published it in 1726 as *An Historical Account of the Small-Pox Inoculated in New England*. It was an almost intimate and certainly personal account of the experiment:[3]

June the 26th, 1721, I inoculated my son Thomas, of about Six, my Negro Man, Jack, thirty six, and Jackey, two and an half Years old. They all complain'd on the 6th Day; upon the 7th, the two Children were a little hot, dull, and sleepy, Thomas (only) had twitchings and started in his sleep. The 28th the Children's Fevers continued, Tommy's twitchings and startings in sleep increased; and tho' the Fever was gentle and his Senses bright, yet as the Practice was new, and the Clamour, or rather Rage of the People against it so Violent, that I was put into a very great Fright.

Six patients—none of them children—were suspected to have died as a result of the inoculation. The 275 who had been successfully inoculated against the dread disease were ignored in the highly charged atmosphere of suspicion and fear, and inoculation failed to gain acceptance. In fact, Cotton Mather was singled out for retaliation; on 14 November 1721, a black pow-

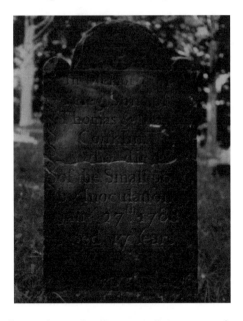

Figure 7.1 Tombstone located in the Fort Hill Cemetery of Huntington, Long Island, in New York (Miller, R. L., *Lancet* 1996; 348:902).

der and turpentine grenade was hurled through the window of his home by a former parishioner and member of a faction that maintained inoculation interfered with God's divine plan. The grenade landed in a guest room and failed to explode. A message from the perpetrator of the crime was found:

Cotton Mather, I was once one of your Meeting; But the Cursed Lye you told of—, You know who, made me leave You, You Dog; And, Damn You I will Enoculate you with this, with a Pox to you.[4]

Inoculation continued to be discussed, evoking passionate attitudes for and against, but it was accepted—and then only grudgingly—only when George Washington ordered inoculated all his Revolutionary War troops.[5] Bitter accusations of malpractice persisted until the end of the century whenever a child died following inoculation (figure 7.1).

Cotton Mather was a pastor–physician (a common phenomenon in the colonies) whose contributions to American medicine extended well beyond his interest in and support for inoculation. It must be acknowledged that his most important book on medical issues was *An Account of the Method and Success of Inoculating the Small-Pox* (1722), which introduced American physicians to the immunizing process. *The Angel of Bethesda* (1724), however, is the more remarkable work in that, very early on, Mather's book furnished an exposition and dissemination of information about a new theory—tiny organisms ("Cells"), seen microscopically in blood, as the cause of infection. Mather's suggestion, that contact and fomites were mechanisms that spread disease, was an original and prescient amplification of the germ theory:[6]

Every Part of Matter is Peopled. Every Green Leaf swarms with Inhabitants. The Surfaces of Animals are covered with other Animals. Yea, the most Solid Bodies, even Marble itself, have innumerable Cells, which are crouded with imperceptible Inmates. As there are Infinite Numbers of these, which the Microscopes bring to our View, so there may be inconceivable Myriads yett Smaller than these, which no glasses have yett reach'd unto. The Animals that are much more than Thousands of times Less than the finest Grain of Sand . . . may insinuate themselves by the Air, and with our Ailments, yea, thro' the Pores of our skin; and soon gett into the Juices of our Bodies. (chap. 7)

Chapter 59 of the *Angel* discoursed on children's common ailments like thrush, whooping cough, seborrhea, and what must be a description of the hyperactive child. Mather called the chapter "Capsula LIX. Infantilin." It was a curious admixture of his fire-and-brimstone pastoral style blended with prescriptions, recipes, and instruction on medical matters. It proffered remedies for the ails of children while inculcating with impassioned rhetoric a heavy dose of guilt in their parents:

Yea, It will be but a Reasonable Thing, for Parents, who see their Infants in Distress, to Enquire, On how many Accounts their Sins may be punished in what befalls their Children; and how far a Righteous God may be now visiting the Iniquity of the Fathers upon the Children.[7]

Mather's citations of recipes from medical texts of the day always were acknowledged and credited. Thrush was treated with a mixture of sage, alum, and honey or "a Frog held unto the Mouth of the Child."[8] Mather suggested standard remedies for teething, reminding the reader that "our first sin was committed with our Teeth. And lo, some of the First Griefs and Pains undergone by our Children, are in Breeding of their Teeth."[9]

"Frowardness" described with warmth and compassion a hyperkinetic disorder in children, and sensible response strategies for "Mothers and Nurses" were imbued with reason and understanding:

Many Mothers and Nurses are Exercised with Froward Children. The Poor Little Creatures are frequently and painfully and noisily out of Order. . . . [W]hen the Children are Froward you don't sett your Witts against Theirs. . . . But lett us now take a Little Care to Quiet the Children.[10]

A decoction of a tea made with nettles, saffron, and honey administered three to four times a day was prescribed for the child, on the presumption that it acted as a calmative. This and other prescriptions were suggested by Mather to treat convulsions, rickets, colic, and gripes.

Two other pastor–physicians who were important contributors to the health of colonial children wrote on diphtheria. During a major epidemic of lethal diphtheria, in which in 1735 alone nearly 5,000 children died,[11] Jabez Fitch (1672–1746) wrote *An Account of the Numbers That Have Died of the Distemper in the Throat Within the Province of New Hampshire* (1736). The epidemic also raged in Massachusetts, where a day of fast and atonement was proclaimed by public broadside. Jonathan Dickinson (1688–1747) published *Observations on That Terrible Disease Vulgarly Called the Throat-Distemper* (1740). Both works were predominantly descriptive, but 30 years later, Bard wrote a text that went beyond simple description.

Samuel Bard (1742–1821), in an *Enquiry into the Nature, Cause and Cure of the Angina Suffocativa*, published in 1771, made observations original to medical literature. Bard recognized that a single disease could be—and was—known by various regional and latinized names.* He then excluded humors as causative factors and emphasized an infective etiology:

The disease I have described appeared evidently to be of an infectious nature, and being drawn in by the breath of a healthy child, irritated the glands of the throat and windpipe. The infection did not seem to depend so much on any prevailing disposition of the air, as upon effluvia received from the breath of infected persons. This will account why the disorder sometimes went through a whole family, and yet did not affect the next-door neighbors; and hence we learn a very useful lesson, namely to remove all the young children in a family as soon as any one is taken with the disease, by which caution I am convinced, many lives have been, and may again be preserved.[12]

Other important new and clinical useful observations accumulated—on scarlet fever, measles, mumps, and the chincough or whooping cough—at a rate that matched and at times surpassed the scientific inquiry being conducted in Europe.

Epidemics of scarlet fever occurred cyclically up and down the eastern coast of the New World, significantly in 1702, in 1735, and—a particularly devastating one—in 1783. Four of Samuel Bard's six children died of the disease.[13]

---

*Canker, throat-distemper, cyanche trachealis, aphthae malignae, phlegmone anginosa, garrotillo, morbus stangulatorius, angina puerorum, angina membranacea, cyanche stridula, soffacatio stidula.

Having attended a large number of scarlet fever patients, Dr. Benjamin Rush (1745–1813)[14] ably described in *Medical Inquiries and Observations*, the disease and its epidemic properties. In a significant contribution to progress in science, Rush dismissed as useless traditional reliance on camphor vapors to prevent the disease, and, serendipitously, he advocated simple hygiene as an efficacious part of treatment:

Camphor has often been suspended in a bag from the neck, as a preservative against this disease. Repeated observations have taught me, that it possesses little or no efficacy for this purpose. I have had reason to entertain a more favorable opinion of the benefit of washing the hands and face with vinegar and of rinsing the mouth and throat with vinegar and water every morning, as a means of preventing this disorder.[15]

Tarwater was a favorite treatment for childhood infections, including scarlet fever and smallpox. A book printed in Dublin by George Lord Bishop of Cloyne in 1744 related:

In certain parts of America, Tarwater is made by putting a quart of cold water to a quart of tar, and stirring them well together in a vessel, which is left standing till the tar sinks to the bottom. A glass of clear water being poured off for a draught . . . [those] who took the tarwater having either escaped that distemper, or had it very favourably. In one family there was a remarkable instance of seven children, who came all very well through the small-pox, except one young child which could not be brought to drink tarwater as the rest had done.[16]

Pertussis, or whooping cough, was characterized in detail by Lionel Chalmers (1715–1777) in *An Account of the Weather and Diseases of South Carolina* (1776). The realism with which he related the suffocating nature of the disease and his inability to suppress the tenacious cough—even with narcotic torpor—still makes for powerful reading:

This disease, commonly begins with a frequent but dry cough; nor have the patients that running at the nose, snuffling or hoarseness, which often ensues from catching cold. The coughing by degrees holds longer, and becomes so severe in a few days, that the sick scarcely have time to breathe during the fits. For so spasmodically affected are the lungs and their appendages, that one interrupted act of violent expiration continues, till the patient, being ready to be stifled, is obliged to fetch breath with all his might in spite of the convulsed condition of these organs. . . . From the shrill or hollow sort of noise, that is made by the rushing of air into the aperture of the windpipe, which is now convulsively constricted, the disease hath the name of hooping-cough. In this distemper, I have tried all sorts of balsamicks and pectorals, without any advantage; oily and other relaxants rather did harm and opiates alone were of but little use. For though I indiscreetly stupified some patients, they nevertheless coughed as often and severely when overwhelmed with sleep as if nothing at all had been given.[17]

Rush and Chalmers both published clinical descriptions of quinsey, or mumps. There were epidemics of the disease in 1744, 1768, and 1786. Measles, of course, was endemic, but especially virulent epidemics struck in 1688, 1713, 1740, 1758, and 1772. The 1772 Charleston, South Carolina, epidemic alone claimed more than 900 children.[18]

During the outbreak of 1713, Cotton Mather's spare diary entries nonetheless reflect the grief and loss that pervaded the general community. The diary cataloged[19] the number of his family and household who died, his wife and several children among them:[20]

November 9. [Referring to his wife] "My dear, dear, dear Friend expired . . . between 3 and 4 in the afternoon."

November 14. [Maid] "Tis a Satisfaction to me, that tho' she had been a wild, vain, airy Girl, yett since her coming into my Family, she became disposed unto serious Religion."

November 17. [His 18-day-old son, a twin] "Little Eleazer . . . about midnight."

November 20. [A daughter, twin to Eleazer] "Little Martha . . . about ten o'clock AM."

November 21. "My lovely Jerusha died on her 17th day of illness, between 9h. and 10h. at Night."

A prominent leader in the community, Mather set aside grief to serve the needs of his parishioners. He wrote *A Letter about the Right Management of the Sick under the Distemper of the Measles*, alerting his congregation to clinical signs heralding the onset of the disease. Clearly, throughout his family's illnesses he had been able to sustain clinical composure, and he shared the personal observations he had made about a disease that had exacted a great personal and tragic toll:

The Unusual Symptoms of an Arrest from the Measles are, an Head-ake; or Troubles in the Eyes; a Dry Cough; an Oppression on the Breast or Stomach; or a pain there, and in the Back and Limbs; and sometimes a Faintness, with Sickness, perhaps Vomiting, or Griping and Purging; A Thirst, with a constant Fever, which is mild at first, but grows high enough before it has done.[21]

Yearly epidemics of summer diarrhea, called "cholera infantum" by Benjamin Rush, dehydrated thousands of infants in large cities, causing their death. There was no scientific study of the "seasonal flux" until Rush published *An Inquiry into the Causes and Cure of Cholera Infantum* in 1777:

By this name I mean to designate a disease, called in Philadelphia, the "vomiting and purging of children." From the regularity of its appearance in the summer months, it is likewise known by the name of "the disease of the season."

It prevails in most of the large towns of the United States. It is distinguished in Charlestown, in South Carolina, by the name of "the April and May disorder," from making its first appearance in those two months. It seldom appears in Philadelphia till the middle of June, or the beginning of July, and generally continues till near the middle of September. Its frequency and danger are always in proportion to the heat of the weather. It affects children from the first or second week after their birth, till they are two years old. It sometimes begins with a diarrhoea, which continues for several days without any other symptom of indisposition; but it more frequently comes on with a violent vomiting and purging, and a high fever. The matter discharged from the stomach and bowels is generally yellow or green, but the stools are sometimes slimy and bloody, without any tincture of bile. In some instances they are nearly as limpid as water.[22]

For sustenance and hydration, Rush prescribed mint and mallow or blackberry teas, and for intestinal spasms and tenesmus, "clysters made of flaxseed tea, or of mutton broth, or of starch dissolved in water, with a few drops of liquid laudanum in them, give ease and produce other useful effects." Like his colleagues, he too resorted to bleeding: "[S]ince the prevalence of the yellow fever in Philadelphia after the year 1793, the cholera infantum has assumed symptoms of such malignancy, as to require bleeding to cure it. In some cases, two and three bleedings were necessary for that purpose."[23]

Both Ruhräh and Abt noted an important American medical observation made in the eighteenth century by Hezekiah Beardsley (1748–1790), who described obstruction of the stomach outlet from a thickened pyloric muscle.[24] It was the first American case report of "congenital hypertrophic stenosis of the pylorus" and was published in the *Medical Society Journal of New Haven* in 1788:[25]

A child of Mr. Joel Grannis, a respectable farmer in the town of Southington, in the first week of its infancy, was attacked with a puking, or ejection of the milk, and of every other substance it received into its stomach almost instantaneously, and very little changed.

"[A]nd very little changed" for the five years of the child's brief life. Beardsley's autopsy findings were included in the report:

On opening the thorax, the esophagus was found greatly distended beyond its usual dimensions in such young subjects; from one end to the other of this tube, between the circular fibers which compose the middle coat, were small vesicles, some of which contained a tablespoonful of a thin fluidlike water, and seemed capable of holding much more. I next examined the stomach, which was unusually large, the coats were about the thickness of a hog's bladder when fresh and distended with air; it contained about a wine pint of fluid exactly resembling that found in the vesicles before mentioned, and which I suppose to have been received just before his death. The pylorus was invested with a hard compact substance, or schirrosity, which so completely obstructed the passage into the duodenum, as to admit with the greatest difficulty the finest liquid.

Business logs kept by colonial physicians suggest that some physicians were better able or more willing to care for sick children. For example, 20 percent of Josiah Bartlett's clinical practice in Kingston, New Hampshire, between 1751 to 1787 was composed of children. In neighboring Kensington, Benjamin Rowe Jr. had only 0.3 percent children in his private practice.[26]

There were few physicians in America. At the time the Continental Congress drew up the Declaration of Independence, their number was estimated to be around 3,500.[27] In most locales a doctor was not available; midwives generally provided services in loco.

There are a number of extant diaries that describe the daily chores and responsibilities of the midwife. Martha Ballard of Maine left a 25-year log starting in 1785. Birthing was her prime responsibility, but she provided general health care to the entire community. In her diary, Ballard described the many times she would sit up at night with a sick child and the diagnoses she made of coughs, fevers, thrashing seizures, and rashes. She recorded both her failures and her successes in her many years of caring for children.[28]

Great distances separated townships, and many communities had neither doctor nor midwife available to them and had small expectations of attracting either to their settlements. Families without access to medically knowledgeable people consulted almanacs on matters concerning health care. *Poor Richard's Almanack* (1763) and *Hutchin's Almanack* (1778), containing guidelines for diagnosis and treatment of adults and children, were indispensable items. Home medical encyclopedias also were available. One such was *Domestic Medicine* by William Buchan (1729–1805), popular in England but not published in America until 1795. Another was the *Primitive Physick* (1747) by John Wesley (1703–1791). Both volumes had extensive sections devoted to children's ailments. Benjamin Franklin (1706–1790) printed *Every Man His Own Doctor, or the Poor Planter's Physician* in 1734, focusing on botanicals and therapeutics that were endogenous and available in the Americas.

Families most often relied on home remedies, concoctions, and plasters from botanicals grown and gathered in their gardens or purchased at the

TABLE 7.1
DRUG CONTENTS OF DR. CRAWLEY'S KIT

Drug	Use
Acid elixir	To curb debility and anorexia
Antimonial drops	As a diaphoretic and emetic
Bark [cinchona]	For fevers
Blistering plasters	For fevers, coughs, asthmas
Calomel [Hg$_2$Cl]	Antihelminthic, antivenereal
Camphor	Antispasmodic, topic analgesic
Cream of Tartar	Cathartic and diuretic
Daffy's elixir	Purgative
Diachylon plaster	For cuts and bruises
Essence of peppermint	Bowel carminative
Febrifuge drops [sal nitre]	For childhood fevers
Fit drops	Vermifuge
Gascoigne's powders	For childhood diarrheas
Goulard's extract	Lead salt astringent wash
Gum plaister [guaiacum]	Childhood cathartic
Hartshorn drops [Ca,PO$_4$]	For stimulation and rickets
Hoffman's drops	For nervousness
Huxham's tincture [bark]	For fevers
Ipecacuanha	Childhood emetic
Jallap	Potent purgative
James's powder	Antimonial antipyretic
Laudanum	Opiate
Magnesia	Mild laxative
Milk of sulphur	For hemorrhoids and pruritus
Musk	For nervous diseases
Nitre [nitrous acid]	Cathartic
Palsy drops	Calminative and antispasmodic
Pectoral drops [ZnCl]	Expectorative
Pile ointment	Antihemmorhoidal
Rhubarb	Cathartic
Rochelle salts	Same as cream of tartar
Salt of wormwood	Antipyretic and antihelminthic
Traumatic balsam [benzoin, aloe]	Expectorant
Turner's cerate	For skin ulcers
Venice treacle	Theriaca
Volatile drops [oil of Cajeput]	Fainting cordial
Worm powder	Antihelminthic
Yellow basilicon	Topical lard and resin for ulcer

nearby apothecary. For those who could afford them, complete medical chests, such as Dr. Crawley's Family Medical Chest (c.1790), were available for purchase. The chests usually had an owner's manual and instructions for use of the contents, which included first-aid dressings, salves, a mortar and pestle, and a compendium of drugs for the most common of ailments. Dr. Crawley's chest contained 38 drugs (table 7.1) and had an adult-dosage schedule.[29] Unfortunately, generally few pediatric guidelines were given, leaving the parents to use their own, at times troubled judgment for certain drugs.

In eighteenth-century Europe, broad and enlightened scientific ideas were being discussed and debated. Giovanni Battista Morgani (1682–1771) of Padua published *De Sedibus et Causis Morborum* in 1761, a treatise on pathology based on 700 dissections describing various congenital heart lesions. Albrecht von Haller (1708–1777) and Aloysio Galvani (1737–1798) refined conduction physiology by separating nerve stimulation from the muscle response. Antoine Laurent Lavoisier (1743–1794) elucidated the nature of respiration in *Experiences sur la respiration des animaux*. . . . Philippe Pinel (1755–1826) in 1794 unchained the insane of Paris's Bicêtre Hospital.

There was significant progress in pediatrics as well—at least in the number of specific publications on children's diseases if not in disease elucidation and improved treatments.[30] A fair number of pediatric treatises—eight major and many minor ones (table 7.2)—appeared in the latter half of the century.

TABLE 7.2
SOME EIGHTEENTH-CENTURY PEDIATRIC PUBLICATIONS

Major		
Nicholas Andry	*L'orthopédie . . .*	1741
Anonymous	*A Full View of All the Diseases Incident . . .*	1742
Jean Astruc	*A . . . Treatise on all Diseases incident to . . .*	1746
William Cadogan	*An Essay upon Nursing . . .*	1748
William Buchan	*De Infantum Vita Conservanda*	1761
N. von Rosenstein	*Underrättelser om Barn Sjukdomar . . .*	1764
George Armstrong	*An Account of the Diseases Most Incident . . .*	1777
Michael Underwood	*A Treatise on the Diseases of Children*	1784
Minor		
Hermann Boerhaave	*Aphorismi de cognoscendis et curanis morbis*	1709
Robert Whytt	*Observations on the Dropsy in the Brain*	1709

Friedrich Hoffman	*Praxis Clinica Morborum Infantium*	1715
Chris. von Hellwig	*Kinder-, Jungfer- und Weiber-Spiegel*	1720
Theodore Zuinger	*Paedo-iatreia Practica*	1722
Richard Conyers	*De Morbis Infantium*	1739
Friedrich Hoffman	*De Praecipuis Infantium Morbis*	1740
Joseph Hurlock	*A Practical Treatise upon Dentition*	1742
Gerald von Swieten	*Commentaries on Boerhaave's Aphorisms*	1743
John Fothergill	*An Account of the Sore Throat attended with Ulcers*	1748
John G. Roederer	*De Pondere et longitudine infantum recens . . .*	1753
M. Brouzet	*Essai sur l'education medicinale des enfans . . .*	1754
J. Desessartz	*Traite de l'education corporelle des enfans . . .*	1760
F. B. de Sauvage	*Tractatus duo pathologici . . . de morbis puerorum*	1760
Verardo Zeviani	*Della cura de' Bambini attaccati . . .*	1761
J. Ballexserd	*Dissertation sur l'education physique des . . .*	1763
J. F. Zückert	*Unterricht von der diaetetischen Erziehung . . .*	1765
Francis Home	*Inquiry . . . Causes and Cure of Croup*	1765
William Heberden	*On the Chicken-Pox*	1767
John Cooke	*A Plain Account . . . Diseases Incident to Children*	1769
Jozsef Csapo	*A Treatise on the Diseases of Little Children*	1771
Hugh Smith	*. . . on Nursing and the Management of Children*	1772
William Farrer	*. . . Rickets in Children . . . and the King's Evil*	1773
Hugh Downman	*Infancy, or the Management of Children*	1774
A. Hume	*. . . Diseases Incident to Women and Children*	1776
J. I. Sampots	*. . . de los recién nacidos anegados . . .*	1777
J. P. Frank	*System einer vollständigen medicinischen Polizey*	1780
William Moss	*Essay on the Management and Nursing of Children*	1781
Andrew Wilson	*Aphorisms . . . Lectures . . . Diseases of Children*	1783
C. J. Mellin	*Der Kinderarzt*	1787
J. B. Matonis	*. . . la feliz dentación de los parvulos*	1788
Benjamin Lara	*. . . Mothers not suckling their own Children*	1791
C. Girtanner	*Abhandlung uber die Krankheiten der Kinder . . .*	1794
C. A. Sturve	*Erziehung und Behandlung der Kinder*	1798
N. Chambon	*Des Maladies des Enfans*	1799

NICHOLAS ANDRY

In 1741, Nicholas Andry (1658–1742) published his best-known work, *L'orthopédie, ou l'art de prevenir et de corriger dans les enfans les difformités du corps, etc.* . . . Illustrated and didactic, it was written in plain prose with practical suggestions for parents to implement at home. Andry focused on ailments he believed altered the symmetry and mechanical function of the body. He associated the development of some deformities with faulty daily routines that ignored children's unique physiology and small stature. For example, about children's rounded shoulders, he wrote:

Nurses, Weaners of Children, and Governesses, who constantly suspend Children by the Leading-string, lifting them up in the Air, make them liable to have the Neck sunk between the Shoulders.

Those Masters and Mistresses who teach Children to read or write upon too high a Table which rises above their Elbows (for it ought to be two Inches lower) expose them to the same Deformity.

It is very proper that Children when they begin to be weaned should eat at the same Table with their Parents. But as the Table is too high for them, they ought to have Seats higher in proportion, and a Footstool beneath their Legs; for they should never be allowed to hang them, as you shall see afterwards.[31]

Andry emphasized the importance of nurturing by parents as well as proselytizing about posture. In many respects his work reflects the influence of Locke's and Rousseau's naturalist views.

In London in 1742, an anonymous editor (speculated to be John Armstrong, the poet–brother of George Armstrong) published a compendium, an anthology of sorts, of the works of the "best Authors who have writ upon the chronicle Diseases of Children."[32] The book, printed for "A. Millar, against St. Clement's in the Strand," claimed to be *A Full View of All the Diseases Incident to Children* (figure 7.2), and, in fact, it was thorough and comprehensive. The preface began:

Children are subject to many Diseases peculiar to the State of Infancy, besides those they are liable to in common with Adults, that I have often wondered they should have been so much over-looked by Medical Authors. But as very young Children have not the Power of Speech to describe their Complaints, which are hardly to be understood otherwise; most Physicians either through Indolence, or the fear of doing Mischief, when the Indications of Cure were not quite so clear as they could wish, have commonly resigned those little Patients to the Nurses and old Women, not scrupling to own their superior Skill in that Branch of Physik.[33]

Its 260 pages had extracts from Harris, Boerhaave, Sylvius, Willis, Andry, Burton, Glisson, Sydenham, and Wiseman, with sporadic interjections of wry footnotes of the editor's own opinion, such as "I should scarce venture so large a Dose of this Medicine to a Child."[34] The book is an important

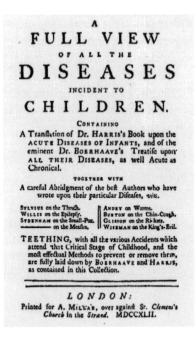

A

FULL VIEW

OF ALL THE

DISEASES

INCIDENT TO

CHILDREN.

CONTAINING

A Tranflation of Dr. HARRIS's Book upon the ACUTE DISEASES OF INFANTS, and of the eminent Dr. BOERHAAVE's Treatife upon ALL THEIR DISEASES, as well Acute as Chronical.

TOGETHER WITH

A careful Abridgment of the beft Authors who have wrote upon their particular Difeafes, *viz.*

SYLVIUS on the Thrufh.	ANDRY on Worms.
WILLIS on the Epilepfy.	BURTON on the Chin-Cough.
SYDENHAM on the Small-Pox.	GLISSON on the Rickets.
——— on the Meafles.	WISEMAN on the King's-Evil.

TEETHING, with all the various Accidents which attend that Critical Stage of Childhood, and the moft effectual Methods to prevent or remove them, are fully laid down by BOERHAAVE and HARRIS, as contained in this Collection.

_____

LONDON:

Printed for A. MILLAR, over againft St. Clement's Church in the Strand. MDCCXLII.

Figure 7.2 Frontispiece of *A Full View of All the Diseases Incident to Children.* Anonymous. COURTESY NATIONAL LIBRARY OF MEDICINE.

forerunner to the modern medical textbook format that also compiles authoritative experts into one volume.

JEAN ASTRUC

Jean Astruc's (1684–1766) *A General and Complete Treatise on all Diseases incident to Children, from their Birth to the Age of Fifteen with particular Instruction to tender Mothers prudent Midwives and Careful Nurses* was published in English in 1746. For the most part unoriginal, it presented common problems with uncommon clarity. Differentiating diarrheas according to presenting symptoms and quality of stools is one such example:[35]

The differences are principally deduced from two heads. 1. The nature of the evacuated matter. 2. The quality and nature of the symptoms which attend the disorder. As to the nature of the evacuations, a Diarrhoea is of four species: 1. Stercoral; 2. Coeliac; 3. Lienteric; and 4. Dysenteric.

Astruc emphasized the inadequacy of the perfunctory, complaint-focused or organ-focused examinations doctors usually made, such as an abdominal examination for a complaint of stomach pain. He advocated—insisted—

that a careful and complete physical examination of the patient be made. He always scrutinized a patient's entire body to ensure a proper diagnosis.

Astruc dismissed superstitious, erroneous, assumptions about the causes of diseases and championed logical and sequential thought regarding etiology. He analyzed, for example, basic mechanisms when considering malnutrition; either the patient did not eat, or food was malabsorbed, or a combination of both factors was the cause:

[N]ot only the good women but also most physicians attributed the source of this disorder to incantation or fascination, because they could discover no other manifest causes of it. Some in general call it macies: But to give a more reasonable account of its causes, they may be reduced to the following heads in general. 1. Because the patients take little or no nourishment. 2. Though they take it in great plenty, yet they dissipate it more abundantly. 3. The combination of both these causes.

The existence of the disorder [wasting] is discovered at first sight. But its causes are more difficult and hidden, since in order to investigate them, the infant's state should be examined.[36]

WILLIAM CADOGAN

In 1754, William Cadogan (1711–1797) was appointed physician to the Bristol Foundling Hospital. In 1768 the Hospital Committee published anonymously a 36-page essay that had been written by Cadogan and sent to one of the governors in 1748. The essay was about the nurture and nutrition of infants and the author's general reflections on society's responsibilities to its children:

Sir,

It is with great Pleasure I see at last the Preservation of Children become the Care of Men of Sense: It is certainly a matter which well deserves their Attention, and I doubt not, the Publick will soon find the good and great Effects of it. . . . The truth of what I say, that the treatment of Children in general is wrong, unreasonable, and unnatural, will in a great measure appear, if we but consider what a puny valetudinary race most of our people of condition are; chiefly owing to bad nursing, and bad habits contracted early. But let any one, who would be fully convinced of this matter, look over the BILLS OF MORTALITY; there he may observe, that almost half the number of those who fill up that black list, die under five years of age.[37]

Feeding customs that hindered breast feeding were deplored; farming out babies to wet nurses was denounced. The author even questioned the common practice of overdressing infants.

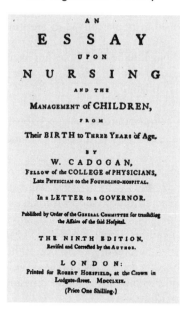

AN

ESSAY

UPON

NURSING

AND THE

MANAGEMENT of CHILDREN,

FROM

Their BIRTH to THREE YEARS of Age.

BY

W. CADOGAN,

FELLOW of the COLLEGE of PHYSICIANS,
Late PHYSICIAN to the FOUNDLING-HOSPITAL.

In a LETTER to a GOVERNOR.

Published by Order of the GENERAL COMMITTEE for transacting
the Affairs of the said Hospital.

THE NINTH EDITION,
Revised and Corrected by the AUTHOR.

LONDON:
Printed for ROBERT HORSFIELD, at the Crown in
Ludgate-street. MDCCLXIX.
(Price One Shilling.)

Figure 7.3 Frontispiece of Cadogan's *An Essay upon Nursing.* COURTESY NATIONAL LIBRARY OF MEDICINE.

There were 10 English editions of this seminal work, called *An Essay upon Nursing and the Management of Children from their Birth to Three Years of Age* (figure 7.3), and several more editions were published in France.

Cadogan strongly believed an infant's first food should be maternal milk. This was a departure from the tradition of feeding some form of pap to infants until maternal colostrum changed to mature milk:

The constant Practice is as soon as a Child is born to cram a Dab of Butter and Sugar down its throat, a little Oil, Panada, Caudle or some such unwholesome Mess. So that they set out wrong and the Child stands a fair Chance of being made sick from the first Hour. It is the Custom of some to give a little roast Pig to an Infant which it seems is to cure it of all the Mother's longings.[38]

Cadogan advised introducing meats to the diet once teeth appeared. If his censure of simple carbohydrates was regarded seriously, he probably prevented many a carie.

As soon as the Children have any teeth, at six or eight months they may by degrees be used to a little flesh-meat; which they are always very fond of, much more so at first, than of any confectionery or pastry wares, with which they should never debauch their taste.[39]

He questioned the morbidity attributed to teething:

Breeding teeth has been thought to be, and is, fatal to many children; but I am confident this is not from nature: for it is no disease, or we could not be well in health 'till one or two and twenty, or later.[40]

Cadogan was most condemnatory about baby farming that deprived infants of biological maternal milk and essential bonding:

I am quite at a loss to account for the general Practice of sending Infants out of Doors to be suckled or dry-nursed by another Woman, who has not so much Understanding, nor can have so much Affection for it as the Parents: and how it comes to pass that People of good Sense and easy Circumstances will not give themselves the Pains to watch over the Health and Welfare of their Children: but are so careless as to give them up to the Common Methods, without considering how near it is to an equal Chance that they are destroy by them. The ancient Custom of exposing them to wild Beasts or drowning them would certainly be a much quicker and more humane way of dispatching them.[41]

He was similarly unforgiving of those who overdressed their babes:

The first great Mistake is that they think a new-born Infant cannot be kept too warm: from this Prejudice they load it and bind it with Flannels, Wrappers, Swathes, Stays etc commonly called Cloaths which all together are almost equal to its own Weight. . . . Shoes and Stockings are very needless Incumbrances, besides that they keep the Legs wet and nasty if they are not chang'd every Hour.[42]

The number of editions of Cadogan's book suggests that his opinions were widely read and, presumably, heeded—despite the condescending tone of his prose. The book did reflect the egalitarian child-rearing practices favored in his times. Cadogan's reference to a reader's miscomprehension of his advice best illustrates his patronizing style and his stinging hauteur:

A Lady of great sway among her acquaintance told me not long ago, with an air of reproach, that she had nursed her Child according to my book, and it died. I asked, if she had suckled it herself? No. Had it sucked any other woman? It was dry-nursed. Then, Madam, you cannot impute your misfortune to my advice, for you have taken a method quite contrary to it, in the most capital point. Oh but, according my direction, it had never worn stocking. Madam, Children may die, though they do or do not wear stockings.[43]

In modern medical circles, Cadogan is sometimes remembered for his *Dissertation on the Gout*, but his fame endures because of the sound medical information he gave in his *Essay upon Nursing*.

WILLIAM BUCHAN

De Infantum Vita Conservanda by William Buchan (1729–1805) was published in Edinburgh in 1761. Buchan served as physician to the Foundling Hospital in Ackworth, where his passion for children's health matured. He endorsed Cadogan's views, and his medical opinions generally paralleled those of his contemporaries. He particularly was zealous about the benefits of exposing infants to fresh air and dressing them with less clothing. His major achievement was in advocating the education of mothers in child care:

It is indeed to be regretted that more care is not bestowed in teaching the proper management of children to those whom Nature had designed for mothers. This instead of being made the principal is seldom considered as any part of female education.[44]

The prescience of Buchan's thinking with respect to inoculation and the potential to apply the concept to other diseases should be mentioned:

No greater boon has ever been discovered for the health of infants than small-pox inoculation; and it is greatly to be hoped that measles, a disease akin to it, may be treated in the same way.[45]

Buchan is best remembered in many circles for his popular book *Domestic Medicine*, which had 19 editions. Although it predominantly was intended as a "home medical handbook," it contained poignant passages revealing Buchan's profound concern about the mortality rates of English children and his belief in the social benefits of a welfare state:

[I]t appears from the annual register of the dead that almost one half of the children born in Great Britain die under twelve years of age. . . . If it were made the interest of the poor to keep their children alive we should lose very few of them. A small premium given annually to each poor family for every child they have alive at the year's end would save more infants lives than if the whole revenue of the Crown were expended on hospitals for this purpose.[46]

NILS ROSEN VON ROSENSTEIN

An Upsala University professor in Sweden, Nils Rosen von Rosenstein (1706–1773), introduced clinical instruction in pediatrics to the curriculum.[47] A series of his lectures over a period of 10 years was considered so outstanding that the Swedish Royal Academy of Sciences reprinted them as a text of pediatrics, called *Underrättelser om Barn Sjukdomar och deras Bote-Model*, published in 1764.[48] Rosen's book was translated into five languages, reaching most of Europe's evolving disciples of pediatric medicine. The English edition by Andrew Sparrman was printed in 1776. Remarkably for the times, Rosen eschewed referring to or quoting the ancients and focused instead on only what he personally had experienced and observed clinically, thus originating a unique feature of clinical care and research. It was a doctrine he urged others to embrace: "[T]herefore physicians ought not to assert any thing, but what they have seen themselves."[49] He carefully annotated his findings and made quite original, incisive deductions, including one, it has been said, that virtually described the process involved in bacterial infections: "The true cause of this disease [whooping cough] must be some heterogeneous matter or seed which has multiplicative power as is the case with smallpox."[50]

One of his statements reflects a unique understanding of acquired immunity—a concept chronologically still in the far future:

A person who has once had the hooping-cough [sic] is as secure from the danger of catching that disorder again as those who have had the small-pox and measles are with regard to those respective diseases. During my practice I never found or heard of any one who has been infected with the hooping-cough more than once.[51]

Rosen was a strong proponent of maternal breast milk, but in the event that "bottle feeding" was necessary, he recommended using the traditional and well-known horn with a leather teat, or *biberon*.[52]

He stressed the importance of immediately treating diarrhea. Rosen also, in an unprecedented moment of enlightened reason, repudiated the usefulness of that sine qua non ingredient, the hoary hare's brain, against the discomforts of teething.

Finally, he had many practical admonitions, such as caution against fireside nursing because of the dangers of cinder burns and smoke inhalation and against eating raw meats and fish because of the possibility of worm parasitoses.

GEORGE ARMSTRONG

George Armstrong (?1712–?1783) was founder of the London Dispensary for the Infant Poor in Red Lion Square in 1769. Between 1769 and 1781 it has been said that he treated more than 35,000 children.[53] Armstrong published his subjective clinical and postmortem observations in his *Essay on the Diseases Most Fatal to Infants . . .* (1767) and enlarged on this work in a now-famous *Account of the Diseases Most Incident to Children from their Birth till the Age of Puberty*, published in 1777. He accurately characterized pyloric stenosis[54] and, as with Cadogan, rejected the idea that teething per se was a mortal danger.

For scrofula, he advocated that city children be sent to the coast for sea air and sea bathing, to be followed by a dry inland climate for a prolonged period of healing—certainly sound advice, given the epidemiology of tuberculosis and the lack of antibacterial agents.[55]

He underscored the importance of learning to decipher children's language of distress—a skill, he added, that was necessary with adult patients as well:

It is common opinion, that the complaints of children are peculiarly difficult to treat on account of the little patients being unable to describe their sensations. But persons actually occupied in the practice of medicine must be aware that it is often no less difficult to sift the truth out of the figurative and theoretical language in which adults are apt to clothe their feelings, than it is to judge of the unadulterated expressions of distress, exhibited by an infant suffering from disease.[56]

Armstrong is cited in medical histories as the founder of the first institution for the treatment of sick children in England. In 1772 his dispensary in Red Lion Square was moved to a larger facility in Soho Square as both a clinic and a hospital:

Several Friends to the Charity has thought it necessary to have a House fitted up for the Reception of such Infants as are very ill, where they might be accommodated in the same Manner as Adults are in other hospitals.[57]

Anecdotally, 100 years later, in 1852, the renowned Hospital for Sick Children on Great Ormond Street was erected a few hundred feet from the site of Armstrong's first dispensary.

When Armstrong became ill, Andrew Wilson (1718–1792) replaced him as director. Wilson also wrote a small tractate based on a syllabus of lectures: "Of the Diseases of Infants and Children" (1783). The syllabus broke no new medical grounds except, as Still[58] notes, that Wilson, importantly, proposed that pediatrics be formally made part of the teaching curriculum:

I have always thought that on account of the importance of the subject both to families and to the public the nature and diseases of infants merited to be treated of in a particular class and course of lectures, as much as any one branch of medicine.

On the Continent, the Viennese Joseph Johann Mastalier established a *Kinderkrankeninstitut* in 1788, a dispensary similar to Armstrong's. These institutions were prototypes of treatment centers—our modern hospitals—for *sick* children, distinct from the hospices or foundling homes that served disadvantaged children,[59] but they were far from being the salvation of the sick child. In Dublin, for instance, the mortality rates of the Dublin Foundling Hospital between 1775 and 1796 compounded to 99 percent! Similar rates were observed in London (75%) and Paris (80%)—eliciting a caustic suggestion from a Parisian critic to inscribe "Ici on fait mourir les enfans" on the portal of the hospital.[60]

MICHAEL UNDERWOOD

In 1784 two volumes entitled *A Treatise on the Diseases of Children* were published by Michael Underwood (1737–1820). There were 10 editions of this important and popular text, the last of them published in 1846. Historian Still was enthusiastic about the book as "manifestly superior to anything that had been written on the subject . . . , [and] with Underwood, pediatrics in England had crossed the Rubicon; the modern study of diseases in childhood had begun."[61]

Underwood was as thorough as the times allowed. He also conjoined his own clinical astuteness with that of prior writers, a union that produced several "new" pediatric insights. Despite the fact that he clung to some old and erroneous notions, such as those regarding teething, the book was, for the most part, fresh and streamlined. Sclerema was described for the first time in English[62] and Underwood consistently acknowledged and credited his sources:[63]

It may be proper in this place to take notice of a peculiar tightness and hardness of the skin over almost the whole body, that sometimes attends that kind of purging when the stools are of a waxey or clayey consistence, and usually takes place in the last stage of the disease, always affording a very unfavorable prognostic. . . . Dr. Denman [1733–1815] first took notice of it in children, and has for some years paid great attention to it.

Recurrent apnea and bradycardia, the "A's & B's" so familiar to today's neonatologist, were first recounted in the pages of the fourth edition of the *Treatise*. Underwood related the treatment of a newborn as had been told to him by Mr. Hey, a surgeon at the Leed's Infirmary:

It had ceased to breathe except now and then giving a gasp, or sob, and was as pale as a corpse. There was however a sensible pulsation of the heart though feeble and slow, but whether the circulation had been kept up all the time previous to his visit could not be ascertained. . . . The child had three other similar attacks in the course of the day, though it had slept composedly between whiles and sucked at the breast. . . .

[Mr. Hey] administered ten drops [of tinctura valerian] in a teaspoonful of a generous white wine, every two hours. The infant was very sensibly refreshed by the first dose and had no return of the disorder except in the slightest degree, and became a very healthy child.[64]

Underwood wrote about a broad, comprehensive range of pediatric topics—congenital jaundice, mastitis, poliomyelitis, the composition of milk, nursery hygiene, infant psychology, cardiac lesions, and so on—as hitherto none had done. His description of congenital heart disease—a first reference—continues to be instructive:

These morbid deviations appearing in different parts have in all the same tendency, viz. in a greater or less degree to obstruct the passage of blood through the lungs, which in some instances have continued nearly the same as in the unborn fetus. The peculiarity is sometimes in the pulmonary artery, which is constricted or closed as it rises from the right ventricle; at others, in the septum cordis, which has an unnatural opening affording a free communication between the two ventricles: sometimes in the aorta, arising equally from the anteriour and posteriour ventricles: and sometimes in the imperfect closure of the foramen ovale or canalis arteriosus.[65]

MINOR PEDIATRIC SCHOLARS

Hermann Boerhaave

Hermann Boerhaave (1668–1738) was a renowned professor of medicine at Leyden, The Netherlands, who attracted pupils from all of Europe and the Russian mainland. His only contribution to pediatrics, however, was *Aphorismi de cognoscendis et curanis morbis*, published in 1709. The book was a compilation of unoriginal characterizations and treatments in a somewhat hazardous order, so an aphorism about meconium, for instance, was followed by a list of reference sources for infantile distress and this, in turn, followed by a statement on convulsions.

It was a difficult source of information to use, but Boerhaave commanded such respect in the medical community that the book had multiple polylingual editions. He was an excellent clinician and, judging by the roster of his students, a superb teacher. He left a great legacy in the persons of his students, including Alex Monro (1697–1767) and Robert Whytt (1714–1766), who brought prominence to the Edinburgh School of Medicine.[66]

Two other students of Boerhaave founded the Vienna School of Medicine: Gerald von Swieten (1700–1772) and Anton de Haen (1704–1776).[67]

Robert Whytt

The postdoctoral training of Scotsman Robert Whytt (1714–1766) in Paris at La Charité and Hôtel Dieu undoubtedly influenced a lifelong study of tubercular meningitis. Whytt actually was a prolific author with varied interests, and he published works on the physiology of sleep and wake states, on the use of cinchona, on fractures, and on earthquakes and volcanic eruptions.

A seminal work written by Whytt was published posthumously. *Observations on the Dropsy in the Brain* (1768) is considered to be his chef d'oeuvre. The study was based on 20 children with acute internal hydrocephalus.[68] Whytt observed that signs and symptoms appeared four to six weeks or more before death: "Children who have water in the ventricles of the brain begin to have many of the following symptoms, four, five, or six weeks, and in some cases much longer, before their death."

He utilized the pulse as a reference point—a course fraught with multiple pitfalls—but nevertheless presented a lucid staging and clear delineation of cerebral tuberculosis. It was a major contribution to the literature.

Whytt divided the process of morbidity and death into three stages:

At first they lose their appetite and spirits; they look pale, and fall away in flesh; they have always a quick pulse, and some degree of fever.

As the pulse changed, Whytt noted, thirst, progressive anorexia, headache, photophobia, and bruxism appeared:

I date the beginning of the second stage from the time the pulse, from being quick but regular, becomes slow and irregular. This sometimes happens about three weeks, often a fortnight or less, before the death of the patient.

Delirium, irritability, and restlessness marked the final stage:

When the pulse (which for sometime was nearly as slow or slower than in a healthful state) rises again to a feverish quickness, and becomes regular, the third and last stage may be said to begin.

Whytt vividly portrayed the fixed brain swelling, or cerebral edema and intracranial hypertension, and a comatose patient with dilated pupils, cerebral posturing, and seizures:

In this stage, the patients are sometimes observed to be constantly raising one of their hands to their head; and are generally troubled with convulsions of the muscles of the arms, legs, or face, as well as with a *subsultus tendinum*. In a girl of thirteen, the day before she died, the hands were strongly bent inwards by a fixed spasm of their muscles.

However elegant his description of tuberculous meningitis, Whytt fell short in elaborating the probable cause of the hydrocephaly. Marie François Xavier Bichat (1771–1802) came closer to the mark (and, ironically, died of tuberculosis):

That the tissues belonging to the brain, by the arachnoid, to the lungs by the pleura, to the abdominal viscera by the peritoneum, it matters not which, may inflame all over in the same manner. Either the hydropsy comes on uniformly or it is subject to a species of eruption miliary-like and whitish, which has not been mentioned, I believe, and which nevertheless merits great consideration.[69]

Bichat's *Traité des membranes* (1799) made early observations conjoining physiology with membrane structure, allowing him to come to such a patho-physiological conclusion.

Friedrich Hoffman (1660–1742) from Halle, Germany, published two works on childhood diseases: *Praxis Clinica Morborum Infantium* (1715) and *De Praecipuis Infantium Morbis* (1740). They were uninspired rewrites of the works of others. Hoffman did publish individual monographs on infantile atrophy (1702), chlorosis (1730), pertussis (1732), and rubella (1740) with some original observations.[70]

Christopher von Hellwig (1663–1721) published *Kinder-, Jungfer- und Weiber-Spiegel* in 1720. The text was personal and at times introspective, containing anecdotes revealing keen observations and sensitivity, such as this description of a depressed child:[71]

I was consulted about a little girl of 9–10 years: she wept constantly and when questioned she could give no other answer than that she herself did not know why she was so depressed. Various things were tried for her, and amongst them this, one hung some of the best saffron[72] over the region of her heart, thereupon in a short time she got over her state of melancholy.

Paedo-iatreia Practica (1722) was written by Theodore Zuinger (1658–1724), a reiteration of traditional knowledge and lore but with several interesting observations as well. The *tussis ferina*, or pertussis, epidemic of 1712 allowed Zuinger to describe the spontaneous hemorrhage associated with violent spastic coughing and the wasting, despite adequate nutrition, that preface the complications of whooping cough.

Zuinger also wrote on *anasarca puerorum*, making a significant correlation between decreased urine and compromised tubules of the kidney. Unknowingly, he described what now is called nephrotic syndrome:[73]

We have seen infants of both sexes in whom not only were the eyelids so swollen that they could not open their eyes, but the genitals also were extraordinarily distended with the serous exudation so that they were almost transparent. . . . Thirst in this disease is intense, the bowels but poorly open, the urine is scanty owing to obstruction or compression of the tubules of the kidney.

An interesting, if narrow, work called *Exanthematologia: Rational Account of Eruptive Fevers* was published in 1730. It was written by Thomas Fuller (1654–1734) and focused primarily on the rashes of measles, chicken pox, and smallpox.[74]

In 1739, Richard Conyers (1707–1759) was appointed physician to Thomas Coram's Foundling Hospital. His uninventive text *De Morbis Infantium* is mentioned only as a part of the pediatric literature of the century. Its influence in the evolution of pediatrics as a discipline otherwise is negligible.

Henry Bracken (1710–?) wrote on midwifery and newborn diseases. In *Midwife's Companion* (1737) Bracken expounded on congenital syphilis and audaciously corrected the widely held views of the venerable Mauriceau:[75]

Of the Venereal lues or French Pox communicated to Infants. Monsieur Mauriceau is of Opinion that a Child afflicted from the Nurse, or bringing the French Disease, as 'tis called, into the World with it, is capable of infecting whole Families and says that such things have been often seen. . . . Therefore I am positive (though a great many bad People would screen themselves by saying they are infected by the Child's sucking their Breasts) that the Venereal Lues, French or Neapolitan Disease, call it which you will, is not many Times, nay very rarely communicated otherwise than by Coition. (chap. 15)

In America, Jabez Fitch (1736) and Samuel Bard (1771) wrote long treatises on diphtheria. In London, John Fothergill (1712–1780) published his clinical observations in *An Account of the Sore Throat attended with Ulcers* in 1748. Fothergill noted the epidemic nature of the disease he assumed was diphtheria:

It began however to shew itself again about 4 or 5 years ago but not very frequently: And tho' some of the Faculty met with it now and then, it remained unknown to Practitioners in general till within these two or three Years. . . . In the Winter of 1746, so many Children died and so suddenly at Bromley near Bow in Middlesex of a Disease that seem'd to yield to no Remedies or Applications, that the Inhabitants began to be alarmed with Apprehensions that the Plague was broke out amongst them; some losing all and others the greater Part of their Children after a few Days Indisposition.[76]

Citing the following passage, Still[77] contends, probably correctly, that Fothergill was not describing diphtheria but scarlet fever:

Generally on the second Day of the Disease the Face, Neck, Breast and Hands to the Finger Ends are become of a deep erysipelatous Colour, with a sensible Tumefaction; the Fingers are frequently tinged in so remarkable a manner that from seeing them only, it had not been difficult to guess the Disease. A great Number of small Pimples, of a Colour distinguishably more intense than that which surrounds them, appear on the Arms, and other Parts.[78]

A brief, but very important work was published by John George Roederer (1727–1763) entitled *De Pondere et longitudine infantum recens natorum* (1753), an accurate study of the average height and weight of a newborn.[79] These early and important parameters of growth and development in children had never been assessed except anecdotally (and inaccurately).

A Plain Account of the Diseases incident to Children with an Easy Method of Curing Them appeared in 1769, written by John Cooke (1705–1777). Cooke readily admitted that he compiled the book's contents from other authors' works and engagingly commented on his own limitations as a writer: "It is impossible to write so as to please all men. I have my oddities as well as my errors, and I believe but few if any are entirely without them."[80] Although Cooke's book comprised current pediatric thinking of the times, his anecdotal style and charm and the pathos of his narrative commend his work.

When discussing colic, for example, with reference to the death of his own child from a narcotic overdose, he wrote:

Opiates with infants ought to be used with the utmost caution. I lost a son above a year old, who was killed instantly, only with eight drops of liquid laudanum, when two drops are sufficient for a babe.[81]

Unnoticed among the cohorts of infants with the usually benign physiological or breast milk–associated neonatal jaundice were newborns with jaundice secondary to sepsis or congenital hepatitis or other equally malignant conditions. Neither Cooke nor his colleagues could prognosticate which infants would die of jaundice, but the common assumption, among wet nurses in any case, was that all would die. Cooke exposed the lack of fostering that wet nurses accorded jaundiced infants—their neglect in either treating or seeking treatment for the infants—and held them responsible for the majority of deaths:

It is much that this distemper is rarely mentioned in practical authors, though a great many newborn babes die of it; most commonly by the neglect of nurses who according to their usual acuteness say, they grow yellow and must die, therefore neither seek for nor try any assistance. Of a hangman and hard-hearted nurse I know not which is the cruelest.[82]

Michael Underwood's description of one type of malignant jaundice, a congenital syndrome that decimated all 11 children born to one family, suggests Crigler-Najjar or a variant syndrome:

Mrs. J. had been the mother of eleven children on nine of which the jaundice appeared a few days after they were born, and they all died within the period of a month after their birth. The tenth child lived six years, was then afflicted with the jaundice and died. In May 1796 Mrs. J. was delivered of her eleventh child: on the third day after its birth the skin became yellow, and the child was at the same time remarkably torpid and sleepy and seemed to be slightly convulsed . . . [he] died on the ninth day.[83]

De la Conservation des Enfans by Joseph Raulin (1708–1784) was published in France in 1768. It was a two-volume work, with Volume 1 covering general aspects of newborn perinatal and preventative care. Volume 2, however, contained extensive discussions of the prevailing wisdom on dry nursing and pap:

[The Germans nourish] their children from their birth with pap composed of the milk of cows or sheep and of barley flour. It is the country which still today uses this method and it is much employed in Upper Germany and in Switzerland and even in France. They give the child this nourishment every four hours and make it drink between times. The most healthy drink, which these people serve is water in which they boil the raspings of a deer horn or ivory and anise seeds. When the ordinary pap seems to incommode the children on account of its sourness and glutinosity, it is replaced by meat juice, the yolk of egg and bread or with toast reduced to powder and mixed with milk or meat juice. (*Nourriture des enfans san le secours du lait*)[84]

An Essay on the Government of Children (1753) by Englishman James Nelson (1710–1794) was profoundly influenced by the writings of Locke and Cadogan. It proffered an opinion about alcohol that remains current:[85]

To give Wine to Infants is a gross Error; and even to those who have pass'd that State, the Practice is very wrong.

Infants, at least for the Year, have no Business with Malt Liquor at all; they ought not to take it; Milk or Water or both together, is their proper Drink.

The surgeon Percivall Pott (1714–1788) wrote a treatise focused on children, called "Remarks on That Kind of Palsy of the Lower Limbs which is Frequently Found to Accompany a Curvature of the Spine . . ." in 1779. His observations have come down to us as Pott's disease or tuberculosis of the vertebrae, resulting in a gibbus, or kyphotic deformity. Pott rendered a clear clinical presentation of the palsy that manifests itself before the spinal deformity:[86]

When it affects a child who is old enough to have already walked, and who has been able to walk, the loss of the use of his legs is gradual, though in general not very slow. He at first complains of being very soon tired, is languid, listless, and unwilling to move much, or at all briskly; in no great length of time after this he may be observed frequently to trip, and stumble, although there be no impediment in his way; and whenever he attempts to move briskly, he finds that his legs involuntarily cross each other, by which he is frequently thrown down, and that without stumbling; upon endeavoring to stand still and erect, without support, even for a few minutes, his knees give way and bend forward.

When a naturally weak infant is the subject, and the curvature is in the vertebrae of the back, it is not infrequently productive of additional deformity, by gradually rendering the whole back what is commonly called humped.[87]

Tetanus neonatorum was a common scourge described as early as the second millennium B.C. in the Edwin Smith papyrus, by Hippocrates in his *Epidemics*, and in the second century by Areteus.[88] Since newborns almost always were born in the home attended by midwives, comments about newborn tetanus were rare, unless a physician happened to attend a parturition of an infant so afflicted. With the advent of obstetrical units and lying-in hospitals, clusters of newborn tetanus began to be observed and studied.

In 1789, Joseph Clark (1758–1834) read a paper before the Royal Irish Academy entitled, "An Account of the Disease which until lately proved fatal to a great Number of Infants in the Lying-in Hospital of Dublin." The author did not exaggerate. In 1792, of 17,650 births, 2,944 died within two weeks of the "nine-day fits." Clark presented the clinical picture:[89]

[S]crewing and gathering of the mouth into a purse accompanied at intervals with a particular kind of screeching . . . in some the agitation is very great, the mouth foams, the thumbs are riveted into the palms of the hands, the jaws are locked from the commencement so as to prevent the actions of sucking and swallowing; and any attempt to wet the mouth or fauces or to administer medicines seems to aggravate the spasms very much; the face becomes turgid and of a livid hue as do most other parts of the body.

Neonatal tetanus persisted until the last years of the nineteenth century. Arthur Nikolaier (1862–1942) and Shibasaburo Kitasato (1852–1931) researched the disease, and Kitasato successfully collaborated with Robert Koch (1843–1910) in isolating the tetanus bacillus. Emil von Behring (1854–1917) developed an antitoxin in 1890.

Christian Wilhelm Hufeland (1762–1836) published a number of pediatric manuscripts, the first of which appeared in 1799; on "hygiene and physical education in children," it was called *A Tract Addressed to Mothers*.

Hufeland was a forceful proponent of smallpox inoculation as well as a zealous believer in the value of hygienic habits. In 1827 he published a prescient book, *Hygiene and Disease of the Fetus in Utero*.[90] Hufeland would marvel at the fetal surgery now performed.

In the midst of advanced and enlightened scientific thinking in the eighteenth century, old beliefs were perpetuated in several short treatises that published inaccurate and fantastical notions. Many were harmless, like those in *The Compleat Housewife* (1753), that recommended this formula for whooping cough: "Take a spoonful of wood-lice, bruise them, mix them with breast milk and take 3 or 4 mornings as you find benefit. It will cure, but some must take longer than others."[91] Others, like gum lancing for teething, were aggressive and invasive.

The subject of teething, now known to produce only two things—drooling and teeth[92]—warrants some attention in these pages since all manner of seizures, madness, and even death once were attributed to this natural phenomenon. Physicians pointed to teething whenever confronted with clinical manifestations they could not otherwise explain. Several treatments for teething were adopted over the centuries, some of them aggressively surgical. Others were nonsensical but essentially harmless, such as wearing coral or applying to the gums a salve made from hare's brain:

To cause children to breed Teeth without pain. Get the head of hare boiled or roasted, and with the brains thereof mix honey and butter, and therewith anoint the childs gums, as often as you please; it softens the gums and makes the teeth cut easy.[93]

A parchment with magical powers also was a popular treatment for sore gums. Around a child's neck was placed an amulet made from a piece of parchment, with the incantation "abracadabra" repeated in an inverted rectangular pattern:[94]

```
A B R A C A D A B R A
A B R A C A D A B R
A B R A C A D A B
A B R A C A D A
A B R A C A D
A B R A C A
A B R A C
A B R A
A B R
A B
A
```

Radical, tortuous lancing of gums also was an applied remedy. The treatment probably originated with the great anatomist-surgeon Ambroise Paré, who, around 1597, offered the following opinion, based on one of his postmortem examinations:[95]

Monseigneur de Nemours sent to fetch me to anatomize his dead son, aged eight months or thereabouts, whose teeth had not erupted. Having diligently searched for the cause of his death, I could not find any, if not that his gums were very hard, thick and swollen; having cut through them, I found all his teeth ready to come out, if only someone had cut his gums. So it was decided by the doctors present and by me that the sole cause of his death was that nature had not been strong enough to pierce the gums and push the teeth out.

In time, virtually universal acceptance of Paré's theory led to the widespread use of a surgical procedure that in fact did little more than deliver pain, infection, and anorexia.

In 1653, Pemell first mentioned gum lancing in the English literature. Almost a century later, in 1742, surgeon Joseph Hurlock, in *A Practical Treatise Upon Dentition*, claimed that "above a tenth part of Infants die in Teething by Symptoms preceding from the irritations of the tender nervous parts of the Jaws."[96]

A footnote in the anonymous *A Full View of All the Diseases Incident to Children* reads,

Mr. Hurlock in his *Treatise on Dentition* is of the Opinion that the Gum ought to be cut as soon it swells: And tho' it should unite again, he apprehends no great Inconvenience from the Cicatrix, which certainly be cut thro' in a Second Operation.[97]

Hurlock, convinced that teething was a pernicious cause of diseases and disorders, lanced his daughter's gums to stop her convulsions. Her coincidental recovery did little to encourage doubt in the procedure:

I quickly catch'd her up, took an instrument from my Pocket and immediately opened her Gums, apprehending this evil from Back-teeth. In the very instant of cutting the Gum she opened her eyes wide . . . and all the convulsive Symptoms of this first fit disappeared.[98]

Scientific-sounding designations, such as *dentitio difficilis* and *dysdontiasis*[99] were given to teething, bolstering medical and general credulity that it was a mortal danger for infants. This opinion was widespread and persisted over for 400 years,[100] and as late as 1910 over 1,600 deaths in England still were ascribed to teething![101]

Gum lancing was advocated in almost all pediatric treatises, those of Cadogan and Armstrong being the exceptions. Some surgeons, such as John Hunter (1728–1793), were convinced of the curative nature of the procedure and advocated repetitive lancing as needed. In *The Natural History of the Human Teeth* (1771), Hunter wrote:

It often happens, particularly when the operation, the lancing of the gums, is performed early in the disease, that the gums will reunite over the teeth, in which case the same symptoms will be produced, and they must be removed by the same method. I have performed the operation above ten times upon the same teeth when the disease had recurred so often, and every time with the absolute removal of the symptoms.[102]

Special lances were designed to perform the procedure, and diagrams demarcating sites for gum cross-cuts were published. Some physicians lanced the gums as often as twice a day![103]

The subject of worm parasitoses, like teething, was widely and often discussed, although treatment changed little through the centuries. Birch juice, raw carrots, mercury clysters, and tobacco smoke enemas[104] were common recommendations. If tobacco smoke enemas failed, other curious methods of vermifuge were suggested.

Tobacco smoke clysters also were used to clear the "peccant humors" that were thought to cause newborn deaths. One midwifery text of 1754 prescribed that tobacco smoke be infused into the rectum of a nearly dead neonate in order to "establish the peristaltic action of the intestines and thus arouse through cooperation of the diaphragm, the action of the heart and lungs."[105]

For *Nabelwurm* (*Vermis umbilicalis*), Theodore Zuinger (c.1720)* recommended a fish be applied to the navel. The thinking was that once worms had their fill of fish, leaving an empty sack of scales and bones, they would be expelled, yielding, it was supposed, a happy child.[106]

Nils Rosen von Rosenstein preferred

tying a string to a piece of fresh pork, introducing it into the intestinum rectum, and pulling it out again after a little time; for a number of these worms will then always follow. This must be done repeatedly, changing the pork at each time, in order to evacuate them all.[107]

The beginning of this chapter recounted the first tentative trials of forms of inoculation against the virulent scourge of smallpox in the first quarter of the

---

*Zuinger also humorously addressed freckles: "Boys and girls alike, if they rejoice in red hair, are particularly powerful in freckles, and so physicians and surgeons are invited to wipe them out. But 'hoc opus, hic labor,' there's the job, to hope to get rid of them; however much you may drive out nature with a pitchfork she will always come back. For this purpose we have tried various things which we thought sometimes the freckles had been dispersed, but they have come back smiling."

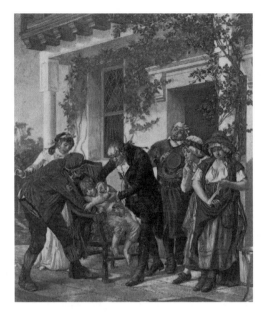

Figure 7.4 Smallpox vaccination depicted by Georges Gaston Melingue. Note the dairymaid wrapping the lesion just abraded to obtain the inoculum. COLLECTION OF THE AUTHOR.

eighteenth century. In the last quarter of the century, Edward Jenner (1749–1823) considered the story of a dairymaid who claimed the cowpox* protected her and her fellow dairymaids from the smallpox. From this crucial piece of information began 23 years of observation and experiments of vaccination, culminating in 1798 with the publication of *Inquiry into the Causes and Effects of the Variolae Vaccinae*.

Jenner performed his first vaccination on 14 May 1796 on eight-year-old James Phipps, with cowpox taken from the hand of dairymaid Sarah Nelmes (figure 7.4). He made two small excoriations on the arm of the boy, onto which he placed pustulous cowpox material from the milkmaid's sores. He sent the boy home and thereafter examined him everyday:

On the seventh day he complained of uneasiness in the axilla and on the ninth he became a little chilly, lost his appetite, and had a headache. During the whole of this

---

*Vaccination stems from *vacca*, a cow. Two hundred years later another animal viral model was to be used for a human vaccine—the rhesus monkey rotavirus was modified to make an effective vaccine for children against rotavirus gastroenteritis (Perez-Schael, L., et al., *N Engl J Med* 1997; 337:1181–87).

day he was perceptibly indisposed, and spent the night with some degrees of rest-lessness, but on the day following he was perfectly well.[108]

Two weeks later, on July 1st, Jenner repeated the procedure, but with smallpox detritus:

Several slight punctures and incisions were made on both his arms, and the matter was carefully inserted, but no disease followed.[109]

Jenner repeated the procedure on several other children, ranging in ages from 11 months to 8 years. All were successfully vaccinated with no seque-lae. In 1853 vaccination was made compulsory by law.

Smallpox was eradicated in the last quarter of the twentieth century. Only one medical and scientific debate on the subject continues—whether or not to destroy the remaining laboratory culture stockpiles of the virus.[110]

The medical achievements of the eighteenth century that contributed to the evolution of the discipline of pediatrics were relatively few in number, but their collective impact was significant. Among the major benefactors of children were Armstrong and his dispensary, Cadogan's essay on nursing, Jenner's vaccination experiment, the elucidation of tubercular meningitis by Whytt and of tetanus by Clark, and a systematic orthopedics for the grow-ing child by Andry.

Two other institutions founded in the eighteenth century reflect the inter-est in and commitment to social issues that dominated the nineteenth cen-tury. In 1785, Valentin Havy (1745–1822) founded a school for blind chil-dren, and in 1784, Charles-Micel de l'Epée (1712–1789) founded a school for the deaf-mute.[111]

NOTES

1. Hugh Downman said of Lady Montague (Downman, 1803, pp. 180–81):

   The triumph was reserved for female hand;
   Thine was the deed, accomplished MONTAGUE!
   . . . . she hath been the cause
   Of heartfelt joy to thousands; thousands live
   And still shall live through her; thy song can please
   None but the sons of Britain.

2. Letter no. 31 in the 1779 edition of *Letters* details the procedure as Lady Montague observed it in Turkey. Clendening, 1960, p. 293.

3. Boylston, 1726, p. 2.

4. *American Heritage* 1996; 47(7):157–59.

5. Duffy, 1979, p. 38.

6. Mather, 1724, chap. 7.

7. Ibid., p. 272.

8. Ibid., p. 273.

9. Ibid.

10. Ibid., p. 277.

11. Duffy, 1979, p. 14.

12. Bard, 1771, pp. 19–20.

13. Ruhräh, 1925, p. 458.

14. Benjamin Rush was one of the signers of the Declaration of Independence.

15. Rush, 1815, pp. 246–47.

16. Jacobi, 1902, pp. 519–20.

17. Chalmers, 1776, pp. 163–65.

18. Jacobi, 1902, p. 463.

19. Cone, 1979, p. 42.

20. Mather experienced a great deal of personal loss in his lifetime. His first wife died of breast cancer and the second, as mentioned, of measles. Of his 22 children, 13 predeceased him—from imperforate anus, "fits," tuberculosis, and 3 from measles. One son died at sea.

21. Cone, 1979, p. 42.

22. Rush, 1815, pp. 215–16.

23. Ibid., pp. 218–21.

24. Ruhräh, 1925, pp. 435–36; Abt, 1945, p. 105.

25. Englishman George Armstrong's report preceded Beardsley's by 10 years (see "George Armstrong" starting on page 166).

26. Allis, 1980, p. 295.

27. Ibid., p. 21.

28. King, 1993, pp. 17–18.

29. Allis, 1980, pp. 380–83.

30. Meissner, 1850.

31. Andry, 1743, pp. 115–16.

32. Anon., 1742, pp. v–x.

33. Ibid., pp. v–vi.

34. Ibid., p. 213. The footnote was attached to Glisson's treatment of rickets with "15 grains of Sweet Mercury."

35. Astruc, 1746, pp. 152–53.

36. Ibid., pp. 224–29.

37. Cadogan, 5th ed., 1773, pp. 3–5. The numbers would, in fact, worsen. Witness some of the statistics as published by Hugh Smith in *The Family Physician* (c.1780) (Still, 1931, p. 455):

Year	Total Births	Deaths<5 years	Deaths<2 years
1762	15,351	10,659	8,372
1764	16,801	9,699	8,200
1766	16,257	10,197	8,035
1768	16,042	10,670	8,229
1770	17,109	10,121	7,994

38. Ibid., pp. 14–15.

39. Ibid., p. 31.

40. Ibid.

41. Ibid., p. 25.

42. Ibid., pp. 8–9.

43. Ruhräh, 1925, pp. 398–99.

44. Buchan, 1807 ed., p. 34.

45. Ibid., pp. 168–69.

46. Buchan, 1825 ed., p. 31.

47. Abt, 1965, p. 122.

48. Vahlquist and Wallgreen, 1964, p. 18.

49. Ibid., p. 27.

50. Ibid., p. 45.

51. Ibid., p. 32.

52. Ruhräh, 1925, p. 440.

53. Ibid.

54. Historians now agree that the earliest known account of pyloric stenosis is that of Patrick Blair in 1717, followed by Christopher Weber in 1758 (Still, 1931, pp. 398–401).

55. Armstrong, 1808, pp. xi–xxx.

56. Ibid., p. xxvii.

57. Still, 1931, p. 420.

58. Ibid., p. 426.

59. Seidler, 1989, pp. 185–89.

60. Abt, 1965, p. 81.

61. Still, 1931, p. 478.

62. Underwood was unaware of a French study of sclerema—*Le'endurcissement des tissus cellulaires ou coagulatión des sucs adipeux* (1782)—written by J. Auvity (1754–1821) and d'Andry (1741–1829) from the Hôpital des Enfants Trouvés.

63. Underwood, 1784, pp. 76–78.

64. Ibid.

65. Underwood, 1841 ed., "Praeternatural Conformations of the Heart," p. 176.

66. Many colonial Americans studied medicine at the Edinburgh School, among them, Benjamin Rush (Hastings, 1974, pp. 74–75).

67. Ackerknecht, 1982, pp. 130–31.

68. Whytt, 1768, pp. 11–24.

69. Ruhräh, 1925, p. 410.

70. Abt, 1965, p. 75.

71. Still, 1931, p. 334.

72. Saffron comes from the dried stigmas of *Crocus sativa*. Many a therapist would wish for such a magical cure from so benign a source.

73. Still, 1931, p. 338.

74. Ruhräh, 1938, pp. 103–6.

75. Bracken, 1737, p. 265.

76. Fothergill, 1748, pp. 27–28.

77. Still, 1931, p. 385.

78. Fothergill, 1748, p. 32.

79. Cone, 1961, pp. 490–98.

80. Cook, 1769, p. ix.

81. Ibid., p. 9.

82. Ibid., p. 22.

83. Underwood, 1842, p. 114.

84. Raulin, 1770, p. 215.

85. Ruhräh, J., *Am J Dis Child* 1933; 46:381–83.

86. Pott, 1779, pp. 10–11.

87. Ibid., pp. 14–15.

88. Hare, 1967, p. 116.

89. Still, 1931, p. 490.

90. Abt, 1945, p. 15.

91. Camp, 1973, p. 51.

92. Teething continues to be blamed for irritability, fever, diarrhea, and insomnia.

93. Glass, 1762, p. 45.

94. Bayne-Powell, 1938, p. 250.

95. Hunt, 1970, p. 121.

96. Hurlock, 1742, p. 11.

97. Anon., 1742, p. 73.

98. Hurlock, 1742, p. 51.

99. Landsberger, 1964, p. 209.

100. In America, physicians subscribed to the view calculating a 4 percent infant mortality due to teething. *American Medical Recorder* 1818; 1:300–301.

101. Dally, 1996, pp. 1710–11.

102. Hunter, 1771, p. 80.

103. Dally, 1996, p. 1710.

104. Vahlquist and Wallgreen, 1964, pp. 46–48.

105. Gordon, M. E., *Am J Gastroenterol* 1993; 88:461–62.

106. Still, 1931, p. 338.

107. Clendening, 1960, p. 266.

108. Jenner, 1798, pp. 31–34.

109. Ibid.

110. This may cease to be debated since recent outbreaks of monkeypox among humans will call for molecular comparisons with the smallpox virus. *Lancet* 1997; 349:1449–50.

111. Abt, 1965, pp. 81–84.

Chapter 8

The Nineteenth Century

In the Age of Revolutions the toppling of the established order in France and America created a climate of unease and uncertainty throughout Europe, leaving as residue severely shaken structures of institutions and traditions. A thorough reappraisal of all human endeavors followed, including an examination of all that pertained to the practice of medicine and medical training.

In the medieval era, Ackerknecht[1] noted, medicine was a library-centered intellectual discipline. During the Renaissance and Reformation periods, the Classical style of bedside teaching was rediscovered and adopted. In the nineteenth century, concepts of the purpose and function of hospitals were redefined, radically altering the centuries-old notion of hospitals as centers of "hospitality and hospice" where the disenfranchised and abandoned poor were taken to die. As Seidler points out, hospitals became centers for medical training, for patient care—the diagnosis, treatment, and cure of patients—and for scientific research in the newly established clinical laboratories.[2]

The institutional setting became the milieu in which the evolution and progression of disease could be studied by student and physician alike and, for the first time, in large numbers. It became possible to catalog and correlate clinical signs and symptoms. Learning continued even with death. The postmortem as a teaching tool once again attained new respect, despite scandals that periodically surfaced about grave robbing.* This was reflected in a quip about cadavers by Scotland's John Hunter (1728–1793) to the father of one of his pupils: "These [cadavers] are the books your son will learn [from] under my direction; the others are fit for very little."[3]

French physicians were the principal innovators in the study and practice of medicine in the first half of the century. The French hospital provided the model for all of Europe as the major resource for education and the primary teaching site. Marie Francois Xavier Bichat (1771–1802) pioneered a new, systematic approach to the autopsy and to pathological anatomy. Claude Bernard (1814–1878) revolutionized physiological studies. Gaspard Laurent Bayle (1774–1816) and Rene Laennec (1781–1826) enhanced the art of clinical auscultation, and Guillaume Dupuytren (1777–1835) enlarged the surgical repertory.

Hospital-based medicine was adopted by physicians throughout Europe: in Ireland by men such as Robert Graves (1796–1853), William Stokes (1804–1878) and Abraham Colles (1773–1843); in England by Richard

---

*The morbid occupation continued through the middle of the nineteenth century. The anatomist's incessant appetite for dissection corpses sustained the booming business of grave robbing all over the continent. The most notorious dealers were William Burke and William Hare of Edinburgh, who, between 1827 and 1829, actually committed murder in order to supply bodies for the anatomy school of Robert Knox.

Bright (1781–1858), Thomas Addison (1783–1843), and Thomas Hodgkin (1798–1864); and in Vienna by Karl Rokitansky (1804–1878) and the renowned Ignaz Semmelweis (1818–1865). In the second half of the nineteenth century, German physicians dominated medical education and practice, and a clinical tool—the glass thermometer—gradually came into common use and ultimately became a universal item in all households.

Since antiquity, fever as an element of illness had been assigned one of the four qualities: *dolor, rubor, tumor et calor*. During the medieval period it became a disease entity and considered a primary ailment, so much so that multivolume manuscripts were written classifying fevers by duration and syndromic associations. Measuring fever by degrees, however, did not occur until Santoria Sanctorius (1561–1636) designed a thermometer that specifically recorded body temperatures. But the clinical significance of body temperature went largely unheeded until Carl Reinhold Wunderlich (1815–1877) wrote *Das Verhalten der Eigenwärme in Krankheiten* in 1868. An English translation of the study was published in 1871 as *Medical Thermometry*. This seminal work expounded on the importance of temperature as a harbinger of disease and, most important, identified a measurable unit—the degree—as a correlate of gravity. Historian Fielding Garrison (1870–1935) commented that Wunderlich "found fever a disease and left it a symptom."[4]

Modern medicine, according to Paul Hastings, began with the practical application of the germ theory[5] in the final decades of the nineteenth century. Certainly, the importance of Louis Pasteur—a basic scientist, not a clinician—in the history of medicine cannot be overstated. Widely known as the originator of a heat-induced partial-sterilization method for wines (and later, for milk), the name of the process—pasteurization—honored its discoverer.

It is, however, from Pasteur's breakthrough studies of infection and their treatment—of anthrax, then rabies—that modern therapeutic practice derives.

Once Pasteur succeeded in immunizing animals against the anthrax germ, he turned his attention to rabies—an even more dreaded, untreatable infection, known at that time to be caused only by mad dogs. In 1882, Pasteur began methodical experiments with laboratory-infected rabbits and dogs, the results of which, by 1885, produced a number of dogs immunized against the rabies virus. Pasteur's work was an astounding research achievement yet to be applied to an infected human—until he was presented with a rabies-infected child. The reality of a stricken boy's inevitable and horrible death proved more compelling to Pasteur than the specter of possibly accelerating the child's death by an injection of the serum from his laboratory.

Pasteur best relates the saga: At 8 A.M. on 4 July 1885, nine-year-old Joseph Meister of Alsace was bitten by a rabid dog:[6]

This child had been knocked over by the dog and presented numerous bites on the hands, legs, and thighs, some of them so deep as to render walking difficult. . . . Joseph Meister had been pulled out from under [the dog] covered with foam and blood.

On 6 July, Pasteur presented the case to his colleagues, who immediately examined the child, counting 14 swollen, tender, and inflamed bites. Their conclusion was that rabies was inescapable:

The death of this child appearing to be inevitable, I decided, not without lively and sore anxiety . . . to try upon Joseph Meister the method which I had found constantly successful with dogs. . . . Consequently, on July 6th, at 8 o'clock in the evening, sixty hours after the bites on July 4th, and in the presence of Drs. Vulpian and Grancher, young Meister was inoculated under a fold of skin raised in the right hypochondrium, with half a Pravaz' syringeful of the spinal cord of a rabbit, which had died of rabies on June 21st. It had been preserved since then, that is to say, fifteen days, in a flask of dry air.

In the following days fresh inoculations were made. I thus made thirteen inoculations. . . . On the last days I had inoculated Joseph Meister with the most virulent of rabies, that, namely, of the dog, reinforced by passing a great number of times from rabbit to rabbit.

The boy recovered. Several months later, Pasteur proved that Meister's was not a chance cure when he effected a like cure, employing the same method of inoculation, to a second rabies-infected patient, a shepherd boy.

The microbial research of Robert Koch (1843–1910) and Emile von Behring (1854–1917) enlarged and bolstered the germ theory. Koch, known to students of science for his Four Postulates,* discovered the tuberculosis bacterium in 1882 and, in 1890, isolated the cholera microbe.

Behring discovered the antitoxin principle. He injected diphtheria antitoxin into guinea pigs and concluded that the antitoxin protected them from lethal exposures to the germ. In 1891, Behring successfully administered the serum to a child who had been dying of diphtheria in a Berlin hospital. The age of specific therapy against infection had arrived.

Pediatrics as a separate field of study became widely recognized and accepted in the nineteenth century, and those who exclusively treated children

---

*To establish the specificity of a pathogenic microorganism: (1) the germ must be identified in all cases of the disease, (2) inoculation of the germ must produce disease in the host, and (3) from the host it must again be obtained, and (4) propagated as a pure culture. New technology, however, has rendered the postulates moot, since molecular methodology now allows the extraction of microbial DNA and RNA from infection sites without culturing and growing the organism. *Science* 1998; 282:220.

TABLE 8.1a
SOME NINETEENTH-CENTURY EUROPEAN PEDIATRIC PUBLICATIONS
PRIOR TO 1850

John Cheyne	*Essays on Diseases of Children*	1802
N. Jahn	*Neues System der Kinderkrankheiten . . .*	1803
Carl Fleisch	*Handbuch uber die Krankheiten der Kinder . . .*	1803
William Heberden	*Morborum Puerilium Epitome*	1804
Jakob von Plenk	*Doctrina de . . . morbis infantorum*	1807
Giuseppe Maruncelli	*Compendio*	1808
Adolp Henke	*Handbook of Pediatrics*	1809
Leopold Gölis	*. . . Physical Training in the First Year of Life*	1811
J. Capuron	*. . . maladies de enfants jusqu'à la puberté*	1813
John Clarke	*Commentaries on . . . Diseases of Children*	1815
John Davis	*Cursory Inquiry into . . . Mortality in Children*	1817
Combes-Brassard	*L'ami des mères*	1819
Robley Dunglison	*Diseases of Children*	1823
P. Bretonneau	*Diphthérite*	1826
Johann Joerg	*Handbook of Pediatrics*	1826
C. Michel Billard	*Traite des . . . enfans nouveaux-nes*	1828
F. Meissner	*Die Kinderkrankheiten*	1828
Gilbert Breschet	*Treatise on Diseases of Children*	1833
	Grundlage der Literatur der Pädiatrik	1850
Emile Berton	*Traite des maladies des enfans . . .*	1837
F. L. Valleix	*Clinique des malades des enfants nouveaux-nes*	1838
F. Rilliet, with Antoine Barthez	*Traite clinique et practique . . . des enfants*	1838
Paul Vanier	*Clinique des Hôpitaux des Enfants*	1841
Francois Barrier	*Traite practique des maladies de l'enfance*	1843
Henry Goodeve	*Hints*	1844
Ernest Bouchut	*Manual Practique*	1845
Alfred D. Donné	*Conseils*	1846
F. L. Legendre	*Anatomisch-pathologische . . . kindlichen Alters*	1847
Charles West	*Diseases of Infancy and Childhood*	1848
	How to Nurse Sick Children	1852

were referred to as "pediatrists." In the first quarter of the century, pediatric issues were the domain of obstetrics, but by 1828, Charles Michel Billard (1800–1832) could and did expound conceptually on pediatrics as a discipline, confident that his ideas would be understood and accepted by his medical colleagues. Child and infant surgery and pediatric orthopedics evolved as distinct disciplines. A renowned German obstetrician, Frederick Meissner, noted in *Grundlage der Literatur der Pädiatrik* (1850) that by 1832 there were 7,000 treatises on pediatric subjects in the literature. A mere 16 of them had been written before the seventeenth century, only 21 during the seventeenth century, and 75 before Rosen's important work on clinical diagnoses (1764). The remaining 6,800 works were published between 1775 and 1832.[7] Tables 8.1 and 8.2 list chronologically the significant European and American pediatric publications of the nineteenth century. A more complete listing can be found in the compilations of Meissner (1850) and Adams (1897).

TABLE 8.1b
SOME NINETEENTH-CENTURY EUROPEAN PEDIATRIC PUBLICATIONS AFTER 1850

Alois Bednar	*Die Krankheiten der Neugeborenen*	1850
Fleetwood Churchill	*Diseases of Children*	1850
Ludwig Mauthner	*Kinder-Diatetik . . .*	1853
	Pädiatrik Lehrbuch	1856
Karl Hennig	*Lehrbuch der Krankheiten des Kindes . . .*	1855
Franz Mayr	*Jahrbuch für Kinderheilkunde*	1857
P. Diday	*. . . Syphilis in New-born Children and Infants*	1858
Alfred Vogel, with Philipp Biedert	*Lehrbuch der Kinderkrankheiten*	1860
A. Trousseau	*Clinique medicale de l'Hotel Dieu*	1861
Carl Gerhardt	*Pädiatrik Lehrbuch*	1861
	Handbuch der Kinderkrankheiten	1887
Johann Steffen	*Klinik der Kinderkrankheiten*	1865
Henri Louis Roger	*Recherches Cliniques*	1867
R. von Rittershain	*Jahrbuch . . . des ersten Kindesalters*	1868
Eduard Henoch	*Contributions to Pediatrics*	1868
	Vorlesungen über Kinderkrankheiten	1881
Paul Guersant	*Surgical Diseases of Infants and Children*	1873
Johann Steiner	*Compendium of Children's Diseases . . .*	1874
Marie Jules Parrot	*Clinique*	1875
Adolf Baginsky	*Central-Zeitung für Kinderheilkunkde*	1877

continued

TABLE 8.1b (continued)

Constant Picot, with Jean d'Espine	*Manuel practique des maladies de l'enfance*	1877
Jules J. Parrot	*L'athrepsie*	1877
Cadet de Gassicourt	*. . . des maladies de l'enfance*	1880
Philipp Biedert	*Die Kinderernährung im Saulingsalter*	1880
J. Uffelmann	*Handbuch . . . Hygiene des Kindes*	1881
Wilhelm Preyer	*Die Seele des Kindes*	1882
Eustace Smith	*A Practical Treatise on Diseases of Children*	1884
F. Criados-Aguilar	*Tratado de las enfermedades de los niño*	1884
James Goodhart	*A Student's Guide . . . Diseases of Children*	1885
F. Copasso	*Osservazioni . . . bambini con applicazioni pratiche*	1887
Edmond Weill	*Traite . . . des maladies du coeur chez les enfants* *Precis de medecine infantile*	1895 1900
Paul Moreau	*Mental Disorders in Children*	1888
S. Tarnier, with J. Chantreuil and P. Budin	*Allaitemente et hygiène du nouveau-né*	1888
Vitale Tedeschi	*Commentari di Practica Pediatrica*	1889
Walter Cheadle, with F. Poynton	*. . . the Artificial Feeding of Infants*	1889
Ludwig Unger	*Lehrbuch der Kinderkrankheiten . . .*	1890
J. W. Ballantyne	*An Introduction to the Diseases of Infancy*	1891
Nil F. Filatov	*Semiotik und Diagnostik der Kinderkrankheiten*	1892
Julius Uffelmann	*. . . Handbuch der Kinderheilkunde . . .*	1893
B. Alvarez-Gonzalez	*Anatomia y fisiologia especiales del niño*	1895
Jules Comby, with J. Grancher and B. Marfan	*Traite des Maladies de l'enfance*	1897
John Thompson	*. . . Examination and Treatment of Sick Children*	1898
B. Marfan	*Traite de l'allaitement*	1899
P. Budin	*Le Nourrisson*	1900

PEDIATRIC HOSPITALS IN THE NINETEENTH CENTURY

One of the more dramatic advances in the history of pediatrics originated in the latter part of the eighteenth century with the establishment of outpatient clinics—a recognition of the need for institutional facilities specific to children's health care. *Ambulatoriums* like George Armstrong's 1769 London Dispensary on Red Lion Square, the 1788 Vienna clinic (Kinderkranken-institut) of Joseph Mastalier, and John Bunnell Davis's 1816 Infirmary were the prototypes.

A seemingly unrelated study of unsanitary conditions of hospitals in France resulted in the eventual establishment of the first children's hospital.

In 1785, King Louis XVI had ordered an inspection of Paris's Hôtel Dieu in response to complaints about the persistent squalor there. Investigators Jacob René Tenon (1724–1816), Pierre-Simon Laplace (1749–1827), and the illustrious Antoine Lavoisier (1743–1794) reported wards accommodating 100 or more patients, with often eight or nine children in a single bed. Their recommendations of one patient to a bed and, importantly, separate hospital facilities for children[8] became part of a new, evolving concept in which hospitals, it was thought, should be centers for science research, medical education, and treatment. The Maison de l'Enfant Jésus in 1802 shifted its function from an orphanage to a children's hospital, modeled after the rapidly increasing number of adult teaching hospitals. The institution, on the rue de Sèvres, was renamed the Hôpital des enfants malades. By 1815 as many as 800 inpatients daily were being admitted to the institution.[9]

Other capitals were slow to emulate this early model—Berlin in 1830, St. Petersburg in 1834, Vienna and Breslau in 1837, Prague in 1842, Turin in 1843, Stockholm in 1845, Copenhagen in 1846, Constantinople in 1847, London in 1852, Edinburgh in 1860, Basel in 1862, and Glasgow in 1883. Between 1850 and 1879, 67 children's hospitals were established in Europe,[10] but the mere foundation of hospitals for children was not an assurance of better care, and mortality rates often remained high. In 1848, Adolf Kussmaul (1822–1902), known for the introduction of gastric intubation, called the Vienna institution a "murder pit." As late as 1890, the Charité in Berlin reported the deaths of 174 of 176 children treated for "atrophia infantium."[11]

St. Anne's Hospital in Vienna—a 12-bed children's teaching hospital founded and funded by Austrian Ludwig Wilhelm Mauther (1806–1858) in 1837—marked the inauguration of formal pediatric instruction in Vienna. In 1842 the hospital moved into a larger building staffed with Sisters of Charity as nurses, and by 1850 it was officially affiliated with the University of Vienna.[12] Mauther was also published, and his three-edition work on children's nutrition was translated into French.

Franz Mayr (1814–1863) succeeded Mauther as director of St. Anne's. His interest was in the treatment of congenital syphilis and measles, and he published a large series of case histories of both diseases. He also wrote a manual on child care. His prominence in medicine is as the first editor, in 1857, of *Jahrbuch für Kinderheilkunde*.

His successor, Herman Wiederhofer (1832–1901), was an exceptional teacher, who for 40 years attracted overflow crowds of students to his lectures. Honored with the first Austrian professorship of children's diseases, his exceptional teaching talent won him renown and established Vienna as a center of pediatric training.[13]

By 1877, child advocates had effected considerable social reform with respect to child labor laws, mandatory education, and routine medical care of children. In this climate of reform and social progress, Karl Rauchfuss's (1835–1915) *Handbuch der Kinderkrankheiten* cited the need for observation and isolation wards, play rooms, physiotherapy facilities, and outdoor activity areas in order to improve overall conditions in children's hospitals.[14]

From her nursing experience in the Crimean War, Florence Nightingale (1820–1910) produced *Notes on Nursing* in 1859. In addition to recommending an organized curriculum for nurse trainees, she advocated separating children and adult patients, albeit for erroneous considerations. Nurse Nightingale believed the cause of infection was a polluted "effluvium" from the sick:

In disease where everything given off from the body is highly noxious and dangerous, not only must there be plenty of ventilation to carry off the effluvia, but everything which the patient passes must be instantly moved away, as being more noxious than even the emanations from the sick.[15]

She perceived children as especially virulent vectors of disease:

[D]o not have children's wards in a general hospital. There at least mix the children with the adults. For a children's ward in a general hospital combines all the disadvantages with none of the advantages of a children's hospital.[16]

The first institution for sick children in the United States was founded in 1855 in Philadelphia. Boston and New York followed suit in 1869 and the District of Columbia in 1871. By 1880, Abraham Jacobi (1830–1919) had been instrumental in the establishment of several hospitals for children in the United States—in Chicago, San Francisco, St. Louis, and Cincinnati— so that, by 1895, there were 26 children's hospitals in America. Jacobi expressed the need for pediatric hospital care:

My plea is for the establishment of children's hospitals. . . . Infants, who are so much more liable to be taken with acute and life-endangering maladies than the class we generally meet with in hospitals, are not admitted. Thus, those who require most aid receive none.[17]

CLINICAL PEDIATRIC SCHOLARSHIP

John Cheyne

The highly regarded work of John Cheyne (1777–1836) at the beginning of the nineteenth century exemplified the increasing professional interest in pediatric subjects. Trained in Edinburgh, Cheyne settled in Dublin and established a flourishing practice. He is best known for his *Essays on the Diseases of Children* (1802) and *Pathology of the Membranes of the Larynx and Bronchia* (1809). His observations in *Essays* on pediatric croup, tubercular meningitis, and cholestasis had never before been so clearly described clinically. The first essay, entitled "Cynanche Trachealis or Croup," totaling 80 pages, relates the historical context:

It may seem strange that a disease so striking with symptoms, so speedy and fatal in the event should not have been clearly described earlier than in the middle of the last century, were it not remembered, that formerly all the ailments of children were much neglected, and that the most eminent physicians, when called to children, went with reluctance, judging their diseases to form a labyrinth for which they had no clew.[18]

In addition to his vivid clinical observations of a patient with croup, Cheyne supplied postmortem findings:

His illness, indeed, does not prevent him from going to sleep, but soon he wakes with a most unusual cough, rough and stridulous. And now his breathing is laborious, each inspiration being accompanied by a harsh shrill noise . . . he tries to relieve himself by sitting erect; no change in posture, no effort gives him relief.[19]

When the child dies after an illness of three, four, or five days, there is found lining the windpipe a white membrane of considerable tenacity.[20]

Cheyne's pronouncements in 72 pages of clinical and pathological descriptions of congenital cholestasis were remarkable for the time. He correctly perceived most instances as congenital cholestasis and a "fatal jaundice," in sharp contrast to the general belief that it was a benign symptom:

[T]he fatal jaundice, such as is described below is not to be removed by emetics, gentle purgatives, and the warm bath, the natural remedies for an obstruction in the ducts. I believe it to be an original and incurable malconformation in the liver. It is a disease peculiar to some families.[21]

William Heberden

In 1804, William Heberden[22] (1767–1845) published *Morborum Puerilium Epitome*, a palm-sized volume of 61 chapters on hygienic measures and descriptions of 52 childhood disorders. The language was concise and pragmatic. The work was reprinted in its entirety by Ruhräh[23] in 1925, with cryptic chapter headings. Chapter 21, on sclerema, was innovative:

1. On the diet and management of children
2. Of emetics
3. Of purgatives
4. Of astringents
5. On the signs of indisposition in children
6. Of those who are born apparently lifeless
7. Of the black colour of infants
8. Of the meconium
9. Of the jaundice
10. Of the thrush
11. Of the hiccup
12. Of acidity and indigestion
13. Of wind on the stomach
14. Of wakefulness
15. Of worms
16. Of vomiting
17. Of the state of the bowel
18. Of the looseness of bowels
19. Of the descent of the fundament
20. Of the erysipelas of children
21. Of a disease attended with hardness of the skin
22. Of the tetanus or locked jaw
23. Of the difficulty of making water
24. Of an incontinence of urine
25. Of ruptures
26. Of hydrocele
27. Of the hydrocephaly
28. Of convulsions
29. Of the teeth
30. Of the disorders of the eyes
31. Of squinting
32. Of bleeding at the nose
33. Of bleeding from private parts
34. Of the flour albus
35. Of a cold in the head
36. Of a cough

37. Of the hooping cough
38. Of the croup
39. Of the ulcerated sore-throat
40. Of the scarlet fever
41. Of the measles
42. Of the small-pox
43. Of the cow-pox
44. Of the chicken-pox
45. Of the infantile fever
46. Of the hectic fever
47. Of the ague, intermittent fever
48. Of the venereal disease
49. Of eruptions
50. Of purple spots
51. Of sore ears
52. Of a chafing of the skin
53. Of chilblains
54. Of the scald-head
55. Of the scrofula
56. Of a white-swelling
57. Of a diseased hip
58. Of the curved spine
59. Of the rickets
60. Of the cleft-spine
61. Of the hare-lip

Heberden's verbal economy, evident in the terse chapters 5, 6, and 23, and his simple and direct approach to clinical issues complement keen observations. Chapter 5 is a succinct primer enabling "pediatrists" to form clinical impressions about infants yet unable to articulate their complaints:

As young children are either not at all, or very imperfectly able to describe their own feelings, it becomes necessary to point out by what marks their disorders may principally be known. These are, wakefulness; restlessness; crying; or, on the other hand, a sullen heaviness; retching, or vomiting; loose, green or slimy stools; loathing of their food; a dry, or foul tongue; convulsions; retraction of the legs; emaciation, or relaxation; a dry and hot skin; eruptions; hiccup; sudden startings from sleep; screaming; hardness and distension of the belly; difficulty breathing; strong pulsations of the arteries in the neck.

Chapter 6 advocated several centuries-old midwives' tactics, including mouth-to-mouth resuscitation:

Children who are born without signs of life, may yet sometimes be saved by timely attention. For this purpose it is useful to throw up injections of any warm liquid; to rub the body either with the hand alone, or with a little brandy; and lastly, to inflate the lungs, by blowing into the mouth.

Heberden was unusual among his colleagues in preferring the use of clysters and water immersion[24] with children, rather than strong diuretics. Appearing in his stunningly brief chapter 23, the reference more likely reflects a predominant lack of understanding of renal physiology:

For a difficulty of making water, the proper remedies are the warm bath, frictions of the belly, and gentle purgatives; also equal parts of milk and warm water injected into the intestines.

Although not encyclopedic, the small volume addressed the more common complaints of children and assuredly was a popular vade mecum for nineteenth-century physicians.

Robert Watt (1774–1819) published *A Treatise on the History, Nature and Treatment of Chin Cough* (pertussis) in 1813. It was predominantly a descriptive work advocating the therapeutic wisdom of the times (liniments, bleeding, tar vapors, purgatives, ipacac, etc.). The appendix to the book, however, lends historical interest to the *Treatise*. In his compilation that spanned 30 years, from 1783 to 1812, Watt annually listed the principal causes of death for Glasgow children under the age of 10 years. With the exception of fatalities due to chincough, the tabulations of the first year markedly contrast with the increased numbers of deaths that Watts recorded in 1812:[25]

	1783	1812
Small pox	155	78
Measles	66	304
Chincough	153	103
Stopping	14	103
W. in head	6	54
Teething	44	45
Bowelhives	107	279
Still-born	42	104
Fevers	118	105
	1,413	2,348

John Clarke

John Clarke (1761–1815), a teaching associate of William Hunter at the London Anatomy School, published a series of essays in 1815 entitled *Commentaries on Some of the Most Important Diseases of Children*. His account of stridor associated with tetany was the book's most useful contribution to clinical diagnosis of the condition:

The child having had no apparent warning, is suddenly seized with a spasmodic inspiration, consisting of distinct attempts to fill the chest, between each of which a squeaking noise is often made; the eyes stare, and the child is evidently in great distress; the face and the extremities, if the paroxysms continue long, become purple, the head is thrown backward, and the spine is often bent, as in opisthotonus; at length a strong expiration takes place, a fit of crying generally succeeds, and the child, evidently much exhausted, often falls asleep. In one of these attacks a child sometimes, but not frequently, dies. . . . Accompanying these symptoms, a bending of the toes downwards, clenching of the fists and the insertion of the thumbs into the palm of the hands, and bending the fingers upon them, is sometimes found, not only during the paroxysm, but at other times.[26]

John Bunnell Davis

In 1816, John Bunnell Davis (1780–1824) founded the London Universal Dispensary for Sick and Indigent Children. Between 1816 and 1821 he compiled the "Annals of the Dispensary," similar to a modern-day "Children's Hospital Bulletin" of case histories.

His most enduring contribution to clinical pediatrics appeared in *A Cursory Inquiry into the Principle Causes of Mortality in Children* (1817). His proposal to send competent volunteers into impoverished London neighborhoods to train poor and ill-informed mothers in nutritional and hygienic standards exhibited remarkable prescience for the time and foreshadowed fundamental concepts that were to become commonplace:

If benevolent ladies could be prevailed upon to form district committees to visit and inspect the health of sick indigent children, much practical good would result from a medical and moral point of view. By such visitations as these it may be predicted that the instances of mortality among children will be quickly diminished; at the same time that such benevolent females corrected the absurd notions and errors of the poor as to the domestic management of their children.[27]

Early French monographs on typhoid fever (1819) and diphtheria (1826) were published by Pierre Bretonneau (1771–1862) in Tours. Bretonneau introduced the use of tracheostomy in the treatment of suffocating *diph-*

thérité in children. Confronted with 100 percent mortality once edema and membranous exudate blocked the airway, Bretonneau's use of tracheostomies was widely adopted despite significant risks, since they at least generally offered a survival rate of approximately 15 percent. Bretonneau actually performed few of these procedures, but his pupil and colleague, Armand Trousseau (1801–1867), performed more than 398 tracheostomies, with an enhanced 22 percent rate of survival.[28] Trousseau was director of the Hôpital des Enfants Malades from 1850 to 1853 and clinical lecturer at the Hôtel Dieu, where his talks on the infections of children were widely attended. He is best remembered for lending his name to the sign of carpopedal spasms associated with infantile tetany. Germain See (1818–1896) succeeded Trousseau at the Hôpital. He was the first to describe observations of chorea associated with endocarditis.

Charles-Michel Billard

Charles-Michel Billard (1800–1832) published *Traités des maladies des enfants nouveaux-nés et à la mamelle* in 1828. Billard's experience as an attending physician at the Hospice des Enfants Trouvés, where he performed autopsies on infants and children, provided the material for the book. His premature demise had an especially unfortunate impact on the advancement of clinical science because his methodology was original and represented an innovative departure from standard clinical observations: "I have written this book with the independence of one who would not draw from existing doctrines anything, however positive, the truth of which could not be proved by established facts or by natural analogy."[29] Historian Garrison considered the system that Billard devised—classifying diseases on the basis of pathology rather than symptoms—the single most significant advance in the understanding of pediatric diseases.[30]

In his book, Billard began with general observations regarding height, weight, skin color, pulse, respiratory rate, and so on. Diseases were classified according to those thought to be congenital in origin and, thereafter, under the anatomical parts affected (skin, intestine, lung, heart, brain, muscle, lymphatic system, eye, blood, etc.).

The following example for diseases of the skin is devoid of etiological concepts but is nevertheless illustrative of his classification system:[31]

 Chapter I: Diseases of the Skin
  Section 1. Malformations
    2. Spots and nevi
    3. Color alterations

4. Inflammations

5. Ecchymosis

6. Tumors

7. Petechiae

8. Erythemas

   Erysipelas

   Measles

   Roseola

   Scarlatina

   Urticaria

   Blisters

   Pemphigus

   Herpes

   Eczema

   Psora

   Variola

   Vaccinia

   Ecthyma

   Acne

   Impetigo

   Tinea

   Lichen

   Psoriasis

   Pityriasis

   Carbuncle

   Burns

Paul Diday (1812–1894) of Lyon wrote a 300-page treatise on syphilis of the newborn in 1841. Translated into English in 1858, the work began with a compelling historical survey of lues and presented all known treatment modalities of the disease. In thorough and comprehensive detail, Diday studied lungs, liver, thymus, heart, kidneys, eyes, teeth, brain, and bones and meticulously described syphilitic skin lesions (figure 8.1).

Diday's comments regarding societal assumptions associated with syphilis have sustained validity and pertinence to this day: "Syphilis is neither always the result of a fault, nor always the consequence of disease in the parent or the [wet] nurse."[32]

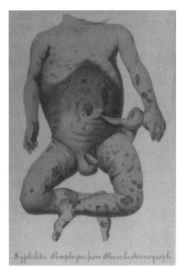

Figure 8.1 Syphilitic newborn, from Diday's *Treatise of Syphilis*, 1841.

A celebrated German obstetrician, Karl Siegumnd Franz Credé (1819–1892) made a major contribution to clinical pediatrics and to the treatment of venereal disease when he introduced the use of silver nitrate solution to prevent gonorrheal ophthalmia of the newborn, a common cause of acquired blindness at the time.[33]

Manuel Tolosa Latour (1857–1919) was attending physician at the Hospital Niño Jesus and founder of the Children's Hospital of Madrid. Latour, however, is best remembered for originating the medical journal *Revista de Enfermedades de los Niños* in 1883.[34]

Pascual Mora, of the Royal College of Medicine in Madrid, published a three-volume work on midwifery, nurture, and diseases of children in 1827. *El hombre en la primera época de su vida o Reflexiones y observaciones acerca de la pubertad, generación, preñez, parto, criaza física, educación moral y enfermedades de los niños* appeared in 1827.[35]

Fredrik Theodor Berg

In 1845, Sweden's Fredrik Theodor Berg (1806– 1877) was appointed professor of pediatrics at the Karoline Institute in Stockholm, the world's first pediatric chair. Berg was an astute observer and clinician, who recorded not only morbid anatomical impressions but also the circumstances surrounding death. Thus, he made early valuable observations on sudden infant death, noting that there was a male predominance and that it commonly occurred at night. At the time, the two common theories about the cause of sudden infant death were "overlaying" and thymic hypertrophy, and Berg disagreed with both. He dismissed overlaying as causative, noting that sudden death also occurred in orphanages. Thymic enlargement, he observed, was evident in infants who died of other causes. "This disease," Berg wrote, "leads to a special irritability in the nervous system in infancy evoking a sudden derangement of life's most important functions. . . . [T]he immature reflecto-motoric action of the nerve system might provide an explanation for this phenomenon."[36]

In 1841 he wrote in detail regarding one of the most common and troublesome infections of infancy—thrush. While Berg was not the discoverer of the fungus responsible for thrush, his thorough description of the organism, conjoined with his study and replication of an artificial medium of its reproductive cycles, was an important contribution.[37]

Berg's lasting contribution to pediatrics was his modernization and realignment of statistical data gathering. In 1858 he resigned the chair of pediatrics to become director of the Central Bureau of Statistics. In that capacity he expanded the bureau's data banks to include not only population but also welfare, agricultural, and industrial data. He founded the journal *Statistisk Tidskrift* in 1869, and in that same year, utilizing parish records, he published a very important paper analyzing infant mortality rates in Sweden.[38]

In Germany, Karl Ludwig von Elsässer (1808–1894) wrote two major works on craniotabes, a softened-skull condition due to metabolic disease. The first, his thesis, appeared in 1837. The second, in 1843, contained a more representative clinical sample of 31 case reports.

Aberrations of the thymus, umbilicus, and genitalia and cephalohematomas were described by Carl Hennig (1825–1911). Hennig was one of the original contributors to Carl Gerhardt's *Handbuch der Kinderkrankheiten* (see below). He published his own text on childhood diseases in 1855.

A Swiss, Frédéric Rillet (1814–1861), wrote monographs on childhood typhoid fever, measles, mumps, and cholera. Additionally, he collaborated with a Parisian colleague, Antoine Charles Ernest Barthez (1811–1891) on the three-volume *Traité clinique et pratique des maladies des enfants*, completed in 1843. Ernest Bouchut (1818–1891) published *Manual pratique* in 1845, the first of six editions that classified childhood ailments and discoursed on hygiene and nutrition. He also published books on nervous diseases of infancy (1860) and on ophthalmoscopy (1876). Bouchut's success in employing intubation in the treatment of diphtheria anticipated by 30 years the adoption of the maneuver made popular by Joseph O'Dwyer.

Alois Bednar (1816–1888), a teacher at the University of Vienna, was the author of a treatise on the newborn (1850), a *Lehrbuch* (1856), and a monograph on the infant's diet (1857). He was considered by Jacobi to be "one of the most original scientific pediatrists of Europe,"[39] but later, memory of his accomplishments was overshadowed by the renown of Carl Gerhardt.

William John Little

In England, William John Little (1810–1894), in a paper published in *Lancet* in 1844, was the first to give a systematic analysis of cerebral palsy, the movement disorder associated with perinatal injury or insult. Little published many other works on deformities and on muscular dystrophies and scoliosis and wrote in support of William O'Shaughnessy's innovation of treating cholera with intravenous saline.* He is best remembered, however, for his work with the spastic diplegia of cerebral palsy:[40]

In many instances the spasmodic affection is produced at the moment of birth, or within a few hours or days of that event. In the majority of the cases of universal contracture of the upper and lower extremities which have fallen under my observation, the subjects were born at the seventh month, or prior to the end of the eighth month of uterogestation. In two cases the birth occurred at the full period of gestation, but owing to the difficulty and slowness of parturition the individuals were born in a state of asphyxia, resuscitation having been obtained, at the expiration of two and four hours, through the persevering efforts of the accoucheurs.

A second, detailed monograph on spastic diplegia, complete with photographs of cerebral-palsied children, appeared nearly 20 years later, in 1862, in *Transactions of the Obstetrical Society of London*. The paper's accurate neurological and somatotypical descriptions and its conclusions—still valid—are noteworthy:

A survey of the history of forty-seven cases, appended, shows that one fact is com-

---

*A major epidemic of Asiatic cholera struck the British Isles in 1831. From the Quay of Sunderland it spread to Scotland, Ireland, and France, where, in Paris, it claimed 19,000 lives. In 1832, London reported 11,020 cases and 5,275 deaths (Apt, 1945, p. 34).

William Brooke O'Shaughnessy (1809–1889), in an 1831 paper published in the *Lancet*, grippingly described the clinical symptoms of a patient with acute cholera, and suggested that intravenous fluids be employed as part of the treatment:

On the floor, extended on a palliasse . . . lay a girl of slender make and juvenile height, but with the face of a superannuated hag. She uttered no moan, gave expression of no pain, but she languidly flung herself from side to side. . . . The colour of her countenance was that of lead—a silver blue, ghastly tint; her eyes were sunk deep into the sockets, as though they had been driven an inch behind their natural position; her mouth was squared; her features flattened; her eyelids black; her fingers shrunk, bent and inky in their hue. All pulse was gone at the wrist, and a tenacious sweat moistened her bosom. . . . [T]he indications of cure . . . are two in number—1st to restore the blood to its natural specific gravity; 2nd to restore its deficient saline matters. . . . [T]he author recommends the injection into the veins of tepid water holding a solution of the normal salts of the blood. (Cosnett, 1989, pp. 768–71)

mon to all the cases of persistent spastic rigidity of new-born children, namely, that some abnormal circumstance attended the act of parturition.[41]

Charles West

Charles West (1816–1898), appointed physician to the London Children's Infirmary in 1842, published the first of seven editions of *Lectures on Diseases of Infancy and Childhood* in 1848. The book was translated into Spanish, French, German, Italian, and Arabic. West wrote that, initially, the book was

founded on the notes of 600 cases and 180 postmortem examinations, which I had observed at the dwellings of the poor in the district where I labored. . . . I have been able in each successive edition to add to the preceding one, and I trust to improve upon it. The present edition embodies the results of 1,200 cases, and nearly 400 postmortem examinations, collected between 30,000 and 40,000 children.[42]

West also published *How to Nurse Sick Children* in 1852 and *A Mother's Manual of Children's Diseases* in 1885. In contrast to Billard, he classified diseases according to the old Salerian system, *a capite ad calcem*.

West is best known for founding the Hospital for Sick Children on Great Ormond Street in 1852. With the help of Henry Bence-Jones (1814–1873), West obtained the erstwhile residence of Richard Mead (1673–1754) and transformed it into a new 10-bed hospital. The drawing room and a larger room, respectively, became female and male wards, and the ballroom was the site of the ambulatory clinic.[43]

All manner of children with all manner of ailments were admitted, but the most common admission diagnosis was that of rickets. In 1865, writing in his *Lectures*, West noted that 30 percent of the patients had signs of rickets. By 1898 that statistic had increased to 50 percent.[44]

Garrison's encomium of West still could be description of a model pediatrician. West, he wrote, was

[one who] took his profession with priest-like seriousness. . . . Children stopped crying and came to him at once. Through a charming ritual, with marvelous toys, of which the drawers of his office desk were full, he had no difficulty in making the most accurate diagnosis. . . . [He] wrote the most palatable prescriptions and never gave a medicine which he had not previously tasted himself.[45]

Fleetwood Churchill

In 1850 an Irishman, Fleetwood Churchill (1808–1878), published a detailed and thorough volume on all aspects of childhood diseases, entitled

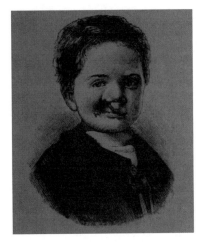

Figure 8.2 Noma. Ashby's *Diseases of Children, Medical and Surgical*, 1889.

On the Diseases of Infants and Children. There is a remarkably long chapter on what commonly was called "noma," also referred to as cancrum oris, gangrene of the mouth, or stomatite gangreneuse (figure 8.2). The term "noma" appears to have first been used in Cornelius Roelan's *Buchlein* (1483)[46] and refers to the devouring gangrene following measles or other debilitating diseases, complicated by scurvy. Churchill's description of septic cellulitis and necrosis is a graphic reminder of the horrific complications that commonly followed routine illnesses before the advent of antibiotics:

In the severe form, the disease always commences in the mucous membrane, preceded by stomatitis, aphthae or ulcerations of the gums, lips, or inside the cheeks . . . the bottom of the ulcer becomes covered with a gray matter evidently gangrenous and the subjacent tissues are swollen and hard . . . from this moment, the ulcerations extend rapidly; at first of a grayish color, they shortly become brown and black, covered with "putrilage" of a fetid odor, and bleeding when touched . . . the portions of the mucous membranes of the mouth in contact with the gangrenous spots become likewise affected, and run the same destructive course. In all directions, the disease extends fearfully, laying bare and destroying the bones.[47]

Herbert Barker

Concerned that "half of all children born in England die before they reach their fifth birthday,"[48] Herbert Barker (1814–1865) in 1859 published *On the Hygienic Management of Infants and Children*:

[T]he newborn infant should be warmly wrapped in flannel. . . . Careful washings should be performed daily. . . . [O]n no account should the infant be submitted to *cold* bathing during the first few weeks of its existence. . . . [T]he early period of infancy is passed in sleep [and] the only natural interruption to repose is the feeling of hunger. . . . There can be no need of artificial food, if, during the first five or six months, the infant is applied to the breast at regular intervals of about three or four hours, by night as well as by day.[49]

In France, Paul Louis Benoit Guersant (1800–1869) served on the surgical staff of the Hôpital des Enfants Malades and in 1864 wrote a text on pediatric surgery that was translated into several languages. It was published in English in Philadelphia in 1873, translated by Robley J. Dunglison (1798–1869), a respected English physician who, in 1824, had accepted Thomas Jefferson's invitation to join the faculty at the University of Virginia.[50] Dunglison by then had already published his own book, *Children's Diseases*.

Guersant's book, *Surgical Diseases of Infants and Children*, 350 pages, covered mixed surgical disciplines from bone to eye to plastic, and so on. A chapter was given over to each condition, yet, unusual in a surgical text, there was not one single illustration. Some of the chapter headings follow:

Cervical adenitis	Coxalgia
Phimosis	Ear foreign bodies
Fractures	Cataracts
Tracheostomy	Hernia repair
Hypertrophy of tonsils	Imperforate anus
Polyps of rectum	Cancer of the eye
Vascular tumor	Club foot
Cysts	Encephalocele
Vesicular calculus	Cephalohaematoma
Hydrocele	Hypospadias
Prolapsed ani	Ranula
Chronic arthritis	Osteitis
Burns	Dislocations
Harelip	Spina bifida
Ozaena (nasal ulcerations)	Gum lancing

A succinct two-page chapter discoursed on both general—chloroform and ether—and local anesthesia:

[W]e make an application either of ice or of the vapour of ether. We pulverize the ice and mix it . . . with a third part of gray salt and place this mixture either in a little gauze bag, or in a gold beater's skin, and apply the bag over the part we wish to render insensible, a result which follows at the end of three or four minutes.[51]

As evidenced by the chapter on gum lancing, anesthesia was not always used:

To perform this operation, it is necessary that an assistant shall hold the child's head firmly; the operator then separates its cheek with a finger of his left hand, hold in his right hand a bistoury.[52]

Marie Jules Joseph Parrot (1829–1883) wrote an extensive work on marasmus called *L'athrepsie* (1877), describing the debilitation and complications of the condition. He also published extensive monographs on congenital syphilis, the most original of which was on pseudoparalysis of newborn lues, written in 1872. He and colleagues Victor Hutinel (1849–1933), Antonin Marfan (1858–1942), and Joseph Grancher (1843–1907) are considered by historian Robert Laplane[53] to be the founders of modern French pediatrics.

In 1884, as sole author, Londoner Eustace Smith (1835–1914) published a singular book of 884 pages—an extraordinary size for a pediatric text. Smith's comprehensive coverage of disorders is illustrated by part 9, on the digestive tract. One hundred pages were divided into chapters on marasmus, gastritis, constipation, diarrhea, hemorrhage, obstruction, typhlitis, peritonitis, tuberculosis, ascites, and parasitoses. Part 10 covered diseases of the liver and was divided into chapters on jaundice, congestion, cirrhosis, amyloid, fatty liver, and hydatid diseases. The book was modern in contents and scope in many respects. With regard to the normal parameters of child health and growth, it was, in company with the literature of predecessors, woefully inadequate, glossing over these aspects in a mere 20 pages.[54]

Harald Hirschsprung (1830–1916), chief physician at the Queen Louise Children's Hospital in Copenhagen, published a monograph on hypertrophy of the colon in the *Jahrbuch für Kinderheilkunde* (1887), using data from autopsies of two babies, 7 and 11 months old:

I will at once present the first specimen. As you see it is a colon, but of surprising size considering it is from a child who died at eleven months of age. As the abdomen was opened there appeared a pair of enormously distended coils of intestine, the S. Romanum and the ever still more dilated transverse colon. The rest of the large intestine was enlarged and the rectum was not only dilated but was the seat of a small constriction. The described parts of the intestine are not only distended but the wall markedly thickened in all its layers and particularly in the muscular part. . . .

What symptoms did this remarkable disease of the colon cause?

Immediately after the birth of the child, which took place in a lying-in institution in Copenhagen, it showed the peculiarity that in spite of various laxatives it had no stool. Only after repeated enemas did the bowels move. The same sluggish action of the bowel continued in the following months and the various remedies had to be used changing from one to the other, but when it was possible to cause a stool it was of a normal consistence and appearance.[55]

Hirschsprung published four case histories of esophageal atresia with tracheoesophageal fistula (1861). His most important report was on controlled hydrostatic reduction of ileocecal intussusception (1876), using enema therapy. Of the 84 children Hirschsprung treated only with enema, 65 (77%) survived. Surgical intervention at the time carried an 80 percent mortality risk.[56]

Carl Gerhardt

Wolfgang Braun (1991) credits the development of German pediatrics to Carl Gerhardt (1833–1902). Gerhardt published two important books: *Pädiatrik Lehrbuch* in 1861 and *Handbuch der Kinderkrankheiten* in 1877. The 16-volume, 7,000-page *Handbuch*, published between 1877 and 1893, with contributions from 56 of the most prominent pediatricians of the time,[57] was the most complete textbook of pediatrics of its era. In volume 7 of his own *Collectanea Jacobi*, Jacobi wrote of the *Handbuch*:

There is hardly any work in any language whatsoever which has advanced practical medicine to so great a degree. Certainly none which has so firmly established the right of pediatrics in the minds and acts of scientists and practitioners.[58]

In a speech before the Pediatric Section of the Gesellschaft für Heilkunde in 1879, Gerhardt cited the need for both the anatomical and physiological study of the child, because "differences between the developing and the developed body are less a question of structure than of function."[59]

Etienne-Louis Fallot (1850–1911) described the congenital heart lesion that bears his name, the tetralogy of Fallot.[60] Marked by pulmonic stenosis, ventricular septal defect, right ventricular hypertrophy, and aortic dextroposition, the French called this lesion the *maladie bleue* because of the intense cyanosis associated with the malformation. Another authority on congenital heart disease was Carl von Rokitansky (1804–1878), who published *Die Defecte der Scheidewände des Herzens* in 1875. Rokitansky was the first to distinguish clearly between ostium primum and secundum defects of the atriae.

Eduard Henoch

Eduard Heinrich Henoch (1820–1910), a student of Johann Schönlein (1793–1864) and Moritz Romberg (1795–1873), directed the pediatric clinic at the Berlin Charité for 20 years. He applied his comprehensive fund of knowledge to a three-volume text on abdominal diseases, published in 1853; the *Beiträge zur Kinderheilkunde* was published in 1861. In 1864 he translated Charles West's textbook into German. Henoch's lectures on children's diseases were published in 1868 and were translated into English, Russian, and French.

Now best remembered by the disease that carries his name, in his time Henoch was a preeminent German pediatrician who published widely and prolifically on the ailments of children. His discussion in *Vorlesungen über Kinderkrankheiten* (1881) on the differential diagnosis of purpura is responsible for its being referred to thereafter as Henoch-Schönlein purpura.[61] This childhood disorder is marked by hemorrhage into the skin, joint pain, colic, and bloody stools and is followed at times by glomerulonephritis:[62]

There is at present no explanation for the undoubted connection of the purpura with the pains and swellings in the limbs and joints. . . . [The] etiological factor is especially absent in a more complicated form, in which, in addition to previously mentioned symptoms, vomiting, intestinal hemorrhage, and colic are also present. I have observed five cases belonging to this variety.

Henoch described the five cases, noting that, after several relapses over a period of a month, all recovered spontaneously. He observed that "serious accidents occurred rarely" but that

These rare cases may terminate fatally after lasting from a month to a year, in consequence of exhaustion complicated by anasarca and dropsy of the cavities or suddenly by hemorrhage into a vital organ, especially the brain.

The successor to Henoch at the Charité was Otto Heubner (1843–1926). Heubner's insights about infectious diseases warrant meritorious mention. His renown among his peers and students, however, derived mainly from the bedside teaching he inaugurated. In 1876, as head of the Leipzig polyclinic, he began visiting the sick in their homes. Gradually, he invited students to accompany him, and they learned to take patient histories, perform physical examinations, record, and prognosticate. Heubner's "hands-on" teaching method at patients' bedsides became so popular that student attendance had to be limited to 25 per semester.[63]

Adolf Baginsky (1843–1918) studied under Rudolf Virchow (1821–1902). He established a polyclinic for children in 1872 in Berlin. He and

Virchow founded the Kaiserin Friedrich Kinderkrankhaus in 1890, considered at the time to be Europe's finest hospital. Baginsky wrote a handbook
on school hygiene (1883), a textbook on children's diseases that had eight
editions, and many monographs. His major contribution to pediatrics is
considered to be the journal he published with the Viennese Alois Monti
(1839–1909)—the *Central-Zeitung für Kinderheilkunde*. Lasting two years,
the journal was followed by another, *Archiv für Kinderheilkunde*, which is
still published.

Johann Theodor August Steffen (1825–1909) was physician-in-chief at
the Stettin Children's Hospital, Germany. He published prolifically, including the book *Klinik der Kinderkrankheiten* in 1895 and extensive monographs on child pathology (1901) and on tumors (1905). He was a contributor to Gerhardt's *Handbuch* and coeditor with Mayr of *Jahrbuch für
Kinderheilkunde*. Steffen was instrumental in the establishment of formal
pediatric curricula in the German medical schools.[64]

Austrian Max Kassowitz (1842–1913) was a major investigator into the
etiology and therapy of rickets. Kassowitz wrote on varicella, variola,
syphilis, dentition, and therapeutics. His magnum opus was a three-volume
study on the aberrant calcification evident in rickets (1881), for which he
proposed phosphorus as a treatment.

As professor of pediatrics at the University of Naples, Francesco Fede
(1832–1913) campaigned for the teaching of pediatrics as a specialty. He
wrote extensively on anemia, marasmus, and kidney diseases, and he established the journal *La Pediatria* in 1893. His compatriot Luigi Somma
(1834–1884) founded another journal of prominence, *Archivio di Patologia
Infantile*, in 1883.

In Bohemia, Alois Epstein (1849–1918) was professor of pediatrics at
Prague University and director of the Infant's Asylum of Prague. He championed asylum reforms and nursery care. Epstein's name is associated with
the small, benign hard-palate retention cysts in the mouths of newborns—
Epstein's pearls. His place in pediatric history, however, is secured by the several outstanding pediatricians he trained, among them Czerny, Moll,
Meyerhofer, and Fischl.[65]

Karl Rauchfuss (1835–1915), the Russian, already mentioned in connection with hospitals for children, became the Tzar's pediatrist. As director of
St. Petersburg's Children's Hospital he organized and taught courses specifically for female medical students.[66] He wrote many monographs on congenital heart disease, arthritis, and croup. Most important, the chapter he
wrote for Gerhardt's *Handbuch* advanced both hospital design and function,
as he insisted on strict isolation protocols for the treatment of infectious children. His Russian colleague Nil Féodorovich Filatoff (1847–1902) was

appointed professor of pediatrics on the Moscow faculty and director of the Chludoff Children's Hospital in 1876. His contributions in infectious diseases were many, but he made his mark in pediatrics as president of the Moscow Society of Pediatrics. In this position he was able to keep children's health issues a major political agenda item for the 10 years of his tenure.

Bernard Jean Antonin Marfan (1858–1942) collaborated with Jacques Grancher (1843–1907) and Jules Comby (1853–1947) on the five-volume work called *Traité des maladies de l'enfance* (1897). Marfan also wrote a book on infantile nutrition called *Traité de l'allaitment* in 1899. To the student of medicine, his name is synonymous with the inherited disorder of connective tissue marked by eye, heart, and skeletal abnormalities—Marfan's syndrome.

Surgical books devoted exclusively to the child started appearing in the latter half of the century. Appropriately, each had a chapter or section given over to anesthesia.

Despite early recognition of the differences between child and adult tolerance and clearance of anesthetic agents, the discipline of pediatric anesthesiology did not come into being until the middle of the twentieth century. Downes cites the first recorded instance of child anesthesia, by Crawford W. Long (1815–1878), nearly 100 years earlier, in 1842:[67]

My third experiment in etherization was made on the 3rd July, 1842, and was on a negro boy, the property of Mrs. S. Hemphill, who resides nine miles from Jefferson. The boy had a disease of the toe, which rendered its amputation necessary, and the operation was performed without the boy evincing the least sign of pain.

Englishman John Snow (1813–1858) began in 1847 to routinely anesthetize children, ages 4 through 16, with ether. Snow experimented with chloroform and by 1857 had successfully anesthetized hundreds of children, among them 186 infants under the age of one year. Snow observed the differences in agent metabolism between adults and children: "The effects of chloroform are more quickly produced and also subside more quickly than in adults, owing no doubt to quicker breathing and circulation."[68]

Alexander Wilson presented sensible guidelines on pediatric anesthesia in a chapter of a book published by Henry Ashby (1845–1908) and surgeon Arthur Wright (1851–1920) in 1889, *The Diseases of Children, Medical and Surgical*:

Cocaine, used subcutaneously, is objectionable from its mode of administration and on account of the symptoms it sometimes causes, and is not recommended for children.

For minor operations nitrous oxide gas is well borne by children; by giving a little ether along with the gas a more prolonged anaesthesia is produced.[69]

Apart from Wilson's innovations in anesthesia, Ashby and Wright's book was a traditional tome, classifying, for example, fever as a disease category rather than as a nonspecific symptom. Scarlet fever, measles, rubella, diphtheria, typhus, varicella, vaccinia, whooping cough, mumps, and malaria all were relegated to Ashby's chapter, "Fevers."

Ashby, an appointed lecturer in physiology at the Manchester Hospital for Sick Children from 1879 until his death nearly 30 years later, is remembered predominantly for his work in preventive medicine and infant welfare and with mentally impaired children.

James Frederick Goodhart

The English pathologist James Frederick Goodhart (1845–1916) published *A Student's Guide to the Diseases of Children*. The first of 10 editions was published in 1885 and translated into French. Somewhat uniquely, Goodhart presented pediatric subjects from a pathological perspective. He defined each disease and presented symptoms, morbid anatomy, prognosis, and treatment. Goodhart described, for example, the anatomical anomalies attributed to cretinism, although the thyroid deficiency that caused the condition was unknown at the time:*

The bones of the skull are thick, the sutures abnormally obliterated, and the various foramina are liable to narrowing. Great importance is attached by some to premature union of the basal suture, by which it is not unreasonably supposed that the growth of the skull, and therefore, of the brain, would be seriously interfered with. The condition of the long bones is also peculiar; their cartilaginous ends being enormously out of proportion to the stunted shafts.[70]

Samuel Gee

Samuel Gee (1839–1911), assistant physician at the Great Ormond Street Hospital for Sick Children and at St. Bartholomew Hospital in London, published a series of monographs in the *St. Bartholomew Hospital Reports* between 1880 and 1888 that are worthy of mention. He studied head-shaking seizures in infants and toddlers, the head-banging syndrome, and what must be the most exquisite description of celiac disease ever written:

---

*The causes and mechanisms of congenital hypothyroidism were unknown. Many children were treated orally with raw, ground thyroid. A quarter lobe of fresh minced sheep thyroid mixed with rice jam was given twice a week to patients. Despite the nauseating effects and wretched vomiting sometimes elicited, this thyroid extract was administered as described until 1893, when Burroughs and Wellcome produced a tablet form (Lomax, 1996, p. 99).

On the Coeliac Affection

There is a kind of chronic indigestion which is met with in persons of all ages, yet is especially apt to affect children between one and five years old. Signs of the disease are yielded by the faeces; being loose, not formed, but not watery; more bulky than the food taken would seen to account for; pale in colour, as if devoid of bile; yeasty, frothy, an appearance probably due to fermentation; stinking, stench often very great, the food having undergone putrefaction rather that concoction. . . .

The patient wastes more in the limbs than in the face, which often remains plump until death is nigh. In the limbs, emaciation is at first more apparent to hand than to eye, the flesh feeling soft and flabby. Muscular weakness great: muscular tenderness often present.

Cachexia, a fault of sanguification, betokened by pallor and tendency to dropsy, is a constant symptom: the patients become white and puffy; the loss of colour sometimes such as to resemble the cachectic hue of ague or splenic disease: the spleen is sometimes enlarged.[71]

While Thomas Barlow (1845–1945) lived well-nigh into the middle of the twentieth century, his major contributions to pediatric medicine occurred before the turn of the century. He was a consulting physician at the Hospital for Sick Children in London and a careful and thorough anatomist who, not uncommonly, performed autopsies immediately after death in the patient's home! He published his meticulous observations in a paper written with Samuel Gee in 1878, in which he demonstrated that purulent meningitis could be separated from the tuberculous form solely on clinical grounds.*

Barlow wrote on a number of topics—pleurisy, syphilis, rheumatism—but his seminal work was on scurvy. In 1883 he published a paper on "acute rickets," in which he proved the condition was combined rickets and scurvy. Barlow reported exhaustive autopsy data on 31 cases. He suggested a simple and easy-to-follow remedy for the condition: fruit juices offered to infants after the age of six months.[72]

Another great pediatric anatomist was J. W. Ballantyne (1861–1923) of Edinburgh, who in 1891 published a three-volume work entitled *An Introduction to the Diseases of Infancy*. A thoroughly original work, there were five chapters on infant pathology. Examining frozen-tissue sections, Ballan-

---

*The use of diagnostic lumbar puncture, today a routine procedure in the assessment and treatment of meningitis, was viewed with suspicion and done with trepidation. Heinrich Quincke (1842–1922) introduced the procedure in 1891 as a treatment for the relief of hydrocephalic pressures. Its value, however, in the diagnosis of purulent meningitis was noted in 1896 by an American, August Caillé (1854–1935), and was performed thereafter primarily for diagnostic purposes.

tyne took notice of the cellular hyperplasia and hypertrophy of the growing organism.[73]

PEDIATRICS IN THE UNITED STATES

Some exchange of medical data between Europe and the United States occurred in the nineteenth century, but generally study, research, clinical application and published materials took place independently. It certainly also can be said that great import was given to data and books of European origin. Nevertheless, original textbooks of pediatrics appeared in significant numbers in America; some are listed in table 8.2.

Samuel Adams (1853–1928),[74] in a paper presented in 1897, credited an anonymous writer, American Matron, with the first comprehensive text on pediatrics in the United States, *The Maternal Physician: A Treatise on the Nurture and Management of Infants . . .*, published in Philadelphia in 1810. In the book, "Matron" acknowledged the authors whom she liberally had quoted (Buchan, Locke, and Underwood among them), but unqualified tribute was reserved for maternal common sense: "[T]hese gentlemen must pardon me if I think, after all, that a mother is her child's best physician, in all ordinary cases."[75]

The book provided a pharmacopeia of "simples"—botanicals—to treat common child ailments and encouraged aggressive invasive procedures, such as routine gum lancing and cutting of the frenulum to prevent "tongue-tie."

Adams attributed the second American treatise on pediatrics to George Logan (1778–1861), who was chief of service at the Charleston Orphan House for 40 years.[76] Logan published *Practical Observations on Diseases of Children, Comprehending a Description of Complaints and Disorders Incident to the Early Stages of Life, and Method of Treatment* in 1825.

Logan, describing the common practice of coagulating the umbilical stump with manure, identified this procedure as the probable cause of newborn tetany. He also dismissed the opinions that climate and "passions" caused the condition. Furthermore, he noted that the condition acquired in adults through puncture wounds was the same as that of newborn tetany. These observations alone assure him a place in Western pediatric history:*

[Tetany] attacks children about the close of the first week, and seldom after the ninth day, and is commonly believed to proceed from unskillful management of the umbilical cord.[77]

---

*Readers will recall that the Chinese recorded this observation in 1156 as *Ch'i feng* (chap. 2).

TABLE 8.2
SOME NINETEENTH-CENTURY AMERICAN PEDIATRIC PUBLICATIONS

American Matron	*The Maternal Physician*	1810
George Logan	*Practical Observations . . . Diseases of Children*	1825
William Dewees	*A Treatise . . . Medical Treatment of Children*	1826
Joseph Flint	*. . . [O]n the Prophylactic Management of Infancy . . .*	1826
M. Page	*An Essay on the Diseases of Children*	1829
John Eberle	*Treatise . . . Diseases and Physical Education*	1833
W. W. Gerhard	*Cases of Rubeola, Followed by Death*	1833
J. T. Lewis	*Diseases and Management of Children*	1837
James Stewart	*Diseases of Children*	1841
D. Francis Condie	*A Practical Treatise . . . Diseases of Children*	1844
John F. Meigs	*A Practical Treatise . . . Diseases of Children*	1848
John B. Beck	*Essay on Infant Therapeutics*	1848
Charles D. Meigs	*Observations on . . . Diseases of Young Children*	1850
Philopedes (J. Stewart)	*. . . [A]bout Sick Children . . .*	1852
Abraham Jacobi	*Contributions to Midwifery . . . Children*	1859
	Therapeutics of Infancy and Childhood	1895
Job L. Smith	*Treatise on Diseases of Infants and Children*	1869
C. H. F. Routh	*Infant Feeding and Its Influence on Life . . .*	1879
Henry Ashby	*The Diseases of Children, Medical and Surgical*	1885
Louis Starr	*Hygiene for the Nursery*	1888
	. . . Diseases of Children by American Teachers	1894
John Keating	*Cyclopedia of the Diseases of Children . . .*	1889
F. Forchheimer	*Diseases of the Mouth in Children*	1892
L. Emmet Holt	*Care and Feeding of Children*	1894
	Diseases of Infants and Children	1896
B. Sachs	*A Treatise on the Nervous Diseases of Children*	1895
Thomas M. Rotch	*Pediatrics*	1895
Bernard Sachs	*Treatise on the Nervous Diseases of Children*	1895

The causes are, punctured wounds inflicted by nails, splinters of wood, &c. near the flexors of the toes, or fingers, or through the tendenious expansions. . . . Writers also mention, cold and moisture applied to the body when heated, as lying in the cool, damp place; as also certain passions of the mind, &c. I have, however, witnessed many cases, and, in every instance, the disease could be traced to one of the first causes only.[78]

Prior to 1815, there had been no large studies or accurate assessments of newborn heights and weights in Europe or America.[79] In reiterating the average measurements of the newborn, Logan reinforced understanding of the normal: "A child, when born, after the full term of uterogestation, will weigh from six to seven pounds, and will ordinarily measure from twenty to twenty-two inches in length."[80]

William Dewees

William Dewees (1768–1841) wrote the first truly comprehensive and authoritative American pediatric work in 1826, called *A Treatise of the Physical and Medical Treatment of Children*. There were eight editions of this popular, straightforward, and practical guide to child care. Although the text did not present groundbreaking concepts or remedies, it was a valuable reference for physician colleagues as they, with temerity, attempted to treat pediatric patients. Dewees did much to dispel their fears:

The belief that the diseases of children almost constantly present nothing but perplexing obscurity or embarrassing uncertainty, has much retarded the progress of inquiry, by engendering doubts of their susceptibility of successful investigation, lucid explanation, or useful arrangement; and of course, that every prescribed remedy has but an uncertain aim; and consequently a contingent, or doubtful effect. We are far from entertaining such opinions; and we are most anxious, so far as our feeble efforts may have power, to banish them from the minds, not only of the medical practitioner, but from all who may entertain them—for they are unworthy of the one, and painful to the other.[81]

American Practitioner

A text published in New Hampshire in 1826 under the pseudonym "American Practitioner" is an example of how closely linked were the disciplines of pediatrics and obstetrics in the first quarter of the nineteenth century. Significant consideration of infant and child ailments often appeared in books on midwifery. Such was the case with the American Practitioner's *London Practice of Midwifery . . . and Principal Infantile Diseases*. William Dewees, as a respected obstetrician and pediatrist, was a constant source reference:

The editor has freely availed himself on the labours of all writers on midwifery, particularly . . . Dewees . . . whose correct and discriminating judgment is unquestioned, and whose opinions are generally received as the best authority, he would acknowledge a special obligation.[82]

The index of the book lists two chapters on child matters:

XIII   1. Food of Infants   2. Symptoms of Health and Disease
        3. Gestures   4. Skin
        5. Respiration

XIV   1. Inflammation of the Eyes 2. Jaundice
        3. Indigestion/Green stools   4. Infantile Fevers
        5. Spina Bifida   6. Abdominal Tumor
        7. Worms   8. Hydrocephalus internus
        9. Scald head   10. Convulsions
        11. Cyanche Trachealis   12. Marasmus

The book offered common wisdom and widely accepted principles of the time intended for use where midwifery and pediatric care were unavailable. The chapters were short, and the references to authorities were extensive. On occasion, differing views were related, as with the treatment of jaundice:

Armstrong, Burns, Underwood and others recommend the treatment to begin with a gentle emetic, but Dewees is opposed to the practice. If repeated and gentle purges of caster oil do not bring down the bilious faeces he gives calomel in small doses until a cathartic effect be produced.[83]

The American Practitioner championed the special needs of infants and children. The chapters on children concluded with a strong appeal to physicians to acquire acumen and experience on child health issues. The admonishments to do so appealed to conscience, pride, and purse:

With this we conclude our account of the diseases of children; and earnestly advise those medical men who have not had much experience in them, to lose no time in obtaining a practical knowledge of their varieties.

The little sufferers are unable to tell us what ails them, and it is not infrequently that the most able and experienced practitioner is deceived in his conjectures. What then must be the perplexity of him, who is nearly ignorant of the diseases of children? He acts with uncertainty and indecision; the friends of the child discover his want of experience, and justly apply to those who are more intelligent in their profession.[84]

Eli Ives

A contemporary of Dewees, Eli Ives (1779–1861) introduced the first formal American academic course in pediatrics[85] at the Yale College of Medicine in 1813. Ives offered the 49 lectures of the course every morning at 10 A.M., six days a week between October and December for 40 years. Several complete sets of handwritten student notes have survived, allowing a composite picture of the materia medica that Ives included. Although Ives was an advocate of polypharmacy and an interventionist, he was not an innovator; and from his lectures, he does not seem to have been an exceptional diagnostician. He had, however, an extensive fund of knowledge, and confidence in his aptitude in treating children. His course began with a strong justification for the need to study the diseases and the treatment of children:[86]

I propose . . . to treat of the habits, diseases and remedies of the infantile state. The subject has received less attention from enlightened physicians than other branches of Medical Science. The causes which have prevented full attention are, in fact, these. From the prejudices that prevail in society, the function of Midwifery has been to a considerable extent, taken from the Physician, and in common with this are the diseases of the infantile state. Nurses have been commonly preferred to regular physicians. Hence, Physicians have paid less attention to the subject. . . .

The difficulty of acquiring a knowledge of the seat of disease in infants arises from their inability to communicate their sensations by language. This has been an excuse (an inadequate one) with some Physicians for neglecting the subject. This very difficulty ought to be an argument in favor of committing the subject to men of science. Although children cannot communicate their sensations by language, yet the symptoms of their diseases are more uniform and more certain in their indications than those of adults. Nothing is concealed by falsehood, reserve, or false modesty, or fear for the event. The Physician does not find, as he sometimes does in the case of adults, the statement of the patient contradicted by the symptoms of the disease. The mind does not, in these cases, react upon the system or the disease to produce nervous excitement.

Two important teachers in early-nineteenth-century America who had won renown were educators of handicapped children.[87] Emulating the example of French educators Havy and l'Epeé, Minister Thomas Hopkins Gallaudet (1787–1851) and ex–naval surgeon Samuel Gridley Howe (1801–1876) devoted their lives to this endeavor.

Gallaudet studied in Paris at the Institut Royal des Sourds-Muet. When he returned to the United States in 1817, he established the first free American school for the deaf, the Connecticut Asylum for the Education and Instruction of the Deaf and Dumb Persons.

Howe served with the Greek navy in a war with Turkey. He returned to Boston in 1831 to direct the New England Asylum for the Education of the Blind. Abandoning the practice of medicine, he became an educator of blind children and a legendary figure. To better understand sightlessness and give students optimum practical instruction, Howe blindfolded himself for hours. Howe's example and success paved the way for a universally accepted goal of education for handicapped children.

John Eberle (1788–1838) published his *Treatise on the Diseases and Physical Education of Children* in 1833. Eberle warned against alcohol ingestion during pregnancy, observing that "the majority of children born of decidedly intemperate mothers, are weak and sickly, and but a few of them arrive at the age of adolescence."[88] He debunked the theory that anomalies were imparted by maternal transference to their young,* and he spurned the cold dipping advocated by Locke:[89]

The *maternal imagination* has been accused of producing the most extraordinary effects on the foetus in utero. During the early and middle ages, it was almost universally believed, that malformations, moles, and other unnatural appearances, were very generally produced by the influence of the imagination of mothers. . . .
Absurdities of this gross and glaring character are now but little entertained even by the most superstitious and ignorant.

Historian Thomas Cone points out that both Benjamin Rush and Eberle made the observation that children developed a craving for salt during the recovery phase after cholera infantum, due, most probably, to hyponatremic dehydration[90]:

The little patient sometimes manifests a most urgent craving, for certain strong and stimulating articles of food, such as salted and smoked herring or shad, old and rancid bacon, and salted beef.[91]

James Stewart (1799–1864) published *Diseases of Children* in 1841. Stewart broke away from the prevailing provinciality of his American colleagues, which had prompted Dewees to comment that some illnesses "are entirely unknown in this country."[92] Stewart looked to Europe for current data, and his was the first American text to publish Laennec's concepts of auscultation and up-to-date postmortem findings as reported in France.

Another of his books, *A Few Remarks about Sick Children and the Necessity of a Hospital for Them*, was published under the pseudonym Philopedes and resulted in the establishment of the New York Nursery and Children's Hospital in 1894 (which subsequently merged with Babies Hospital).

---

*Some physicians themselves promulgated superstitions. As late as 1900, obstetrician Emma Drake advised the *enceinte* to "look at beautiful pictures, study perfect pieces of statuary and forbid as far as possible the contemplation of unsightly and imperfect models . . . [so as to produce] beautiful, vigourous children" (Camp, 1973, pp. 19–20).

David Francis Condie (1796–1875) published *A Practical Treatise on the Diseases of Children* in 1844. Its popularity was extensive and lasted beyond 1868, when the sixth edition was issued.

Some confusion indubitably resulted from the appearance, in 1848, of another popular text with the same title. Of the two, the book written by John Forsyth Meigs (1818–1882)[93] was the more significant and original. By the author's own admission, the contents were largely derived from Rilliet and Barthez, and "the author has constantly consulted the works of Underwood, Dewees, Eberle, Stewart, Condie, Billard, Barrier, Berton, Bouchut, Breachet, and Valleix."[94] However, Meigs devised an ordered, descriptive classification system, unique in his time and now commonplace: the study of diseases classified by definition, synonym, frequency of occurrence, causes, pathology, symptoms, diagnosis, treatment, and prognosis.

In 1848, John Brodhead Beck (1794–1851) published *Essay on Infant Therapeutics*, in which he described the effects of opium (which was in common use) on infants and children. Beck strongly recommended against its use:

With regards to the effects of opium on young subjects, there are two facts which seem to be well established. The first is, that it acts with *much greater energy* on the infant than it does on the adult; the second is, that it is more *uncertain* in its action on the infant than the adult. . . . [I]ts use should be avoided as much as possible in the young subject . . . great caution should be exercised in the *form* in which it is administered. No preparation should ever be used, which is not of a known and determined strength.[95]

Of mercury, most commonly given as calomel (Hg_2Cl_2) he cautioned:

The too common practice of giving calomel as an ordinary purge, on all occasions, is certainly unjustifiable . . . in very young children, mercury ought never to be used as a cathartic, unless there is a special reason for resorting to it.[96]

Beck's wariness regarding the bloodletting of pediatric patients was expressed as a "great caution":

Great caution should be exercised in bleeding children to the point of syncope. . . . [T]o determine the precise amount of blood proper to be drawn, is a matter of much greater necessity; and involves more serious consequences in the child than in the adult. . . . From uncertainty in estimating the quantity of blood lost by leeches,[97] and the dangers attending the loss of too much from them in children, too great caution cannot be exercised in their use.[98]

Abraham Jacobi

The first children's clinic in New York was established by Abraham Jacobi (1830–1919) in 1860. A quintessential teacher and clinician, Jacobi was, as already mentioned, instrumental in the establishment of children's hospitals in the United States. A professor of pediatrics in New York for nearly half a century, his appointment as professor of infantile pathology and therapeutics at the New York Medical College is believed to have been the first academic pediatric appointment in America.

In 1880, Jacobi organized the Pediatric Section of the American Medical Association (AMA). Emphasizing the need for specific and systematic training in pediatric medicine, Jacobi wrote:

There are anomalies and diseases which are met within the infant and child only. . . . Therapeutics of infancy and childhood are by no means so similar to those of the adult that the rules of the latter can simply be adopted to the former by reducing doses. The differences are many.[99]

Jacobi presciently foresaw the emergence of pediatric study as an integral component of medical education:

Every future improvement in general medical education will favor the study of pediatrics. There will be a time in the near future when the student in medicine will be aware that he will have to pass an examination in the subjects connected with the physiology and pathology of the young. There will be another time when the medical courses will be both long and numerous enough to permit the clinical instruction in the diseases of children being given three or six times a week, and another in which there will be bedside teaching.[100]

In 1909, Jacobi's published works were organized into eight volumes. Among the more important monographs were studies on diphtheria and intubation, intestinal obstructions, and infant nutrition. A prolific writer, Jacobi published books on teething, intestinal diseases, the thymus gland, and a three-edition book on infant diet. He also was a contributor to Gerhardt's *Handbuch*. His greatest academic achievement, however, was lobbying Congress to appropriate funds for the printing of the *Index Medicus*,[101] compiled by John Shaw Billings (1838–1913).*

Clinically, Jacobi advocated the insufflation of air to treat intussusception, a modality of treatment that fell into disfavor but now is back in vogue. He

---

*Jacobi was a good friend of Billings, who in 1865 became director of the Library of the Army Surgeon General. Billings spent 30 years expanding the collection of what would become the National Library of Medicine of the National Institutes of Health.

devised a handheld mirror for indirect laryngoscopy, and he was the first American doctor to make use of the new roentgen ray.[102] He was an ardent opponent of unnecessary tonsillectomies and the routine and heavy use of calomel.

Jacobi, a social and political activist, used the bully pulpit to agitate for reform. With reference to a boy he had treated for pneumonia, he said:

A boy of 12 should not work in a coal mine at 4 cents an hour and the 4 cents withheld from him and his starving family on account of a debt incurred by his father who was killed in the same coal mine. Perhaps you can convince the commonwealth more if you doctors would go into politics.[103]

Jacobi was named first chair of the AMA section on pediatrics in 1871 and president of the New York Academy of Medicine in 1885. A founding member of the American Pediatric Society in 1888, he became president of the AMA in 1912. In the words of his friend and colleague Jerome Leopold, Jacobi was one "who has done more than any other physician to place pediatrics in American on a firm and lasting basis."[104] He was, in no small measure, the Father of American Pediatrics.

Job Lewis Smith

Job Lewis Smith (1827–1897),[105] a contemporary of Jacobi, was named professor of morbid anatomy in 1861 at Bellevue Hospital and in 1876 was appointed professor of diseases of children.

Smith wrote over 160 monographs, and his experience and fund of knowledge in anatomy and pediatrics allowed him to assert in the preface to his book, *The Treatise on the Diseases of Infants and Children*:

While the author has respected the opinions of previous writers, and has adopted them, so far as they appeared to be correct, he has depended much more for the material of his treatise on clinical observations and the inspection of the cadaver.[106]

The first of eight editions was published in 1869, and the book was translated into Spanish. In the 1869 edition there was a first reference to the application of thermometry to children.

Smith was an impressive innovator: he treated croup with steam inhalations and used potassium chlorate and ammonia muriate as expectorants rather than calomel. Importantly, he voiced the self-limited nature of most infectious diseases, advising that they primarily be treated supportively and expectantly.

Smith was attending physician to several hospitals in New York. He organized the American Pediatric Society in 1888. In his later years he championed the drive for certified milk (see below).

Curiously, despite his stature as a scholar and keen observer of pathology, Smith accepted outmoded concepts of the origins of fetal deformities:

It is the popular belief, and the belief of many physicians, that vivid mental impressions sometimes have a direct effect on the development of the foetus. Many cases are on record in which infants were born with marks or deformities, corresponding in character with objects which had been seen and had made a strong impression on the maternal mind at some period of gestation. . . . [T]he mother and foetus have a distinct existence as regards their nervous systems and even their blood. Still, the multitude of facts which has accumulated justify the belief that deformity or other abnormal development of the foetus sometimes, is due to the emotions of the mother.[107]

Joseph O'Dwyer

The procedure *tubage de la glotte*, introduced by Ernest Bouchut in 1858, had been rejected by the French Academy and had fallen into disuse. Twenty-three years later, in 1881, after tracheostomy had failed as a clinical measure, Joseph O'Dwyer (1841–1898) reintroduced intubation to treat suffocating diphtheria.

O'Dwyer's first intubation was performed on a three-year-old child. The child died 16 hours later, but of toxemia, without respiratory failure, and O'Dwyer was encouraged to persevere. A second patient, a four-year-old, survived the choking diphtheria. After several modifications of his equipment and four years spent perfecting the technique, O'Dwyer was able to report a 35 percent rate of survival of children who ordinarily would have died of respiratory failure. O'Dwyer published a detailed paper on the procedure in the *New York Medical Journal* in 1885.[108]

Jacobi, a colleague of O'Dwyer, who had participated in over 2,500 tracheostomies, commented, "After 1887, I rarely ever operated, and my friends stopped tracheostomy when O'Dwyer taught us all intubation."[109]

O'Dwyer researched an alternative to the invasive procedure in collaboration with Emmet Holt (1855–1924), William Northrup (1851–1935), and Samuel Adams (1853–1928). In 1896, O'Dwyer described the results of the treatment protocol in *The Report of the American Pediatric Society's Collective Investigation into the Use of Antitoxin in the Treatment of Diphtheria in Private Practice*. The American experiment confirmed the results of a French study that had been presented at the 1894 Budapest Congress by Emile Roux (1853–1933), Claude Martin (1843–1911), and Auguste

Chaillou (1866–1915), in which patients with suffocating diphtheria had been treated with antidiphtheria serum—and mortality rates had dropped from 73 percent to 14 percent.[110]

O'Dwyer and his colleagues documented[111] a staggering 5,794 cases[112] of diphtheria treated with antitoxin. The mortality rate of 12 percent was compared to an 1892 study of 5,546 children in which the mortality rate had been 70 percent.[113]

William Northrup (1851–1935), professor of pediatrics at Bellevue Medical College, was the most experienced gross pathologist of the time, having conducted hundreds of infant autopsies. In addition to his contribution to O'Dwyer's study of diphtheria antitoxin, Northrup wrote on emphysema, empyema, sclerema, and scurvy and is best remembered for his studies on respiratory pathology.

Just as a change in body temperature became recognized as an indicator of disease and/or recovery, a deviation from expected height and weight signaled a clinical problem. As mentioned, in 1825, George Logan wrote on normal birthweight and length of full-term infants.

In the 1830s Adolf Quetelet (1797–1874) of Belgium studied growth measurements and was among the first to document normal physiological weight loss during the first week of life and the discordance in height and weight during adolescence.

In 1829, Louis René Villermé (1782–1863) published data on the effects of poor nutrition and poverty on growth and development, showing that growth rates were lower among the poor population.[114]

Edwin Chadwick (1800–1890) compiled data with that of Quetelet's early studies for the Statistical Society of London. Chadwick's study was the first to meticulously examine and chart children's growth. Like Villermé, Chadwick's goal was to determine the impact of impoverished living conditions and child labor on the overall health and growth of children. In 1833 and again in 1837, Chadwick's measurements of the heights and weights of boys and girls working in the Manchester textile factories indicated growth at the third percentile,[115] an affirmation of Villermé's conclusion of the negative effects on children of an adverse environment.

In Scotland the Interdepartmental Committee of Civil Servants conducted a study that also documented the negative effects of inferior nutrition on the growth of working-class children. The committee recommendation to provide free balanced meals was initiated in 1906, and the recommendation to provide routine physical examinations of schoolchildren was implemented in 1907.[116]

In America, Henry P. Bowditch (1840–1911) published the first detailed American study that examined and established normal-growth baselines

(1875), data that, surprisingly, had not been produced before that time.[117] The study, conducted at the behest of the state of Massachusetts, charted 24,000 bits of data from all students of the Boston public schools. The baseline statistical analysis conducted by Bowditch remains valuable to this day.

Four major American pediatric textbooks appeared in the late nineteenth century, written by Keating, Starr, Rotch, and Holt.

John Keating (1852–1893) produced a four-volume work entitled *Cyclopaedia of the Diseases of Children, Medical and Surgical* in 1889. An ambitious compilation of articles written by Canadian, English, and American authors, it contained first-rate anatomical illustrations of healthy and diseased tissue and postmortem photographs and was admirably inclusive of all disciplines that related to pediatrics.

In the introduction, Jacobi wrote, "Upon me has been conferred the honor of introducing to the medical public the essays of all the distinguished men contributing to this great work."[118]

George McClellan wrote on anatomy, Angel Money, on the physiology of the infant, E. O. Shakespeare produced a thorough chapter on the evolving discipline of bacteriology, and Thomas Morgan Rotch predictably expounded on his favorite topic—infant feeding. Samuel Adams discussed the weaning of infants. There was an astonishing 26-page chapter on teratology, written by William Dabney, that supported the notion of maternal impressions as the cause of deformities.

Louis Starr (1849–1925) wrote a very popular book for parents in 1888, *Hygiene for the Nursery*. His second book appeared in 1894 with a decidedly chauvinistic title: *An American Text-Book for the Diseases of Children by American Teachers*.

Thomas Morgan Rotch (1849–1914) published *Pediatrics* in 1895. It was written in the first person, referred only to his own cases, and featured his own illustrations. There were five editions of the book. It is remembered primarily for the rigid nutritional formulas he devised, based on exacting percentage ratios. The percentage method was first developed by Philip Biedert (1847–1916) in *Die Kindernährung in Säuglingsalter und die Pflege von Mutter und Kind* (1880). It was an attempt to approximate human milk by using cow milk and compounding the protein, sugar, and fat (cream) contents.

Rotch devoted 133 pages of his text to infant feeding, including four pages[119] of complex equations for reducing the casein contents of milk to produce (as it was called for the first time) an infant "formula." An example of the method is as follows:

$$P = C/Q \times b + \text{whey}/Q \times b'$$
$$F = C/Q \times a + \text{whey}/Q \times a'$$
$$C = Q(F-a')/a-a'$$

where

C	=	total quantity of cream
Q	=	total quantity of mixture
F	=	prescribed percent of fat
P	=	prescribed percent of protein
a and a'	=	known percent of fat in cream and milk
b and b'	=	known percent of protein in cream and milk
c and c'	=	known percent of sugar in cream and milk

Howard Pearson quotes Oliver Wendell Holmes's (1809–1894) quip on the matter: "A pair of substantial mammary glands had the advantage over the two hemispheres of the most learned professor's brain in the art of compounding a nutritious fluid for infants."[120]

As the turn of the century approached, the feeding of babies had become embroiled in muddled "scientific controversy," leaving mothers wary of their common sense and the collective maternal experience of millennia. In addition to Rotch's novelties, several books and monographs were full of myriad advice on the "proper" diet for a newborn.

An amusing anonymous rhyme [strongly suspected to have been the work of John Ruhräh (1872–1935)] was written on the topic:

Soranus, he of ancient Rome,
He had a simple trick
To see if milk was fit for sale,
He merely dropped it on his nail
To see if it would stick;
Yet spite of this the babies grew
As any school boy'll tell to you.

Good Metlinger in ages dark
Just called milk good or bad
No acid milk could vex his soul
He gave it good, he gave it whole
A method very sad;
Yet babies grew to man's estate
A fact quite curious to relate.

Time sped and science came along
To help the human race,

Percentages were brought to fame
By dear old Rotch, of honored name,
We miss his kindly face;
Percentages were fed to all
Yet babies grew both broad and tall.

The calorie now helped us know
The food that is required
Before the baby now could feed
We figured out his daily need
A factor much desired;
Again we see with great surprise
The babies grow in weight and size.

The vitamin helps clarify
Why infants fail to gain,
We feed the baby leafy food
Which for the guinea pig is good
A reason very plain;
And still we watch the human race
Go madly at its usual pace.

We have the baby weighed today
The nursing time is set,
At last we find we are so wise
We can begin to standardize
No baby now need fret;
In spite of this the baby grows
But why it does God only knows.

Away with all such childish stuff
Bring chemists to the fore,
The ion now is all the rage
We listen to the modern sage
With all his latest lore;
And if the baby fret or cry
We'll see just how the ions lie.

A hundred years will soon go by
Our places will be filled
By others who will theorize
And talk as long and look as wise
Until they too are stilled;
And I predict no one will know
What makes the baby gain and grow.[121]

Luther Emmet Holt

The first major publication of Luther Emmet Holt (1855–1924) was *The Care and Feeding of Children: A Catechism for the Use of Mothers and Children's Nurses* in 1894. The book comprised the material he had prepared for nurses in lectures on newborn care at New York's Babies Hospital.[122] Initially it was a compact 66 pages. There were 12 revisions and 75 printings, and the book, ultimately expanding to 200 pages, was translated into Spanish, Russian, and Chinese.

Holt's advice was aimed at American middle-class mothers. The book— and its influence—spanned the first quarter of the new century and returned child-rearing practices to strict and spartan principles. Crying, even screaming babies were not to be embraced and soothed; infants were not to be rocked, played with, or kissed:

Playing with young children, stimulating to laughter and exciting them by sights, sounds, or movements until they shriek with apparent delight, may be a source of amusement to fond parents and admiring spectators, but it almost invariably an injury to the child. This is especially harmful when done in the evening. It is the plain duty of the physician to enlighten parents upon this point, and insist that the infant shall be kept quiet, and that all such playing and romping as has been referred to shall, during the first year at least, be absolutely prohibited.[123]

Holt maintained that habits were formed early on, and therefore parents were admonished to begin training their young in infancy:

Training in proper habits of sleep should be begun at birth. From the outset an infant should be accustomed to being put into his crib while awake and to go to sleep of his own accord. Rocking and all other habits of this sort are useless and may even be harmful. An infant should not be allowed to sleep on the breasts of the nurse, nor with the nipple of the bottle in his mouth. Other devices for putting infants to sleep, such as allowing the child to suck a rubber nipple or anything else, are positively injurious.[124]

Holt's militancy on the point of self-gratifying thumb sucking or the use of pacifiers led to the extreme: he advocated elbow splints during the day and arms tied down at night. Toddlers playing with food was another forbidden activity.[125]

Holt expounded his theories in his 1896 medical textbook for physicians, *Diseases of Infants and Children*. There were 11 editions of this text, and it was translated into Spanish, French, German, Italian, and Chinese. Currently in its 20th edition, it has evolved into *Rudolph's Pediatrics* and easily outdistances all pediatric textbooks as the one longest in continuous print.

Holt believed in percentage-feeding techniques and formulas of certified cow's milk. He took Rotch's data on formulas and zealously modified and adjusted the sequential percentages according to the age of the infant.

In 1901, Holt succeeded Jacobi as professor of pediatrics at the College of Physicians and Surgeons, Columbia University. He was founder and editor of both the *Archives of Pediatrics* and the *American Journal of Diseases of Children*. Holt's effective bedside teaching technique prompted two of his pupils to reminisce:

[A student] would present the case before the group and, on Holt's question, "Doctor, what is your diagnosis?" give it and outline his treatment. Holt would then ply him with questions, often leading towards pitfalls, designed to test his observations and thought. The questions were practical, directed to bring out some useful point, impersonal but kindly. Prognosis was never neglected. (When one of us worked as a student at the Babies Hospital in 1903, Holt had an envelop placed at the head of the bed in which each member of the staff was required to enter his prognosis in writing.) As we look back on these clinics, conducted in the Socratic fashion, they were rarely equaled.[126]

New titles of medical journals in all disciplines proliferated in the nineteenth century. Some of the pediatric titles are listed in table 8.3 and are confirmation that pediatrics had come into its own as a specialty. Historian Garrison[127] cataloged a total of 157 journals of pediatrics, of combined obstetrics and pediatrics, and those of a new discipline, child advocacy.

The new discipline of child advocacy emerged as concerns about public health, hygiene, and the detriment of poverty conditions became more commonplace. In Europe, Rudolph Virchow, Edwin Chadwick, and Hermann Cohn campaigned for preventive-medicine measures and public-health inspection of schools and hospitals.[128]

Early infant welfare advocates were Louis René Villermé (1782–1863) and Johann Peter Frank (1745–1821).[129]

Villermé's statistical studies of mortality in Parisian arrondissements established the correlation between poverty and crowding with early infant and childhood mortality. Frank, of the University of Padua, was a pioneer in school hygiene. Between 1777 and 1788 he wrote an exhaustive four-volume tome, *System einer vollständigen medicinischen Polizey*, on public-health issues as they pertained to nearly all aspects of life- and health-care delivery, including school health. No element escaped his scrutiny. He emphasized the importance of proper lighting, heating, and ventilation in schools and even analyzed the proper angles and heights of the desks and seats for optimum visual acuity.[130]

More than 98 years transpired before the topic was addressed again. Hermann Cohn (1838–1906) of Breslau, Silesia, published in 1866 a report

TABLE 8.3
SOME PEDIATRIC JOURNALS OF THE NINETEENTH CENTURY

Bibliothek für Kinderärzte	Vienna	1792
Analekten über Kinderkrankheiten	Stuttgart	1834
Clinque des hôpitaux des enfants	Paris	1841
Journal für Kinderkrankheiten	Berlin	1843
Jahrbuch für Kinderheilkunde	Vienna	1867
Archiv für Kinderheilkunde	Stuttgart	1880
Revista de enfermedades de niños	Madrid	1883
Archivio di patologia infantile	Naples	1883
Revue mensuelle des maladies de l'enfance	Paris	1883
Archives of Pediatrics	New York	1884
Baby	London	1887
Transactions American Pediatric Society	Philadelphia	1890
Mére et l'enfant	Montreal	1890
Pediatrics	New York	1896
Dietskaya Meditsina	Moscow	1896
Maternity and Child Welfare	London	1897
Medicina de los niños	Barcelona	1900

on children's myopia caused by poor lighting and inappropriate school desks. Rudolf Virchow (1821–1902), also from Silesia, published a book in 1869 supporting Cohn's conclusions. In 1871, Edwin Chadwick (1800–1890) wrote *On Schools as Centres of Children's Epidemics*, emphasizing the acute need for school hygiene policies. In France, Louis René Villermé's 1829 paper in the *Annales d'hygiene publique*, discussing the correlation between growth and poverty conditions,[131] marked the advent of the science of auxology—the study of growth and development. Villermé further enlarged his study in a two-volume text, *Tableau de l'etat physique et moral des ouvriers employes dans les manufactures de coton, de laine et de soie . . .*, published in 1840.

The high incidence of infant mortality was related directly to squalid social conditions in post–industrial revolution societies. Families were forced into makeshift, unsanitary housing in crowded urban areas. Working mothers in workshops were among the least able to care for their infants, who rarely were nursed. Fatigue, illness, or simply abject misery and ennui contributed to egregious neglect. It was not until 1844 that French officials were jarred into action. A Parisian mayor of the First Arrondissement, Firmin Marbeau (1798–1875), founded a *crèche*,[132] an institution where working mothers could leave their infants with supervising nuns and "rockers" and where physicians paid daily visits.[133] A Societé des Crèches was formed. Although nine additional crèches were successfully established in Paris within the next three years, they were inadequate to the need. Therefore, the centuries-old, ingrained custom of giving over infants to wet nurses prevailed. In 1860–1861, the infant mortality rate in France was 22.3 percent, compared to Sweden's 14.1 percent, Scotland's 14.9 percent, and England's 17 percent.[134]

In England, the Life Protection Act, passed in 1872, sought to register and license all facilities of long-term day care—"farming out," as it was called. In France, Theophile Roussel (1816–1903), a physician and a member of the French Parliament, sponsored legislation enacted on 23 December 1874—the *loi Roussel*—that required government inspection of all places where infants were farmed out, including the crèches and factory nursing rooms. A related law prohibited the employment of women for a statutory period before and after parturition. Similar statutes were enacted in Switzerland (1877); Hungary (1884); Austria (1885); Holland and Belgium (1889); England, Germany, and Portugal (1891); Norway (1892); Spain (1900); and Sweden and Denmark (1901).[135]

Obstetrician Pierre Budin organized, in Paris, the first postnatal clinic, where newborns were examined and weighed (1892). Women at the clinic routinely were instructed, pre- and postpartum, in nutrition and hygiene. Perinatal traumas,[136] such as congenital facial palsy secondary to forceps delivery, were described by Antoine Dubois (1756–1837). Brachial plexus paralysis was reported and assessed by obstetricians William Smellie (1697–1763) in 1756, Duchenne de Boulogne (1806–1875) in 1872, and Wilhelm Erb (1840–1921) in 1874.

Despite physicians' long understanding that prematurity contributed to infant mortality, there was initial resistance to using incubators. One physician, a proponent of Social Darwinism, wrote:

It is maintained by some that it is inconsistent with the best physical development of the men and women of our nation to rear these little creatures, it being assumed that they will have impaired physical vigor and transmit this to their offspring.[137]

But the success of the new science in sustaining premature life was compelling, and several physicians designed incubators. In Germany, Karl Franz Credé (1819–1892) used a fixed model, and American Thomas Morgan Rotch (1849–1914) designed a mobile version. In France, obstetricians Stephane Tarnier (1828–1897) and Pierre Budin (1846–1907) designed a simple incubator that was nothing more than a vented box warmed by hot-water bottles (figure 8.3). Of their contribution to pediatrics, historian Cone commented:

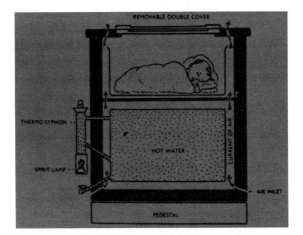

Figure 8.3 Tarnier's incubator. Budin, 1907. COURTESY NATIONAL LIBRARY OF MEDICINE.

Both men were obstetricians by training, and although both were among the foremost French obstetricians of their day, their contributions to pediatrics . . . were of even greater and lasting importance.[138]

The Tarnier incubator was designed to hold two infants and was somewhat cumbersome, but Tarnier's associate, Pierre Auvard (1855–1941), designed a model to hold one infant.

In 1856, Tarnier instituted rigorous prophylactic antiseptic measures in the Maternité that reduced maternal mortality due to puerperal fever from 17 percent to 1 percent. In 1878 incubators and gavage feedings were introduced by Tarnier in the nursery, contributing to higher rates of survival. In 1880, Tarnier reported an impressive decrease in mortality from 66 percent to 38 percent among infants who weighed a little over four pounds—less than 2,000 grams. Tarnier's pupil, Budin, instituted a postnatal weekly visit program to examine newborns and instruct mothers on hygiene and nutrition. The popular program evolved as the *consultationes de nourissons*, and was adapted all over France, resulting in increased survivals of the *desdébiles*.[139] By 1890 infant mortality in France fell to 15.4 percent, a reduction directly attributable to overall efforts in France to improve the welfare of infants.[140]

The germ theory and its elucidation contributed to the reduction of infant and child mortality in several ways. Epidemiology was understood, for the first time, and focus on disease prevention became a true possibility. As early as 1874, Otto von Bollinger (1843–1909) had demonstrated that milk could carry tuberculosis.[141] Moreover, ignorance and poverty contributed to appalling habits of hygiene. In common use at the time were large, 16-ounce

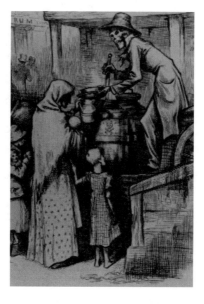

Figure 8.4 "Toxic Milk" by Thomas Nast (1878). COURTESY NATIONAL LIBRARY OF MEDICINE.

nursing bottles fabricated from blown glass, pewter, or pottery. They had nipples of chamois or pickled calf teat until 1840, when rubber nipples were manufactured.[142] These feeding devices harbored bacteria contaminated milk that caused infectious diarrheas, a leading cause of illness and death in children. Cows' milk and the devices in which milk was served became recognized as disease vectors that posed a high infection risk for infants.

After Pasteur discovered that heat destroyed bacteria contaminating and souring wine, the German chemist Franz von Soxhlet (1848–1926) successfully applied Pasteur's process to milk. "Pasteurization," inspection and monitoring of milk-handling sanitation rendered milk "disease free" without altering the product.

It took the tenacious efforts of several individuals to effectively control the epidemics associated with tainted milk. In America, a campaign to clean and certify milk was spearheaded by Henry Coit (1854–1917), who worked doggedly for years to educate the public, influence a change in public opinion and attitudes, enlist the interest and energy of the medical community, and encourage lawmakers to enact and enforce effective legislation.

As late as the first decade of the twentieth century, milk in America continued to be sold over the grocery counter by dipping into five-gallon cans of unrefrigerated milk (figure 8.4).

A paper read at the meeting of the pediatric society in 1901 examined the quality of such milk with respect to summer epidemics of diarrhea:

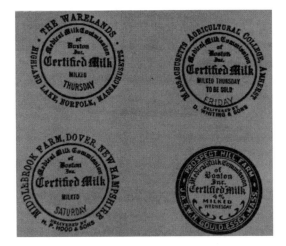

Figure 8.5 Certification seals from various milk stations. Waserman, M. J., Henry Coit and the certified milk movement (*Bull Hist Med* 1972; 46:359).

It should be remembered that most market milks show hundreds of thousands of bacteria to the cubic centimetre, and that as delivered in large cities, many of them show millions. . . . Such figures demonstrate the retched and dangerous hygienic conditions that attend the production and sale of most market milks.[143]

Henry Chapin (1857–1942) presented a paper at a scientific meeting in 1893, in which he described milk that was studied after being centrifuged: "the detritus was found by microscopic examination to contain pus and blood corpuscles, dirt and hair."[144]

Some dairies fed their cows residuals from distillery mash for economic reasons. These cows produced "swill milk," which commonly was believed to produce infant intoxication.[145] To increase the yield or to alter the quality and appearance of milk, corrupt dealers added molasses, chalk, and even plaster of Paris. A New York Commission of Health reported in 1902 that 53 percent of more than 2,000 samples of milk tested were adulterated.[146]

Many medical and social professionals vocalized complaints about the public health need to control the handling and processing of milk, but it took the wealth and influence of philanthropist Nathan Straus (1848–1931) to effect meaningful change. He established over 300 certified milk stations (figure 8.5) in the United States[147] and Europe.* Straus addressed the Board of Aldermen of New York City in 1907:

---

*Gaston Variot (1855–1930) and Leon Dufours (1860–1934) introduced similar innovations in France. These centers, the Dispensaire del Belleville and Goutte de Lait, were the first to offer certified milk for sale in France. Huard and Laplane, 1981; 3:195. Variot, G., *L'Hygiene infantile; allaitement maternal et artificiel* (Paris, 1916).

Under ideal conditions of production, the milk may be free from danger. To say that it is possible for inspectors to control conditions on thousands of farms, so as to make them ideally perfect, does not seem ordinarily reasonable. I welcome the good that may come from inspection, but protest most emphatically against leaving people of this city with no other protection than inspection. . . . Direct all your efforts towards securing proper scientific pasteurization of such of the milk supplies as has not been certified. I warn you that every day's delay is a crime against the health of this community.[148]

From one milk station opened by Straus on Randalls Island, New York City, a reduction in the rate of infant mortality from 51 percent to 18 percent was realized in the first year of operation.[149]

When pasteurized milk became commonly available and it was widely established that careful cleaning and sterilization of containers and feeders were essential to eradicating microbial contamination, public-health officials reported a dramatic drop in rates of infant mortality. In New York, for example, from 1898 to 1911 the infant death rate fell from 20.3 to 12.0 per thousand—nearly 40 percent—and milk-associated contagious diseases fell by 43 percent.[150]

Some pediatricians contended that pasteurization might decrease bacterial content, but the final product still was contaminated milk. Others believed that heating milk destroyed its nutritional value. The popular press swayed public opinion and silenced the skeptical by reporting that home pasteurization devices produced disease-free milk with normal taste, texture, and nutrition. Mothers opted for pasteurization, and physicians' opposition disappeared.[151]

NOTES

1. Ackerknecht, 1982, p. 146.

2. Seidler, 1989, pp. 181–97.

3. Strauss, 1968, p. 135. Inspired by the Paris model, William and John Hunter built an amphitheater in 1767 for their private anatomy school on Great Windmill Street in Soho, London. The facade still stands, and the building now houses the Lyric Theater.

4. Garrison, 1929, p. 431.

5. Hastings, 1974, pp. 79–84.

6. Pasteur, L., *Compt. Rend. Académie des Sciences*, trans. D. H. Clendening (Paris, 1885).

7. Ballabriga, 1991, p. 4.

8. Radbill, 1955, p. 415.

9. Lomax, 1996, p. 15.

10. Ballabriga, 1991, p. 6.

11. The remaining two patients also died but were listed in the subsequent year's statistics. Landsberger, 1964, p. 207.

12. Abt, 1945, p. 76.

13. Abt, 1965, p. 96.

14. Seidler, 1989, pp. 189–90.

15. Nightingale, 1859, p. 13.

16. Ibid., pp. 125–26.

17. Bremner, 1971, 2:831.

18. Cheyne, 1801, pp. 11–12.

19. Ibid., p. 16.

20. Ibid., p. 18.

21. Ibid., pp. 8–10.

22. Heberden's father, William the elder (1710–1801), also is well known to students of medicine for his description of *digitorum nodi*—small pea-size growths overlying osteoarthritic finger joints—appropriately called Heberden's nodes.

23. Ruhräh, 1925, pp. 524–55.

24. The hydrostatic pressures of water immersion at 22 torr/ft. result in redistribution of blood volume, central hypervolemia, and marked natriuresis (40 uEq/min) and diuresis (1.5 ml/min/1.73 m^2). Colón, 1990, p. 22.

25. Watt, 1813, pp. 193–314.

26. Clark, 1815, p. 97.

27. Davis, 1817, p. 30.

28. Abt, 1945, p. 24.

29. Billard, 1839, p. 432.

30. Abt, 1965, p. 87.

31. Billard, 1839, pp. v–viii.

32. Diday, 1851, p. 177.

33. *Die Verhütung der Augenentzündung der Neugeborenen*, 1884.

34. Vilaplana Satoree, 1934, p. 188.

35. Ibid.

36. Norvenius and Randers, 1997, p. 446.

37. Abt, 1945, p. 92.

38. Norvenius and Randers, 1997, p. 447.

39. Abt, 1965, p. 92.

40. *Lancet* 1844; 1:319.

41. *Trans Obstet Soc Lond* 1862; 3:293.

42. West, 1850, pp. v–vi.

43. Abt, 1945, p. 38.

44. Lomax, 1996, p. 94.

45. Abt, 1965, p. 90.

46. Radbill, 1976, p. 754.

47. Churchill, 1850, pp. 397–410.

48. Dunn, 1994, pp. 228–29.

49. Ibid.

50. Abt, 1945, p. 108.

51. Guersant, 1873, pp. 279–80.

52. Ibid., pp. 339–40. A bistoury (c.1500) was a probe-pointed lancet.

53. Laplane, 1991, p. 45

54. Smith, 1884.

55. Ruhräh, J., *Am J Dis Child* 1935; 50:472–75.

56. Touloukian, 1995, pp. 914–15.

57. Gerhardt, 1877. A partial list of the book's outstanding scholars and their chapter contributions is as follows:

Karl Hennig (1825–1911)	Sclerema, thymus
Johann Steffen (1825–1910)	Diseases of the brain
Johann Rehn (1831–1918)	Rickets, rheumatism
Karl Binz (1832–1913)	Therapeutics
Heinrich Bohn (1832–1888)	Diseases of skin and mouth
Wilhelm Henke (1834–1896)	Anatomy
George F. Thomas (1838–1907)	Kidney diseases
Oswald Kohts (1844–1912)	Meningitis, osteomyelitis
Herman Wiederhofer (1832–1901)	Bronchus, intussusception
Alois Monti (1839–1909)	Croup, diphtheria
Rudolph Demme (1836–1892)	Thyroid diseases
Oskar Wyss (1840–1911)	Typhus, pneumonia, TB
Karl Rauchfuss (1835–1915)	Hospital design
Abraham Jacobi (1830–1919)	Hygiene, diphtheria

58. Jacobi, 1909, p. 499.

59. Braun, 1991, p. 24.

60. Historians now recognize the first complete description of this lesion to have been made in the 1672 *Acta Medicine et Philosophia* by Neils Stensen. Acierno, 1993, pp. 161–62.

61. Many of Schönlein's views were disproved long ago. Among his beliefs were that stress soured a mother's milk, leading to infantile convulsions; that older mothers had poor milk, responsible for marasmus; that rickets and tuberculosis were one disease; that brain tuberculosis was due to gonorrhea and that gonorrhea was the first stage of syphilis. Abt, 1945, p. 55.

62. Henoch, 1882, pp. 317–18.

63. Abt, 1945, pp. 62–63.

64. Abt, 1965, p. 94.

65. Kagan, 1952, p. 358.

66. Abt, 1945, p. 97.

67. Downes, 1994, pp. 1–2.

68. Snow, 1858, p. 49.

69. Ashby, 1889, p. 651.

70. Goodhart, 1885, p. 468.

71. Ruhräh, J., *Am J Dis Child* 1934; 48:159–64.

72. Barlow, 1957, pp. 20–28.

73. Abt, 1945, pp. 19–20.

74. Samuel Adams held the second full-time American Professorship in Pediatrics at Georgetown University in 1898. He wrote several monographs on infectious diseases, especially on diphtheria and typhoid. In 1897 he was elected President of the American Pediatric Society and, at his inauguration, presented an informative historical review of American pediatrics.

75. Adams, 1897, p. 10.

76. Radbill, 1976, p. 758.

77. Logan, 1825, p. 34.

78. Ibid., pp. 180–81.

79. Cone, 1985, p. 3.

80. Logan, 1825, p. 15.

81. Dewees, 1829, p. vi (preface to pt. 2).

82. American Practitioner, 1826, p. iv.

83. Ibid., p. 254.

84. Ibid., p. 279.

85. Recall that in Sweden Nils Rosen von Rosenstein had given formal pediatric lectures as early at 1761.

86. Pearson, 1986, pp. 45–46.

87. Cone, 1979, pp. 87–90.

88. Eberle, 1833, p. 8.

89. Ibid., pp. 12–13, 52–53.

90. Cone, 1979, p. 80.

91. Eberle, 1833, p. 297.

92. Cone, 1979, p. 79.

93. Meigs's father, Charles Dulucena Meigs (1792–1869), an obstetrician, wrote a pediatric text, *Observations on Certain Diseases of Young Children*, in 1850.

94. Meigs, 1848, p. x.

95. Beck, 1849, pp. 10–17.

96. Ibid., p. 50.

97. The practice of bloodletting dates back millennia. In the middle of the twentieth century, leeches could still be purchased in American drugstores and at this writing are still used throughout the Third World. They are also under research study for their anticoagulant proteins.

98. Beck, 1849, pp. 76–81.

99. Bremner, 1971, pp. 817–18.

100. Ibid.

101. Abt, 1965, p. 108.

102. Leopold, 1957, p. 15.

103. Haggerty, 1997, p. 465.

104. Leopold, 1957, p. 13.

105. Cone (1979) asserts that Smith was a very close second to Jacobi as a "father of American pediatrics" (p. 104).

106. Smith, 1872, p. v.

107. Ibid., pp. 21–22.

108. Ruhräh, 1938, pp. 176–80.

109. Abt, 1965, p. 108.

110. Laplane, 1991, p. 44.

111. Charles Chapin (1856–1941) of Providence, Rhode Island, established the first Health Department bacteriology laboratory in 1888. Cases could now be confirmed by culture, and by late 1890, release from quarantine was dependent on a negative culture.

112. King, 1993, pp. 77–78.

113. Cone, 1979, p. 110.

114. Tanner, 1992, p. 106.

115. Ibid., 1992, pp. 107–8.

116. Other growth studies in Europe were conducted by Francis Galton (1822–1911) and Luigi Pagliani (1847–1932). Hamilton, 1981, pp. 241–42.

117. Cone, 1974, pp. 67–76.

118. Keating, 1890, p. v.

119. Rotch, 1903, pp. 112–245.

120. Pearson, 1994, p. 3.

121. Veeder, 1957, p. 154.

122. Park and Mason, 1957, pp. 37–38.

123. Holt, 1916, p. 5.

124. Cable, 1972, pp. 165–66.

125. Holt, 1916, p. 6.

126. Park and Mason, 1957, p. 43.

127. Abt, 1965, pp. 125–30.

128. Ibid., p. 84.

129. Ballabriga, 1991, p. 1.

130. Baumgartner and Ramsey, 1934, pp. 69–72.

131. Abt, 1965, p. 117.

132. The concept subsequently was adopted in Austria, Italy, and Germany.

133. Holt, 1916, p. 900.

134. Ibid., p. 151.

135. Abt, 1965, pp. 153–56.

136. Huard and Laplane, 1981, 1:86.

137. Baker, 1991, pp. 654–55.

138. Cone, 1985, p. 38.

139. Ibid., p. 39.

140. Baker, pp. 655–56.

141. Abt, 1945, p. 69.

142. Scheffel, 1993, p. 27.

143. Faber and McIntosh, 1966, p. 62.

144. Ibid., p. 30.

145. Cone, 1979, p. 141.

146. Ibid., p. 142.

147. As of 1905, less than 1% of American milk was certified. King, 1993, p. 113.

148. Bremner, 1970–1971, p. 870.
149. Cone, 1979, p. 144.
150. Faber and McIntosh, 1966, p. 86.
151. King, 1993, pp. 115–16.

Chapter 9

The Twentieth Century

1900	Boxer rebellion
1901	Inception of the Nobel Prize
1906	San Francisco earthquake
1909	Orthodontia introduced
1912	*Titanic* sinks
1914	World War I
1916	Irish Easter rising
1917	Russian Revolution
1918	Spanish influenza pandemic
1921	Banting and Best isolate insulin
1927	Lindberg crosses the Atlantic
1929	Electroencephalography
1932	Sulfa drugs make appearance
1934	Adolf Hitler becomes Führer
1936	Spanish Civil War
1939	Paul Müller develops DDT
1946	Nuremberg trials
1948	World Health Organization
1949	NATO formed
1952	Elizabeth II enthroned
1953	Hillary and Tenzing on Everest
1959	Ascent of Fidel Castro
1961	Yuri Gagarin in space
1968	Barnard's heart transplant
1969	Man on the moon
1971	Computerized axial tomography (CAT scan)
1983	Last case of smallpox on earth
1990	PCR technology comes of age

There is an anecdote that places the Chinese chairman, Deng Xiao Ping (1904–1997), in Paris to celebrate the bicentennial of the French Revolution. When asked by a reporter how he believed the Revolution had affected world history, Deng replied, "It is too soon to tell." So it is with medical "revolutions." They require time—and distance—before enduring, valid assessments can be made of the impact of technological innovations, treatment protocols, newly developed medicines, and even the pathophysiology of disease. The cure of one year may be exposed as the scourge of the following year—and vice versa.

Thalidomide comes to mind in this context. Those of us over 50 years of age recall that the drug was used extensively in Europe to assuage nausea in early pregnancy until it was named as a causal agent of thousands of horrific fetal abnormalities and its use was banned. After more than 40 years, the drug has proved in experiments to be effective as an immunosuppressant and is being considered for use again.

Corticosteroid treatment was hailed in the early 1940s as a cure for rheumatoid arthritis, when, as it turns out, it is at best palliative. In some patients it had disfiguring side effects with mortal complications.

Some diseases have disappeared. Reye's syndrome is a case in point. Undiagnosed and untreated, it was a lethal illness in children, who disproportionately died from liver failure and brain swelling. In the view of expert physicians, the potential for epidemics was strong, and indeed, several communities experienced a number of cases within a brief period of time. Reye's became a footnote in the history books after the causative viral-toxin connection—salicylates (especially in aspirin)—was discovered and made widely known.

These few examples illustrate the difficulty in justly evaluating progress in twentieth-century medicine. A narrowed focus does allow unquestionable and indisputable areas of progress to be reviewed with confidence, and this chapter will discuss those. It is also possible, as in appendix 9.1 at the end of this chapter, to list a selective catalog of the names of twentieth-century medical giants in the field of pediatrics. Historians in the future, however, will be much better able to separate the substantial and seminal advances in medicine from the merely ephemeral. They certainly will have at their disposal copious amounts of data to sift through. It is the hope of the author that this text will be a useful guide for them in their research.

In my view, the history of pediatrics in the twentieth century can be called the "Age of Confidence." Following a lull in medical research during the years of the First World War, in which basic science progressed little, there was an explosion of research activities and the excitement of discovery among scientists. Enthusiasm about and trust in the future were restored.

The study of human growth and development evolved into a science of eugenics. Medical schools formally began to establish departments of pediatrics. Microbiology research led to vaccines, antimicrobials, and insecticides, all of which moderated the spread of epidemics. An understanding of dietary deficiencies, vitamins, and metabolism enhanced nutrition. The mechanisms of depletion and dehydration shock were studied. Parenteral therapy was proposed. Pain was controlled by the use of new drugs. X-rays allowed noninvasive diagnostic studies to be made. The chromosomal code was broken. Preventive medicine, prophylactically sustaining health in the healthy, became an achievable goal.

Medicine had fissured into several areas of specialized care—in adult medicine, surgery, and pediatrics. By midcentury, subspecialists were being trained in all disciplines. Research protocols rendered unprecedented scientific insights on a colossal scale and were responsible for countless new clinical treatment modalities. Optimism and confidence about the health of future generations and especially about the world's children have been, therefore, the prevailing themes in twentieth-century medicine.

In America, the discipline of pediatrics received further enhancement and legitimacy through the body of research and publications appearing in almost logarithmic numbers. Many of these researches were published in the *Transactions* of the American Pediatric Society (APS), which had been founded in 1888.[1] Until 1938 the *Transactions* remained the major medium of publication for researchers engaged in the study of childhood diseases. The APS, however, remained a small club, confining membership to only 110. Thought was given to forming a new society, with open-membership doors to any physician trained in pediatrics. Planning for this society started at the Portland meeting of the American Medical Association (AMA) in 1928, but in the end the catalyst for the new society, the American Academy of Pediatrics, was a political and philosophical one.

The Sheppard-Towner Act of 1921, with a federal appropriation of $7 million, aimed to reduce infant and child mortality by providing state-planned and -administered health clinics for prenatal and preventive pediatric care and public-health nurses to instruct mothers on nutrition and child care. Senator James Reed of Missouri considered the Act a harbinger of socialized medicine and was one of many dissenting voices regarding the legislation, claiming that "the fundamental doctrines on which the bill is founded were drawn chiefly from the radical, socialistic, and bolshevistic philosophy of Germany and Russia."[2] In 1922, at its annual association meeting, however, the pediatric branch of the AMA supported the Sheppard-Towner Act. There was much rancor and berating; and before the day was over, the AMA House of Delegates vindictively condemned the Act. The conflict and disagreement continued to fester for years; and in the end, after intense lobbying by various groups, including the AMA, the law was repealed in 1929. A year later, in 1930, no longer able to tolerate fundamental philosophical differences, a schism group of AMA members, strong advocates of children's rights, established the American Academy of Pediatrics.[3]

In this new Age of Confidence, pediatric research in *nutritional and metabolic sciences* marked the first areas of intensive investigation. Traditionally— and economically—maternal breast milk with pap and panada supplementation had been mainstays of infant nutrition. Pap consisted of flour or bread crumbs cooked in water or milk, and panada added meat broth and eggs to these basic ingredients. Recipes had existed for centuries that were simple and affordable, such as those of Vallambert (c.1565):

[PAP]

The flour of which it is made nowadays the greater part of the nurses pass simply through a sieve without other preparation. Others cook it in the oven. . . . The milk mixed with the flour is commonly from the goat or cow, that of the goat is better. When one intends to add more nourishment one adds finally an egg yolk, when one wishes to guard against constipation one adds honey.

[PANADA]

One grates a crumb of bread very small, then one puts it in a bouillon of good flesh in a small glazed earthen pot and puts it to cook on a small charcoal fire without smoke. Sometimes it is cooked in a bouillon of peas or other legumes, with oil or butter and more often it is cooked with goats or cows milk or milk of sweet almonds. Others mix with the panada an egg yolk or the entire egg.[4]

In the twentieth century, breast feeding, for the first time in history, fell into disfavor, and the numbers of nursing mothers precipitously declined as bottle-feeding became the vogue. Pap, too, was replaced, by commercial baby foods. Historians Apple[5] and Bullough[6] have formulated several reasons for the phenomenon: an increase in hospital births, growing availability of wholesome milk, the changing roles of women, commercial alliances between the food industry and medicine, and improvements in the rubber nipple. Bullough noted that wet-nurse advertisements disappeared from the newspapers.[7]

Milk processing had become common, and by 1910 home iceboxes made the safe storage of milk universally possible. By 1927, William McKim Marriott (1885–1936) was recommending the use of evaporated milk in preparing formulas, further assuring microbe-free and storage-safe milk for those homes still without refrigeration.

A soy formula, first used in the United States by John Ruhräh (c.1909), and solid food were recommended for infants at ever-earlier ages.[8] In 1897 the recommended age for the introduction of vegetables was 36 months. By 1916 it was down to one year, and in 1950 it was four months. In 1928 both *beikost* and commercial canned baby food arrived on the American grocery shelf.

Formula feeding became more and more popular in America despite governmental efforts to promote the health benefits of maternal breast milk. Analysis of data from the 1900 and 1910 census reveals that those children breast-fed the longest had mortality rates 40 percent lower than their formula-fed peers.[9]

Unexpectedly, as breast feeding diminished, the incidence of scurvy increased. Formulas as yet had no vitamin fortification. Alfred Hess (1875–1933) in 1914 recorded greater instances of scurvy among toddlers in the New York Hebrew Infant Asylum when orange juice no longer was served. In 1928, Albert Szent Györgyi[10] (1893–1986) isolated hexuronic acid, which, in 1932, was identified by biochemists Waugh and King[11] as the antiscorbutic factor of citrus. Thereafter, fruit and juices were added to the diet, and disease rates decreased dramatically.

Cod liver oil had been recommended for rickets as early as 1824, but causative factors and cures eluded the medical community until the twentieth century. The near absence of rickets from sunny countries such as Egypt and fish-consuming countries such as Japan made little impression. In 1909, Georg Schmorl (1861–1932) of Denmark examined the bones of infants who had died between the ages of 2 and 48 months. He ascertained, to the astonishment of all, that nearly 90 percent of those studied had evidence of rickets.[12]

Finally, a series of monographs published between 1908 and 1912 by Isidore Schabad (1870–?) in Russia established that cod liver oil prevented rickets as well as cured it. In Berlin, in 1919, Kurt Huldschinsky (1883–?) used artificial heliotherapy to treat rickets, and in New York the research of Alfred Hess confirmed Huldschinsky's findings.

Basic biochemical defects of rickets continued to be studied. The research of John Howland (1873–1926) and Benjamin Kramer (1887–1972) paved the way for a cure. They developed a semimicro method for serum calcium measurements in children, taking careful note of calcium and phosphate levels. With the advent of the x-ray, they were able to study the evolution and progress of the osteopathy. Edward Parks (1877–1969) and Elmer McCollum (1879–1967) picked up on Howland's and Kramer's research and further refined it, using rats as animal models and studying dietary as well as osteopathic factors.[13]

At the 1921 APS meeting sunlight and cod liver oil as antirachitic factors were discussed, triggering a cascade of research into the solar irradiation of dermal provitamins. Vitamin D finally was identified as the curative agent, found in the barely palatable cod liver oil. When Philip C. Jeans (1883–1952), in 1936, persuaded the Commission on Foods and the AMA to mandate that supplemental vitamin D be added to cow milk, future generations of children were spared the disagreeable taste of cod liver oil.[14] Hector DeLuca in 1968 and E. Kodicek (in 1968–1970) shared their research findings, which defined the active metabolites in vitamin D.[15]

With the gradual scientific understanding of the function of the major vitamins—A, B-complex, C, D, and folic acid—incidences of scurvy, rickets, tetany, xerophthalmia, beriberi, pellagra, and macrocytic anemias began to wane. The nutritional status of children in developed countries improved so dramatically that new growth-curve standards became necessary.

In the Third World, childhood malnutrition continued unabated, sadly providing researchers with ample material to study the pathophysiology of starvation.

As early as 1865, F. Hinojosa published in Mexico a vivid description of protein malnutrition,[16] but the first formal study of the aberrant physiology and basal metabolic rates in marasmics was made by Fritz Bradley Talbot (1878–1964) in 1921.[17]

Cicely Williams (1893–1992) introduced in 1935 the terminology of *kwashiorkor*,* and in 1945 Eugen Kerpel-Fronis (b.1906) defined the limits of recovery from severe marasmus.[18] Emilio Soto (1908–1980) demonstrated that emergency rehydration of the malnourished child in tropical countries could be accomplished with readily available coconut water.[19] In 1948, John C. Waterlow (b.1916) referred to the fatty liver of malnutrition,[20] and in 1959, Derrick B. Jelliffe (b.1921) refined the clinical descriptions and observations of both protein and protein-calorie malnutrition.[21]

While basic nutrition and deficiencies were being elucidated, metabolic energy and requirements were being studied. Max Rubner (1854–1932) delineated the energy value of the major food groups, establishing that one gram of dry protein yielded 4.1 calories; one gram of fat, 9.3 calories; and one gram of carbohydrate, 4.1 calories.[22] He formulated the relationship between metabolic rate and body surface area, the latter being of seminal importance in the nutritional treatment of infants and children.[23] Formerly, the dosage treatment of children had been haphazard, arbitrary. Some doc-

---

*"The name 'kwashiorkor' indicates the disease the deposed baby gets when the next one is born, and is the local name in the Gold Coast for a nutritional disease of children associated with a maize diet" (Williams, C. D., *Lancet* 1935:2:1151–52).

tors prescribed half the adult dose; others based dosage on anecdotal observations. Rubner's use of body surface area provided a consistent and universal understanding of the ratio between body water and energy requirements and a dosing parameter.

Rubner and Johann Heubner (1843–1926) calculated the compensatory as well as the normal energy requirements for the malnourished child. Heubner then simplified the concept and facilitated its application by introducing daily caloric requirements based on kilogram body weight.

An understanding of the acidosis of dehydration was advanced by John Howland and William McKim Marriott, in a paper presented in 1915 before the APS. Howland and Marriott proved that the dyspnea, agitation, and torpor that accompanied severe childhood summer diarrhea were due to base loss, not to metabolic "alimentary intoxication," as had been suggested by Heinrich Finkelstein (1865–1942). Finkelstein had theorized that sugar and salt intoxication produced the torpor, for which *eiweissmilch*, or albumin milk, was prescribed.[24] Howland and Marriott's studies led to the treatment of this life-threatening process with intravenous fluids and bicarbonate. Their findings were elegantly duplicated and confirmed by Oscar Schloss (1882–1952).

Several decisive renal and gastrointestinal physiology studies resulted in the successful treatment of acidosis of dehydration from acute diarrhea, a major killer of children. In 1923, James Gamble (1883–1959) defined renal acid excretion and extracellular fluid composition (ECF). Daniel Darrow (1895–1965) in 1935 determined the osmotic pressure of ECF and, in 1950, with Clifton Govan (b.1917), advocated the addition of potassium to the intravenous solution.[25] Homer W. Smith (1895–1962) established the glomerular filtration rate with inulin clearance.

Infectious diseases constituted the next major threat to childhood health. The nineteenth-century observations of Theodor Escherich (1857–1911) on the normal bacterial flora of infants established baselines against which abnormal flora and intestinal symptoms could be compared. Escherich demonstrated that infant gut flora was established after birth, from oral contamination acquired in passing through the birth canal and during nursing. Paul Ehrlich (1854–1915) showed that maternal milk countered the effects by transmitting immunity against infection to the infant.[26]

Once diphtheria and tetanus antitoxins proved successful, immunological and diagnostic advances continued at breakneck speed. Anitsera for scarlet fever and meningococcemia were developed. Emil von Behring (1854–1917) introduced an immunizing mixture of diphtheria antitoxin with toxin. This was followed by formalin inactivation of the toxin (which did not affect antigenicity), allowing for a safer vaccine.[27] Bela Schick (1877–1967) devised a test that monitored diphtheria susceptibility, thereby identifying children at risk.

It was found that congenital syphilis could be prevented by treating the infected mother during pregnancy. Additionally, the introduction of routine and mandatory premarital testing identified mothers at risk, and the incidence of congenital syphilis declined dramatically. Blindness resulting from gonorrhea ophthalmitis also was reduced substantially by the prophylactic instillation of silver nitrate, introduced by Carl Seigmund Franz Credé (1819–1892) in 1881 but not popularized until the turn of the century.

In 1899, using the tobacco mosaic model, Martinus Beijerinck (1851–1931) produced the first evidence of a filterable viral particle. In 1935, Wendell M. Stanley (1904–1971) crystallized the particle as an RNA protein, triggering a cascade of investigations into smaller and smaller particles.

Gilbert Dalldorf (b.1900) and Grace Sickles (1898–1959) isolated the coxsackievirus in 1947, while John F. Enders (1897–1985), Thomas H. Weller (b.1915), and Frederick C. Robbins (b.1916) cultured the polio virus in 1949, opening the doors for Jonas Salk (1914–1995) and Albert Sabin (1906–1993) to produce vaccines in 1955 and 1956, respectively. Sabin's oral vaccine—portable, easily administered, and inexpensive—was used by preference globally, and by 1992, having witnessed the demise of smallpox, scientists began to discuss the eradication of polio from the Western hemisphere.[28]

Table 9.1 lists major contributors to scientific advances against infectious diseases, and table 9.2 is a list of milestones in the evolution of pediatric immunology. Table 9.3 catalogs the introduction of the antimicrobials, beginning with sulfonamide drugs, and the antibiotics—a colossal advance in the annals of medical history.

Taken as a whole, these achievements enabled public-health prevention programs on an unprecedented scale. Worldwide vaccination programs against diphtheria, tetanus, pertussis, smallpox, measles, mumps, and polio and campaigns against insect-borne diseases (with DDT) and parasites such as hookworm and *Schistosoma* were mounted and successfully executed in many parts of the world.

TABLE 9.1
SOME TWENTIETH-CENTURY CONTRIBUTORS TO THE SCIENCE OF INFECTIOUS DISEASES AND THEIR AREAS OF RESEARCH

Alexander, Hattie (1901–1968)	*Hemophilus* influenza
Avery, Oswald (1877–1955)	Pneumococcal polysaccharides
Bordet, Jules (1870–1961)	Cultured *Bordetella* pertussis

continued

Bradford, William (b.1898)	Developed wireloop for pertussis Nasopharyngeal culture
Christie, Amos (b.1902)	Pulmonary histoplasmosis
Debré, Robert (1882–1978)	Cat-scratch fever
Dubos, Rene (1901–1982)	Natural ecology of gut flora
Bordet, Jules (1870–1961)	Cultured pertussis agent
Gajdusek, Carlton (b.1923)	Slow viruses
Jones, T. D. (1899–1954)	Hemolytic streptococcus Rheumatic fever
Krugman, Saul (b.1911)	Rubella and hepatitis
Lincoln, Edith (1891–?)	Tuberculosis
Noguchi, Hideyo (1876–1928)	Cerebral syphilis
Paul, John (1893–1972)	Rheumatic fever, infectious mononucleosis
Rammelkamp, Charles (1911–1981)	Streptococcus glomerulonephritis
Seibert, Florence (1897–?)	Purified protein derivative of TB
Shope, Richard (1901–1966)	Swine influenza A
Topping, Norman (1908–1997)	Developed typhus vaccine
Wannamaker, Lewis (b.1923)	Streptococcus rheumatic fever
Zahorsky, John (1871–1963)	Roseola infantum

TABLE 9.2
RESEARCH ACHIEVEMENTS IMPACTING ON PEDIATRIC IMMUNOLOGY

1900	Landsteiner describes ABO blood groups
1902	Richet and Portier describe anaphylaxis
1903	Von Pirquet coins "allergy"
1911	Noon and Freeman evolve concept of immunotherapy
1912	Schloss develops the scratch test
1921	Prausnitz and Kunster show passive transfer of antibodies by serum
1930	Donnally demonstrates transfer of antibodies in maternal breast milk
1937	Cooke and Loveless evolve concept of blocking antibodies
1939	Tiselius and Kabat show antibodies are gamma globulins
1944	Medawar and Burnet present graft rejection principles
1947	Levine and Stetson describe the Rh system
1950	Good refines immunological principles and demonstrates the role of the thymus in animals

1950   Glanzman and Riniker report agammaglobulinemia associated with disappearance of lymphoid tissue

1952   Bruton describes congenital agammaglobulinemia

1959   Smythe works on the immunosuppression of malnutrition

1961   Hanson begins work on the protective aspects of breast milk IgA

1962   Barandum prepares intravenous gammaglobulins

1964   Dausset elucidates HLA antigens

1965   DiGeorge defines the human model of immunodeficiency associated with thymus absence

1968   Gatti performs stem cell immunological transplant

TABLE 9.3
ADVANCES IN ANTIBIOTICS THERAPY

1912	Neosalvarsan	Ehrlich and Hata
1928–1940	Penicillin	Fleming, Florey, and Chain
1935	Sulfonamides	Domagk
1943	Bacitracin	Johnson
1944	Streptomycin	Waksman
1947	Chloramphenicol	Waksman
1948	Tetracycline	Duggar
1952	Erythromycin	McGuire
1954	Nystatin	Dutcher
1956	Vancomycin	McCormick
1957	Kanamycin	Umezawa
1963	Gentamicin	Weinstein
1966	Clindamycin	Magerlein

Wilhelm Konrad Roentgen's (1845–1922) development of the x-ray in 1895 was appreciated immediately as a great achievement for mankind—adult and child. This noninvasive diagnostic tool eliminated the need for painful manipulations and palpations or surgical incisions for diagnostic purposes. A new science, *radiology*, had been introduced. As early as 1896 a crude prototype was in use: a 14-year-old boy injured while skating on the Connecticut River lay for a twenty-minute exposure on an emulsion-coated glass plate that revealed a fractured ulna.[29]

A radiology pioneer, Francis H. Williams (1852–1936) published *The Roentgen Rays in Medicine and Surgery* in 1901. Around 1897, Williams and

Walter B. Cannon (1871–1945) used the technology to study swallowing mechanisms, peristalsis, and gastric emptying by feeding children bread and milk mixed with bismuth subnitrate.[30]

In 1910 the first textbook on pediatric radiology, *Living Anatomy and Pathology: The Diagnosis of Diseases in Early Life by the Roentgen Method*, was published by Thomas Morgan Rotch (1849–1914). Paul Reyher (1876–1934) published *Das Röntgenverfahren in der Kinderheilkunde* in 1912, and Herbert Assmann (1882–1950) wrote *Die Röntgendiagnostik der Inneren Erkrankkungen* in 1921. Gordon Stoloff (1898–?) published *The Chest in Children* in 1930, and Stephen Engle (1878–?) and Ludwig Schall published *Handbuch der Röntgendiagnostik und Therapie im Kinder* in 1933.

During the 1920s and 1930s the radiological criteria of scurvy, rickets, lead poisoning, anemias, syphilis, hemophilia, tumors, and other diseases were established. Radiology also was responsible for a controversy in which status thymicolymphaticus was deemed a disease requiring treatment.[31] Infants who had succumbed to sudden infant death were found, on posthumous x-ray, to have enlarged thymuses. It was hypothesized that death was secondary to thymic compression of vessels in the mediastinum. Healthy infants therefore were prophylactically x-rayed, and, in the presence of a large thymus, they were irradiated to shrink the organ. In fact, the infant thymus is normally large, and Edith Boyd (1895–1978) made efforts to debunk the fallacious theory, but it persisted until the 1960s.

The bible of pediatric radiology, *Pediatric X-ray Diagnosis* by John Caffey (1895–1978), appeared in 1945. Caffey contributed revolutionary descriptions and analyses of bone changes in avitaminoses, bone aging, osseous disease, and tumors and, importantly, made possible the correlation between subdural hematomas with healing fractures as evidence of child abuse.[32]

Edward Neuhauser (1908–1987) elucidated the pulmonary changes of cystic fibrosis, the appearance of vascular rings, and the radiological signs of Hirschsprung's disease.

Urography, myelography, pneumoencephalography, and angiocardiography defined more and more congenital as well as acquired diseases, leading to new modalities of treatment.

In the last quarter of this century, ultrasound, computerized tomography, magnetic nuclear resonance, and nuclear radiography, of course, were introduced, rendering obsolete many former types of diagnostic studies in children (table 9.4).

When *anesthesia* became a routine part of *surgery*, subterfuge and surprise no longer were necessary to subdue an unsuspecting child requiring a surgical procedure for which there was no safe sedation. After the turn of the century, moreover, sophisticated anesthesia and greater understanding of the

TABLE 9.4
SOME RADIOLOGIC STUDIES NOW OBSOLETE IN CHILDREN[33]

Skull x-rays for calcification

Pneumoencephalography

Ventriculography

Intravenous cholangiogram

Oral cholecystography

Oblique chest x-rays

Tomography

Cardiac fluoroscopy

Lymphangiography

Myelography

Umbilical aortography

physiological concepts of heat loss, blood volume depletion, postoperative nutrition, fluid and electrolyte management, and antibiotics made longer operative time and more complex pediatric surgeries possible. Surgeons, using noninvasive radiological measures, facilitated by modern anesthesia, could correct complex anomalies, make repairs, excise malignancies, drain infections, and alleviate pain.

The father of pediatric surgery was William E. Ladd (1880–1967) of Boston Children's Hospital, where he established clinical and training programs for infant and child surgery. In 1913, Ladd employed the x-ray to diagnose intussusception. In 1933 he described small-bowel obstruction secondary to malrotation, as well as a simple procedure for relieving the duodenal compression.[34] In 1939 he performed the first successful staged repair of esophageal atresia. N. Logan Leven, in St. Paul, Minnesota, performed the same procedure at about the same time.

Ladd and Robert Gross (1905–1988) published their textbook *Abdominal Surgery of Infancy and Childhood* in 1941.

Advances in pediatric anesthesia and microsurgical techniques encouraged attempts to treat lesions once thought unapproachable, particularly those of congenital heart disease. Robert Gross, Ladd's successor, in 1939 performed the first ligation of a patent ductus arteriosus (PDA). Together with Charles Hufnagel (1916–1989) in 1945, Gross devised an experimental approach for repair of aortic coarctation. In Sweden that same year, C. Crafoord (b.1899) performed a coarctation repair. In 1949, Gross first used a homologous graft to correct a coarctation aneurysm. Gross published

Surgery of Infancy and Childhood in 1953, and *An Atlas of Children's Surgery* in 1970.

The study of heart malformations always had been conducted along anatomical lines until Maude Abbott (1869–1940) and Helen Brooke Taussig (1898–1986) reexamined the discipline and reclassified cardiac anomalies along pathophysiological lines, which broadened thinking regarding surgical intervention. Abbott wrote her *Atlas of Congenital Cardiac Diseases* in 1936, and Taussig published *Congenital Malformations of the Heart* in 1947.

Pediatric cardiovascular surgery truly came into its own as a result of a palliative procedure developed by Taussig and Alfred Blalock (1899–1964). The Blalock-Taussig procedure for tetralogy of Fallot and pulmonary stenosis was done first in 1945. Taussig's own words regarding one of her patients are worth quoting:

[One] operation was on an utterly miserable, small, 6-year-old boy who had a red-blood-cell count of 10 million and was no longer able to walk. When Dr. Blalock first removed the clamps, the blood welled up in the child's chest. Dr. Blalock quickly controlled the hemorrhage and poured in plasma. Suddenly Dr. Merrill Harmel cried, "He's a lovely color now," and I walked around to the head of the table and saw his lovely normal pink lips! The child woke up in the operating room and asked, "Is the operation over?" When Dr. Blalock said "Yes," the child said "May I get up now?" From that moment on he was a happy and active child.[35]

R. C. Brock (b.1914) repaired a stenosed pulmonary valve in 1948. In 1954 open heart surgery via cardiopulmonary bypass was done for the first time at the University of Minnesota.[36] Other milestones of pediatric surgery are listed in table 9.5.

Mention of *pediatric endocrine disorders* such as cretinism or precocious puberty can be found in older texts but only as descriptions of appearance with little understanding of their nature or causes. It was not until the middle of the twentieth century that the subdiscipline of pediatric endocrinology was established. Lawson Wilkins (1894–1963), with his textbook *The Diagnosis and Treatment of Endocrine Disorders in Childhood and Adolescence* (1950) and his array of national and international fellows, was largely responsible. The discipline's underpinnings[37] began with the expositions of Claude Bernard (1813–1878) and Charles Brown-Séquard (1817–1894) on secretions, which William Bayliss (1860–1924) and Ernest Starling (1866–1927) later named hormones. Viennese Artur Biedl's (1869–1933) text *Innere Sekretion* (1910) was, essentially, endocrinology's "incunabulum."

In 1922, Frederick Banting (1891–1941) and Charles Best (1899–1978) published their seminal work on insulin, and in the 1940s Edward C.

TABLE 9.5
PEDIATRIC SURGERY MILESTONES

1905	Froehlich: *Etudes de chirurgie infantile*
1906	Kirmisson: *Précis de chirurgie infantile*
1908	Holmgren: *Om innerörats variga sjukdomar*
1912	Ramstedt procedure for pyloric stenosis
1914	Griffith describes bleeding Meckel's diverticulum
1926	Abt and Strauss correct bleeding Meckel's diverticulum
1929	Forssmann introduces cardiac catheterization
1930	Drachter and Gossmann: *Lehrbuch der Chirurgie des Kindesalters*
1936	Katherine Dodd defines meconium ileus
1944	Ombredanne: *Précis clinique et opératoire de chirurgie infantile*
1948	Swenson devises the pullthrough
1951	Dennis uses venous diversion for atrial septal defect (ASD) repair
	Campbell: *Clinical Pediatric Urology*
1953	Gibbon introduces the heart-lung machine and Lewis uses hypothermia for ASD correction
1954	Merill and kidney transplantation
1964	Mustard does a two-stage correction for transposition
1965	Glenn devises shunt for hypoplastic right ventricle
1966	Rashkind develops balloon septostomy
1968	Rastelli makes aortic homografts for complex lesions
1971	Fontan performs a caval–pulmonary artery shunt

Kendall (1886–1972) and Tadeus Reichstein (b.1897) discussed corticosteroids. Progress in endocrinology, however, was not possible until a facile method was developed by which to identify, measure, and study hormones. This occurred as a result of the work of Nobel laureates Solomon Berson (b.1918) and Rosalyn Yallow (b.1921), who, in the 1950s, defined and refined the radioimmunoassay methodology. The process made possible the identification and quantification of very specific molecules often found circulating in nanogram concentrations. Significant achievements that had an impact on pediatric endocrinology are listed in table 9.6.

The field of *gastroenterology* blossomed with the availability of the x-ray, which facilitated the study of peristalsis and functional anatomy; manometry for measuring pressures; biopsy technology to study tissue and enzymol-

TABLE 9.6
SOME MILESTONES THAT TOUCH ON PEDIATRIC
ENDOCRINOLOGY AND METABOLISM

1850	Chatin shows that some cretinism can be prevented by iodine
1856	Brown-Séquard demonstrates adrenals necessary for life
1874	Kausmaul breathing described
1896	Vassale and Generali reveal tetany secondary to parathyroidectomy
1898–1904	Adrenaline isolated
1901	Froehlich syndrome described
1905	Bulloch and Sequeira describe adrenogenital syndrome
1908	Von Reuss describes galactosemia
1909	Garrod's *Inborn Errors of Metabolism*
1910	Apert describes the adrenogenital syndrome
1914	Erdheim demonstrates compensatory parathyroid hyperplasia in rickets, and thyroxin is isolated by Kendall
1915	Keaton and Koch work on the nature of gastrin
1917	Marine and Kimball give iodine to schoolgirls for the prophylaxis of goiter
1920	Dubreuil and Anderodias show hyperinsulinemia in the newborns of diabetic mothers
1922	Banting and Best work on insulin
1927	Medes described tyrosinosis
1928	Kamm isolates vasopressin
1929	Action of thyroid stimulating hormone (TSH) described
1931	Androsterone is isolated by Butenandt and Fanconi continues work on dwarfism and renal rickets
1933	Feldberg and Gaddum elucidate acetylcholine role in nerve conduction
1934	Folling reports on phenylketonuria
1937	Bakwin studies newborn tetany and hypoparathyroidism
1937–1952	Adrenal cortical hormones isolated
1938	Reilly uses I^{131} to study the thyroid in children
1942	Talbott calls attention to increased androgens in the adrenogenital syndrome
1945	Beadle presents the one gene–one enzyme concept
1950	Lee works with cadaveric growth hormone extracts Wilkins's . . . *Endocrine Disorders of Childhood* . . .
1954	Bickel treats phenylketonuria with a special diet Menkes reports on maple sugar urine disease McQuarrie describes infantile idiopathic hypoglycemia
1957	Winters works on hypophosphatemic rickets
1972	Mandatory screening for infantile hypothyroidism
1985	Genetech introduces recombinant growth hormone

ogy; immunoprotein assays to study antigens and antibodies; and noninvasive ultrasound and radionuclides. With the advent of fiberoptics and ever smaller devices, even newborn imaging became possible. Achievements in pediatric gastroenterology appear in table 9.7.

TABLE 9.7
SIGNIFICANT MILESTONES IN PEDIATRIC GASTROENTEROLOGY

1888	Gee	Celiac affliction
1894	Swaine	Corrects first biliary cyst
1900	Gilbert	First example of metabolic liver dysfunction
1913	Ylppö	Concept of immaturity of biliary metabolism
1927	Ladd	First surgical cure of biliary atresia
1929	Freudenberg	*Physiology and Pathology of Digestion in Infancy*
1935	Gross	Describes inspissated bile
1935	Knaver	Describes cystic fibrosis (CF)
1938	Blackfan	Abnormal glucose metabolism of CF
1944	Farber	Describes exocrine gland inspissation of CF and suggests term "mucoviscidosis"
1947	Dicke	Bread and biscuits worsen celiac disease
1949	McMahon, Taunhauser	Describes intrahepatic biliary atresia
1950	Weigers, Van de Kamer	Wheat-free diet in celiacs decreases steatorrhea
1950	Dean	Large-scale testing on fluorides for caries
1951	Schwachman	Gelatin test for CF; popularizes term "mucoviscidosis"
1952	Illingworth, Cori, Cori	Series of papers describing glycogen storage disease
1952	Crigler, Naggiar	Metabolic familial jaundice
1953	diSant 'Agnese	Finds elevated sweat sodium in CF
1953	Cole, Lattle	Glucuronyl transferase immaturity
1954	Hsia	Micromethod for bilirubin
1954	Jelliffe	Veno-occlusive disease
1956	Astley	*Alimentary Radiology of Children*
1956	Isselbacher	Congenital galactosemia
1959	Gibson, Cooke	Pilocarpine iontophoresis for CF
1959	Kasai	Biliary atresia surgery
1963	Reye	Visceral steatosis and encephalopathy
1963	Starzl	Transplantation
1967	Scriver, Larochelle	Hereditary tyrosinemia
1964	Rubin	Mucosal changes of celiac disease
1968	Sharp	α_1-Antitrypsin liver disease
1971	Peden	Total parenteral nutrition (TPN) cholestasis
1971	Silverman, Roy, Cozetto	*Clinical Pediatric Gastroenterology*

continued

1973	Alagille-Watson	Arteriohepatic dysplasia syndrome
1973	Goldfischer	Peroxisome/mitochondrial defect
1983	Balistreri, Huebi, Suchy	Physiological cholestasis concept
1983	Alagille, Colón, Mowat	First texts of hepatology in France, United States, and England

As a consequence of growing awareness of the importance of prenatal and antenatal care, *neonatology* evolved as a distinct discipline (table 9.8). The concept of antenatal attention had begun with Edinburgh obstetrician John Ballantyne, who had studied the effects on newborns of maternal infection—syphilis, tuberculosis, and typhoid—and toxic exposures to alcohol and opiates. His findings resulted in a published appeal in 1901 for the establishment of maternity hospitals.[38] At the time, more than 95 percent of babies were born at home. Accurate statistics with respect to birthrates and mortality were virtually impossible. Viable prematures, for example, often were cited as stillborns by families who had neither the means nor the psychic energy to nurse a premature into survival. Except in parish baptismal books, even healthy full-term newborns commonly were not registered.

TABLE 9.8
HIGHLIGHTS IN NEONATOLOGY

1903	Hochheim	Description of hyaline membrane disease
1914	Von Reuss	*Diseases of the Newborn* (English, 1922)
1915	Grulee	Research into the feeding of prematures
1917	Newman	*The Biology of Twins*
1922	Hess	*Premature and Congenitally Diseased Infants*
1927	Scammon	Compiled data on fetal and newborn growth
1929	Ylppö	Studies on prematures
1931	Farber	Hyaline membrane disease
1935	Brock	*Biologische Daten für den Kinderarzt*
1937	Bakwin	Hypoparathyroid tetany
	Gesell	Studies in developmental medicine
1938	Darrow, R.	Erythroblastosis and maternal antibodies
1940	White	*Physiology of the Fetus*
	Bundesen	Started premature transport service in Chicago
	Windle	*Physiology of the Newborn*
1941	Hess and Lundeen	*The Premature Infant: Its Medical and Nursing Care*
	Clifford	Description of the postmature
	Gregg	Description of congenital rubella syndrome

1941	McCance	Newborn metabolic and renal function studies
	Smith	*Physiology of the Newborn*
1942	Terry	Suspected oxygen >40% in retinopathy of prematurity (ROP)
1943	Day	Studies of newborn respiratory metabolism
	Kanner	Infantile autism
1944	Helfrick and Abelson	First documented report of infant TPN
1946	Barcroft	*Researches on Prenatal Life*
	Wallerstein	Exchange transfusion for erythroblastosis
1947	Dean	Newborn renal maturation studies
1948	Dunham	*Premature Infants: A Manual for Physicians*
	Parmelee	*Management of the Newborn*
	Schaffer	*Diseases of the Newborn*
	Diamond	Exchange transfusion for erythroblastosis
1950	Widdowson	Newborn chemical composition and growth
1951	Royce	Indwelling nasogastric tube for nutrition
1951–1954		Oxygen toxicity and retrolental fibroplasia
1953	Apgar	Newborn perinatal score; national cooperative study of oxygen toxicity and ROP
1954	Pick	Placental abnormalities and newborn stigmata
1959	Avery	Relationship of surfactant to respiratory distress syndrome (RDS)
1961	Lenz and McBride	Association of thalidomide and phocomelia
1963	Lubchenco	Publishes intrauterine growth curves
	Freda	Anti-D Rh immunoglobulin for erythroblastosis
1964	Dawkins	Fat thermogenesis in the newborn
1967	Northway	Describes bronchopulmonary dysplasia
1968	Dudrick	Long-term infant TPN
1971	Gregory	Respiratory distress and continuous positive airway pressure (CPAP) treatment
	Gluck	Phospholipid analysis for fetal lung maturity
1977	Dubowitz	*Gestational Age of the Newborn*

Exact cumulative statistics of mortality and morbidity of newborns and mothers began in America around 1915. The appalling figures stimulated attempts to shift the accouchement site from the home to the more sanitary environment of the hospital. It was a gradual process.

Obstetricians began to defer to their pediatric colleagues, whose skills in nurseries caring for tiny infant bodies were widely appreciated and allowed obstetricians to focus attention on postpartum care of mothers.[39] By the end of the 1930s the partnership between the two disciplines was well established.

Incubator design became more complex and sophisticated. In the early twentieth century, inexpensive models for home use as well as for hospital units were advertised. Home models relied on electric hot plates or carbon filament bulbs for heat and wet sponges for humidity. Hospital units had glass tops or sides and wheels for mobility; they used hot water for heat. By the 1930s and 1940s incubators—"isolettes"—were made of Plexiglas, electrically heated air warmed and humidified, and the salvage of the small newborn had become a routine occurrence.*

Technological advances supplied the means to sustain premature newborns as well as to treat specific and often life-threatening problems: micromethodology requiring very little blood, exchange transfusions, radiant warmers, respirators, microsurgery, newborn pharmacodynamics, and other elements of care for tiny bodies were given exacting attention. Feeding was greatly facilitated by the introduction of the rubber catheter for gastric suctioning and gavage. Neonatologists worked in this setting, rendering newborn intensive care to highly compromised new life. The statistic for newborn mortality, nearly 100 per 1,000 in 1915, had been lowered to 9 per 1,000 by the late 1970s.

Social activists, such as American crusaders Josephine Baker (1873–1945) and Lillian Wald (1867–1940), played an important concomitant role in reducing infant mortality. Baker earned her medical degree in 1898 and in 1908 became director of the Division of Child Hygiene in New York City. She instituted programs instructing mothers on how to deal with summer diarrheas, promoted enforced licensing of midwives, and organized the Little Mothers' League, an educational program for the older sisters of beleaguered families who cared for younger siblings. At the end of her tenure in 1923, the city had the lowest infant mortality rate of any city in Europe or America.[40]

---

*Public awareness regarding the use of incubators for premature infants increased as a result of the publication of magazines and journals on mothering. And "incubator-baby side shows" (bizarre as they sound) made even the uninterested curious. In 1896, Martin Couney (?1860–1950) had been asked by his old mentor, Pierre Budin, to arrange an exhibit of incubators for the Berlin World Exposition in the hope of enlisting public support for their use in hospitals. Couney obliged with six incubators, a group of nurses and six tiny babies from the Berlin Charité in a public display called *Kinderbrutanstalt*. Daily, large crowds paid to see the "human hatcheries," and Couney got a whiff of a windfall. He repeated the exhibit in London (1897), Omaha (1898), Paris (1900), Buffalo (1901), and St. Louis (1904) and finally made the show an annual fixture at Coney Island, New York. Thousands of dollars were generated by as many as 3,000 patrons a day who wanted to see premature babies in incubators. Couney's exhibit was on display in San Francisco in 1915, Chicago in 1933, and at the New York World's Fair in 1939! (Silverman, 1979, pp. 127–40).

Wald directed the Visiting Public Health Nursing Association, which operated out of the Henry Street Settlement in New York and watched over new mothers and their babies during home visits.

Two more tables remain. The penultimate table (table 9.9) in this chapter is a list of all the winners of the E. Mead Johnson Pediatric Research Award given to those individuals whose lifetime of study and investigation into diseases of children has been exceptional.

The final table (appendix 9.1) in this chapter is a beadroll of personages who have made significant contributions to the discipline of pediatrics during the twentieth century. Collectively, their works contributed to dramatically reduced rates of child morbidity and mortality worldwide.

The world's children face an uncertain future. The twenty-first century will begin with many serious unresolved problems—political, social, and medical. Pediatricians treat patients whose medical conditions have roots in the complicated social issues of the times, and they spend a great deal of time addressing these as well as rendering medical care.[41] Teenage pregnancies, child abuse, AIDS, violence, drugs and alcohol, starvation, and environmental toxicities present unique and often insurmontable challenges.

Teenage pregnancies—children having children—are at the root of several child-nurturing problems. These pregnancies commonly lead to prematurity, low birth weights, poor nutrition, poor parenting, child abuse, even infanticide.[42] In the United States alone, 15 of every 1,000 children are victims of abuse or neglect, and nearly 80 percent of the perpetrators are parents.[43]

Child abuse occurs at the hands of parents and, in many countries, results from exploitation in the workplace. In political wars, children commonly are helpless pawns and victims of warring factions. Illiteracy, starvation, maiming, disease, and death are their only destinies.

The world's AIDS epidemic will continue to engulf tens of thousands of children. One of every hundred persons on this earth is human immunodeficiency virus (HIV) positive. Most live in countries that cannot afford the new drugs being developed to combat HIV.

Measles and malnutrition remain scourges worldwide. Case fatality rates vary from 5 percent to 25 percent in developing nations.[44] These deaths are from preventable plagues—malnutrition and starvation callously inflicted as a political weapon, and measles for want of simple vaccination. The old Arabic proverb "Count your children after the measles has passed" still applies today.

The world's environment remains threatened as nations strive to achieve industrial advancements regardless of the cost to the planet. Pesticides, herbicides, polyhalogenated biphenyls, heavy metals, emission gases, acid rain, and radiation are major hazards now and in the foreseeable future.

In the foreseeable future, however, are also many exciting prospects. Several protocols already are in place that, when fully realized, will contribute most positively to the world and its children. More and more disease entities will disappear as research breakthroughs make cures possible. The human genome will be completed. Gene therapy and plenipotent cellular transplant are in the offing. Finally, the "brave new world" of space colonization is at hand. Current speculation about the future and health of children in space[45] will in time defer to our grandchildren's reports of their trips to the new frontier. They will be fascinating sagas!

TABLE 9.9
E. MEAD JOHNSON AWARD RECIPIENTS

1939	Frederic Gibbs	EEG and epilepsy
	Dorothy Anderson	Cystic fibrosis research
1940	Robert Gross	Surgical management of the patent ductus arteriosus (PDA)
	Lee Farr	Serum proteins in nephrosis
1941	Rene Dubois	Development of antibacterials
	Albert Sabin	Nutrition in CNS viral infections
1942	David Bodiam	Pathophysiology of polio
	Howard Howe	
	Harold Harrison	Parathyroid metabolism
	Helen Harrison	
1943	Hattie Alexander	Treatment of Haemophilus influenza
	Philip Levine	Erythroblastosis and Rh factor
1944	Fuller Albright	Causes of osteomalacia
	Josef Warkany	Nutrition and congenital malformations
1945	No awards	
1946	Horace Hodes	Transmission of Japanese B encephalitis
	Paul Harper	Malaria in the South Pacific
1947	Helen Taussig	Tetralogy of Fallot research
	Louis Diamond	Exchange transfusion in the newborn
1948	Wolf Zuelzer	Hematology research
	Benjamin Spock	Teaching of pediatrics
1949	Nathan Talbot	Practical endocrinology
	Henry Barnett	Newborn kidney function
1950	Charles May	Research into cystic fibrosis
	Henry Shwachman	
	Gertrude Henle	Prevention of mumps
	Walter Henle	

1951	William Wallace Victor Najjar	Physiology of intracellular fluid Metabolism of bilirubin
1952	Seymour Cohen Ovar Swenson Edward Neuhauser	Research on bacterial viruses Treatment of congenital megacolon
1953	Frederick Robbins Thomas Weller Margaret Smith	Viral tissue cultures Research into bacterial infections
1954	Robert Cooke Vincent Kelley	Renal regulation of body composition Pituitary-adrenal axis
1955	Robert Good	Disturbances of gamma globulin system
1956	David Gitlin Arnall Patz	Serum protein metabolism Oxygen in retrolental fibroplasia
1957	Alfred Bongiovanni Walter Eberlein Albert Dorfman	Steroid biogenesis Metabolism of connective tissue
1958	William Silverman Norman Kretchmer	The premature Amino acid metabolism
1959	C. Henry Kempe Barton Childs	Smallpox and vaccination studies Genetics and metabolic disease
1960	Robert Aldrich Irving Schulman	Disorders of pyrrole metabolism Regulation of platelet production
1961	Lytt Gardner Donald Pickering	Physiology of the adrenal gland Research on childhood hypothyroidism
1962	Park Gerald Robert Vernier	Hemoglobin structure Renal disease of childhood
1963	Carleton Gajdusek Richard Smith	Children in primitive cultures Immunology of the newborn
1964	Robert Chanock Abraham Rudolph	Pediatric respiratory diseases Postnatal circulatory adjustments
1965	David Hsia Stanley James	Phenylketonuria research Acidosis of birth asphyxia
1966	William Tooley Robert Winters	Pulmonary blood flow of the newborn Acid-base balance
1967	Henry Kirkman Henry Meyer Paul Parkman	G-6-PD deficiency Live attenuated rubella vaccine
1968	Mary Ellen Avery Charles Scriver	Newborn pulmonary physiology Amino acid cellular transport

continued

1969	Frederick Battaglia	Fetal physiology
	Gerald Odell	Neonatal hyperbilirubinemia
1970	Myron Winick	Brain growth and development
	Joseph Bellanti	Anti-viral antibodies
1971	Paul Quie	Antibacterial host defenses
	Fred Rosen	Human complement system
1972	Chester Edelmann	Developmental renal physiology
	Frank Oski	Newborn red cell metabolism
1973	Henry Nadler	Amniocentesis and cytogenetics
	James White	Platelet physiology
1974	Andre Nahmias	Childhood infectious diseases
	E. Richard Stiehm	Immunology research
1975	John Robbins	Research on Haemophilus influenza
	David Smith	
	Rawle McIntosh	Immunology of renal disease
1976	Haig Kazazian	Molecular biology of hemoglobin
	David Rimoin	Hereditary cartilage-bone metabolism
1977	Arthur Ammann	Pediatric immunology
	Michael Miller	Mechanisms of inflammatory response
1978	Samuel Latt	Cytogenetics and chromosome replication
	Pearay Ogra	Immunologic mucosal barriers
1979	Philip Ballard	Fetal glucocorticoid receptors
	Harvey Colten	Complement deficiency
1980	R. Michael Blaese	Disorders in immunodeficient children
	S. Michael Mauer	Glomerular diseases in children
1981	Robert Desnick	Inherited metabolic diseases
	Erwin Gelfand	Mechanisms of T-cell activation
1982	Larry Shapiro	X-chromosome inactivation
	Jerry Winkelstein	Complement in host defense
1983	Laurence Boxer	Granulocyte function research
	Samuel Lux	RBC membrane in spherocytosis
1984	Jan Breslow	Genetics of atherosclerosis
	John Phillips	Genetics of polypeptide hormone disorders
1985	Russell Chesney	Pediatric nephrology research
	A. Joseph D'Ercole	Hormonal control of growth
1986	Raif Geha	Allergy and immunology research
	Alan Jobe	Surfactant in RDS physiology
1987	Donald Anderson	Leucocyte biology
	Stuart Orkin	Clinical molecular biology
1988	Barry Wolf	Biotinidase deficiency

1988	Jeffrey Whitsett	Molecular biology of pulmonary surfactant
1989	Steven Reppert	Research on fetal clocks
	Robert Yolken	Rapid methodology of viral identification
1990	Gregory Grabowski	Human lysosomal disorders
	Arnold Strauss	Mitochondrial enzyme disorders
1991	Louis Kunkel	Molecular basis of muscular dystrophy
	Ronald Warton	
1992	Ann M. Arvin	Herpes and varicella infection studies
	Francis Collins	Molecular genetics of cystic fibrosis
	Lap-Chee Tsui	
1993	Edward McCabe	Molecular basis of pediatric diseases
	Alan Schwartz	Receptor-mediated endocytosis
1994	David Williams	Hematopoietic stem cell biology
	David Permutter	Molecular biology of α_1-antitrypsin
1995	Margaret Hostetter	Pathogenesis of candidiasis
	Alan Krensky	Transplant rejection studies
1996	Perrin White	Molecular genetics of steroid diseases
	Huda Zoghbi	Inherited neurological syndromes
1997	Donald Leung	Chronic allergic diseases
	Elaine Tuomanen	Mechanisms of bacterial pathogenesis

NOTES

1. The roster of founding members is a who's who of twentieth-century pediatrics: Job Lewis Smith, Samuel Adams, Alexander Blackader, William Booker, August Caillé, Francis Huber, Abraham Jacobi, Henry Koplik, Thomas Latimer, Arthur Meigs, Charles Putnam, Thomas Rotch, August Seibert, Louis Starr, and William Watson. Faber and McIntosh, 1966, pp. 7–11.

2. Hawes, 1991, p. 56.

3. Huges, J. G., *Pediatrics* 1993; 92:469–70.

4. Fildes, 1986, pp. 224–30.

5. Apple, 1980, pp. 402–17.

6. Bullough, 1981, pp. 257–59.

7. Ibid.

8. By 1941 the American Food and Drug Administration (FDA) had ordered infant food labeled for water, calorie, protein, fat, carbohydrate, calcium, phosphorus, iron, and vitamin content. Powdered formulations did not appear until the second half of the century when technology facilitated the economical and practical reduction of electrolytes in which to make a quality protein source with reduced salts. In 1980, Congress passed the Infant Formula Act, which placed the regulation of formulas under the control of the FDA (Filer, 1993, pp. 285–86).

9. Preston, 1994, pp. 126–27.

10. Szent Györgyi, A., *Biochem J* 1928;22:1387.

11. Waugh, W. A., King, C. G., *J Biol Chem* 1932;97:325.

12. Harrison, 1991, p. 163.

13. Shipley, P. G., Park, E. A., McCollum, E. V., et al., *J Biol Chem* 1921;45:343–48.

14. Jeans, P. C. *JAMA* 1936;106:2066–69.

15. Blunt, J. W., DeLuca. H. F., and Schones, H. K., *Biochemistry* 1968;7:3317–22. Kodicek, E., *Lancet* 1974;1:325–29.

16. Hinojosa, F., *Gac Med Mex* 1865;1:139–44.

17. Talbot, F. B., *Am J Dis Child* 1921;22:358–70.

18. Kerpel-Fronius, E., *J Pediatr* 1945;30:244–49.

19. Soto, E., et al., *Am J Dis Child* 1942;64:977–95.

20. Waterlow, J. C., *MRC Report*, no. 263, 1948.

21. Jelliffe, D. B., *J Pediatr* 1959;54:227–56.

22. Lusk, 1932, p. 130.

23. Swyer, 1991, p. 206.

24. Abt, 1965, p. 136.

25. Cone, 1979, p. 205.

26. Silverstein, 1996, pp. 1–3.

27. Grundbacher, 1992, pp. 188–89.

28. De Quadros et al., 1992, pp. 239–52.

29. Griscom, 1995, p. 1399.

30. Singleton, 1995, p. 108.

31. Not for the first time. Felix Platter (1536–1614) spoke of *mors thymica*. Ruhräh, 1925, p. 239.

32. Downes, 1995, pp. 1409–10.

33. Ibid., p. 1417.

34. Abt, 1965, pp. 248–49.

35. Taussig, H. A., *J Am Med Wom Assoc* 1981;36:43–44.

36. Moller, 1994, p. 2479.

37. Prader, 1991, pp. 97–103.

38. Ballantyne, J. W., A Plea for a Pro-maternity Hospital. *Br Med J* 1901;1:813–14.

39. Desmond, 1991, pp. 314–17.

40. Bendiner, 1995, pp. 68–71.

41. Colón, 1989, p. 45.

42. Overpeck, M. D., et al., Risk Factors for Infant Homicide. *N Engl J Med* 1998;339:1211–16.

43. *Child Health, USA*, Maternal and Child Health Bureau, 1997.

44. Belamarich, P., Measles and Malnutrition. *Pediatrics in Review* 1998;19:70–71.

45. Colón, A. R., and Colón, P. A., 1992, pp. 5–20.

APPENDIX 9.1
SOME PROMINENT FIGURES OF 20TH-CENTURY PEDIATRICS

ABT, Isaac (1867–1955): editor of *Pediatrics* (1923) and *Pediatric Year Book*; first president, American Academy of Pediatrics

ACUNA, Mamerto (1875–?): *Manual Practico de Alimentación de Lactantes*

ALBRIGHT, Fuller (1900–1960): 19 eponymic syndromes

ALDRICH, C. Anderson (1888–1949): *Babies Are Human Beings* (1938)

ALEXANDER, Hattie (1901–1968): research on *Haemophilus influenzae* meningitis

AMBERG, Samuel (1874–?): with Helmolz, *Diseases of the Genito-Urinary System in Infancy and Childhood* (1930)

ANDERSON, Dorothy (1901–1963): pathology of cystic fibrosis (1938), trypsin assays (1942)

ANDERSON, Henning (1916–1978): Danish pioneer pediatric endocrinology

APERT, Eugene (1868–1940): characterized acrocephalosyndactyly; *Précis des maladies des enfants* (1909)

APGAR, Virginia (1909–1974): devised a newborn stability scale

ARENA, Jay (b.1909): advocate of studies in childhood poisoning

BABONNEIX, Leon (1876–1942): with Nobécourt, *Traite de Médecine des Enfants* in five volumes (1933)

BAGINSKY, Adolf (1843–1918): editor of *Archiv für Kinderheilkunde*

BAKWIN, Harry (1894–1972): researched newborn water metabolism; with Ruth Bakwin, *Behavior Disorders in Children* (1953)

BARCROFT, Joseph (1872–1947): *Researches on Pre-natal Life . . .* (1946)

BATTEN, J. de (1861–1918): pediatric neurologist to the Hospital for Sick Children in Great Ormond Street

BENDIX, Bernhardt (1863–?): with Jules Uffelmann, *Handbuch der Kinderheilkunde*

BESSAU, Georg (1884–1944): worked on intravenous treatment of septic shock

BIEDERT, Philip (1847–1916): pioneer in calorimetric method of infant nutrition

BINET, Alfred (1857–1911): developer of psychometrics (1905)

BLACKFAN, Kenneth (1883–1941): devised methods of intraperitoneal fluid administration for babies

BLOCH, Carl Edward (1872–1952): Danish pioneer in pediatric pathology

BOKAI, Janor (1822–1884): *Die Geschichte der Kinderheilkunde*

BOURNEVILLE, Desire (1840–1909): pediatric neurologist to the Bicetre

BRAZELTON, T. Berry (b.1918): child development and behavioral scale

BRENNEMANN, Joseph (1872–1944): *Practice of Pediatrics* (1936)

BROWN, Dennis (1892–1967): devised new surgical techniques and conducted research on congenital anomalies

BRUIN, J. de (1861–1927): *De Voeding van het Kind in het eerste Levensjaar* (1905)

BRÜNING, Hermann (1873–?): with Schwalbe, *Handbuch der allgemeinen Pathologie und der pathologischen Anatomie des Kindersalters* (1912)

BRUNS, Ludwig (1858–1916): *Handbook of Nervous Diseases of Children* (1912)

BUDIN, Pierre (1846–1907): *Manual pratique de l'allaitment* (1905)

BUTLER, A. M. (1894–1986): metabolic balance studies; developed methods for sodium and plasma protein determinations

CALMETTE, Albert (1863–1933): with C. Guerin introduced the BCG tuberculosis vaccine (1926)

CAMERER, Wilhelm (1842–1910): studied composition of human milk and infant growth

CAMERON, Hector (1878–?): *Diet and Diseases in Infancy* (1915)

CARONIA, Guiseppe (1884–1977): worked on childhood leishmaniasis

CARPENTER, George (1859–1910): *Congenital Syphilis in Children in Everyday Practice* (1901)

CARR, Walter (1859–1942): devised a "premature unit" without incubators

CASAMAJOR, Louis (1881–1962): pediatric neurologist

CATHALA, Jean (1891–1969): *L'hygiène et la clinique de la première enfance*

CATTANEO, Cesare (1871–?): *Terapia delle malattie dell'infanzia . . .* (1901)

CAUTLEY, Edmund (?–1944): *Diseases of Children* (1910)

CERVESATO, Dante (1850–1905): founder of the school of pediatrics in Bologna

CHAPIN, Henry Dwight (1857–1942): *Theory and Practice of Infant Feeding* (1902)

CHAPPLE, Charles (1903–1979): refined the incubator, allowing fresh air from outside and closely regulating temperature and humidity—the "isolette"

CHOREMIS, Konstantinos (1900–1966): *He phymatiosis ton paidon* (1928)

CHURCHILL, Frank (1864–1946): first editor of *American Journal of Diseases of Children* (1911)

COCKAYNE, Edward (1880–1956): *Inherited Abnormalities of the Skin and Its Appendages* (1933)

COMBY, Jules (1853–1947): with Marfan and Grancher, *Traite des maladies de l'enfance*

CONCETTI, Luigi (1853–1920): founded *Rivista di clinica pediatrica*

CONE, Thomas E. (1915–1998): historian of American pediatrics

COOKE, Robert (b.1920): renal electrolyte function in children

COOLEY, Thomas (1871–1945): one of the founders of the American Academy of Pediatrics; described thalassemia major

CROSS, Mary (1902–1973): *The Premature Baby*

CZERNY, Adalbert (1863–1941): *Der Arzt al Erzieher des Kindes* (1908); *Sammlung klinischer Vorlesungen über Kinderkeilkunde* (1948)

DARGEON, Harold (1897–?): *Tumors of Childhood* (1940)

DAVISON, Wilbert (1892–1972): *The Compleat Pediatrician*

DAY, Richard (1905–1989): studied newborn thermoregulation

DEBRE, Robert (1882–1978): described congenital adrenal hyperplasia with salt loss and hypophosphatemic renal tubular acidosis; with Rajschman, founded UNICEF; with Edmond Lesne and Paul Rohmer, *Pathologie Infantile* (1943); infant hematology

DeLANGE, Cornelia (1871–1950): early clinical geneticist; *Het Kind*

DENY, Pierre (1903–1969): bacteriology of childhood diseases

DeTONI, Giovani (1895–1973): auxology of Italian children

DIAMOND, Louis (b.1902): founder of pediatric hematology

DICK, George (1881–1967) and Gladys (1881–1963): research on toxins of *Streptococcus*

DICKE, W. D. (1905–1962): demonstrated the ill effects of wheat in celiac disease

DRAPER, George (1880–1959): *Acute Poliomyelitis* (1916)

DUKES, Clement (1845–1925): defined the exanthem of rubella

ECKERT, Hans (1873–?): *Grundriss der Kinderheilkunde*

ECKSTEIN, Albert (1891–1950): wrote on encephalitides of children

ENGEL, Stefan (1878–?): with Marie Baum, *Grundriss der Sauglingskunde*

ESCHERICH, Theodor (1857–1911): worked on intestinal flora of infants; counted among his students, Moro, von Pirquet, Pfaundler, Jehle, Schick

FANCONI, Guido (1892–1979): renal tubular disorders and textbook, *Lehrbuch der Pädiatrie*, with Wallgren (1950)

FARBER, Sidney (1903–1973): established pediatric oncology, chemotherapy

FEDE, Francesco (1832–1912): founder of the school of pediatrics in Naples

FEER, Emil (1864–1955): *Lehrbuch der Kinderheilkunde* (1911)

FELDMAN, William (1879–1939): *The Principles of Antenatal and Postnatal Child Physiology* (1920)

FINDLEY, Leonard (1878–1947): worked on the etiology of rickets (1908); *The Rheumatic Infections in Childhood*

FINKELSTEIN, Heinrich (1865–1942): *Lehrbuch der Säuglingskrankheiten* (1912); proponent of isolation wards and recording daily temperatures, weight, intakes and outputs; described the physiological anemia of newborns (1911)

FISCHL, Rudolf (1862–?): *Die Ernährung des Sauglings in Gesunden und Kranken Tagen* (1903)

FISHER, Louis (1864–?): *Diseases of Infancy and Children* (1907)

FLEXNER, Simon (1863–1946): introduced the serum treatment of meningococcemia

FORD, Frank (1892–1970): *Cerebral Birth Injuries and Their Results* (1927); *Diseases of the Nervous System in Infancy, Childhood, and Adolescence* (1937)

FORSYTH, David (1877–1941): *Children in Health and Disease* (1909)

FOURNIER, A. (1832–1914): researcher in congenital syphilis

FRANGENHEIM, Paul (1876–1930): *Diseases of the Osseous System of Childhood* (1913)

FRASER, F. C. (b.1920): geneticist; collated malformations associated with specific genes

FREUD, Sigmund (1856–1939): wrote on childhood diplegias

GALTON, F. (1822–1911): conducted statistical studies on heredity

GARRAHAN, Juan (1893–1965): *Précis de Medecine Infantile*

GARROD, Archibald (1857–1936): biochemical geneticist; with Batten and Thursfield, *Diseases of Children* (1913)

GERSTENBERGER, Henry (1881–1954): powdered infant formula (1915)

GESSEL, Arnold (1880–1961): researched psychometrics and development

GILBERT, Augustin (1858–1917): described a familiar jaundice

GLANZMANN, Edouard (1887–1959): *Einführung in die Kinderheilkunde*

GLUCK, Louis (1924–1998): pioneer in perinatology, focusing on L/S ratio

GODIN, Paul (1859–1935): applied baselines to auxology

GOLDBLOOM, Alton (1890–1968): *Care of the Child* (1928)

GOMEZ-SANTOS, Federico: *Boletín médico del Hospital Infantil*

GORDON, Harry (1906–1988): defined some infantile developmental norms

GORTER, Evert (1881–1954): school of pediatrics of Leyden

GROB, Max (1901–1976): introduced operative artificial hypothermia; pioneered some cleft lip and palate procedures

GRULEE, Clifford (1880–1962): studied infant nutrition

GUÉNIOT, Alexandré (1832–1935): first defined prematurity based on weight

GUEST, George (1898–1967): studied the red blood cells of infants

GYORGI, Paul (1893–1976): conducted research on nutrition, vitamins biotin, riboflavin, and B_6

HAMBURGER, Franz (1874–?): *Children's Diseases* (1926)

HAMILL, S. McClintock (1864–1948): White House Conference on Child Development (1930)

HARRIS, Harry (1919–1994): *Human Biochemical Genetics* (1959); detected allelism by protein electrophoresis

HEMPLEMANN, Theodor (1885–1943): research on roseola (1921)

HENRY, Charles E. (b.1915): *Electroencephalogram of the Normal Child* (1944)

HERTER, C. A. (1865–1910): *On Infantilism from Chronic Intestinal Infection* (1908)

HERWERDEN, Marianne (1874–1934): cytogeneticist and advocate of eugenics

HESS, Alfred (1875–1933): researched the steroids and radiation therapy of rickets

HESS, Julius (1876–1955): established the first premature-care ward in the United States (1922)

HEUBNER, Johann (1843–1926): described caloric requirements (1901); *Lehrbuch des Kinderheilkunde* (1903)

HOCHSINGER, Carl (1860–?): *Gesundheitspflege des Kindes im Elternhause* (1903)

HODES, Horace (1907–1989): symposiums in pediatric immunology

HOOFT, Carlos (1910–1980): school of pediatrics in Belgium

HOWLAND, John (1873–1926): prominent educator; established the Harriett Lane House

HUTINEL, Victor (1849–1933): *Les maladies des enfants* (1909)

IBRAHIM, Yussof (1877–1953): isolated enterokinase in the infant

JANEWAY, Charles (b.1909): immunological research on children

JOBLING, James (1876–1961): worked with Flexner on meningiococcemia

JOCHIMS, Johannes (1899–1965): *Die Bedeutung der Nahrungsfette in der Pediatrie*

JONES, T. Duckett (1899–1954): hemolytic strep and rheumatic fever

JOSIAS, Albert Henri (1852–1906): *Therapeutiques Infantile* (1906)

JUNDELL, Isak (1866–1945): editor of *Acta Paediatrica*

KAREWSKI, Fredinand (1858–1923): *Surgery of Childhood*

KASSOWITZ, Max (1842–1913): introduced cod liver oil into the treatment of rickets; wrote on newborn syphilis

KELLER, Arthur (1862–1934): with Czerny, *Des Kindes Ernährung . . .* (1906)

KEMPE, C. Henry (1922–1984): pioneer in battered-children syndrome

KENNEDY, Roger (1897–1966): first American protocol for penicillin in children (1944)

KLEINSCHMIDT, Hans (1885–?): *Therapeutisches Vademekum für die Kinderpraxis* (1919)

KNOEPFELMACHER, Wilhelm (1866–?): conducted nutritional studies; early in 1898 recognized disturbances caused by cow milk

KNOX, John (1872–1951): leader in public health and maternal–child health programs

KOPLIK, Henry (1858–1927): redescribed pathognomonic measles "spots"; *Diseases of Infancy and Childhood* (1902)

KRABBE, Knud (1885–1961): neuroembryologist

KRUSE, Walter (1864–?): coeditor with Paul Selter of *Child Health and Hygiene* (1914)

LACHAPELLE, Séverin (1850–1913): founder of the Crèche in Montreal

LAMY, Maurice (1895–1975): early leader in genetics; *Affections congénitales et héréditaires* (1946)

LANGSTEIN, Leopold (1876–1933): crusader for child nutrition and hygiene programs

LANNELONGUE, Odilon (1840–1911): *Affections congenitales*

LEE, Pearl (1871–1945): worked with Cooley on thalassemia

LEFETRA, Linnaeus (1868–1965): developed a "premature room" environment without incubators

LEINER, Karl (1871–1930): dermatology of children

LELONG, Marcel (1892–1973): *La puériculture* (1957)

LESNÉ, Edmond (1871–1962): researcher in rickets

LEVINE, Samuel (1895–1971): conducted infantile metabolic studies

LEVINSON, Abraham (1888–?): *Examination of the Child* (1923); *Cerebrospinal Fluid in Health and Disease* (1919)
LIND, John (1909–1983): worked on fetal circulation and neonatal physiology
LOMBARDINI, Luigi (1831–1898): *Sulla Placenta: Ricerche*
LOMBROSO, Cesare (1836–1909): *Ricerche sull cretinismo in Lombardia*

MACOUZET, Roque: *Arte de criar y de curar a los Niños* (1910)
MACY, Icie (b.1892): *Nutritional and Chemical Growth in Childhood*
MANTOUX, Charles (1877–1947): intradermal tuberculosis test (1908)
MARFAN, Antonin (1858–1942): *Clinique des maladies de la premiere enfance* (1928)
MARRIOTT, William (1885–1936): acidosis researcher; *Infant Nutrition* (1930)
MASSON, Raoul (1875–1928): organizer of Hôpital Sainte Justine
McCOLLUM, Elmer (1879–1945): experimental rickets research
McKUSICK, Victor (b.1921): *Hereditary Disorders of Connective Tissues* (1956)
McNUTT, Sarah (1839–1930): studied the neuropathy of birth injuries
MEDIN, Karl (1847–1927): reported first large epidemic of polio
MENEGHELLO, Julio (b.1915): worked on nutritional diseases; pediatric education throughout South America; textbook *Pediatria* in fifth edition
MEYER, Ludwig (1879–?): leader of Israeli pediatrics; *Die Sauglingsernährung . . .* (1930)
MILLER, Nickolay (1847–1897): introduced <2500 grams as criteria for the premature in Russia
MITCHELL, A. Graeme (1889–1941): with Crozer Griffith, *Textbook of Pediatrics* (1933)
MONTESSORI, Maria (1870–1952): child development and education, *Casa di Bambini*
MORO, Ernst (1874–1951): infantile reflex, bactericidal powers of maternal milk
MORQUIO, Luis (1867–1935): *Gastrointestinal Diseases of Infancy*; known for work on osseous dystrophy
MORSE, John (1865–1940): *Textbook of Pediatrics* (1923)
MOSER, Paul (1865–1924): described antistreptococcal serum (1902)
MOURIQUAND, Georges (1880–1966): researched vitamins and nutritions
MYA, Guiseppe (1857–1911): founder of the school of pediatrics in Florence
MYERS, Bernard (1872–?): *A Practical Handbook on the Diseases of Children*

NADAS, Alexander (b.1913): *Pediatric Cardiology* (1957)
NASSAU, Erich (1888–?): with Meyer, *Ernährungstörungen in Saulingsalter* (1923)
NELSON, Waldo (1898–1997): the "Green Bible," *Textbook of Pediatrics*
NETTER, Arnold (1855–1936): bacterial infectious diseases
NEUMANN, Hugo (1858–1912): *Uber die Behandlung der Kinderkrankheiten*
NEURATH, Rudolf (1869–?): researched the physiological maturation of children; *Die pubertät; Physiologie, Pathologie* (1932)
NEWMAN, George (1870–1948): *Infant Mortality* (1906)

NIEMANN, Albert (1880–1921): *Kompendium der Kinderheilkunde* (1920)

NOBÉCOURT, Pierre (1871–1943): *Precis de medecine infantile* (1907)

ONODI, Adolf (1857–1920): *Accessary Sinuses of the Nose in Children* (1911)

OSKI, Frank (1932–1996): hematologist and researcher in RBC enzymes; advocate of child-centered legislation

PAGLIANI, Luigi (1847–1932): conducted studies on growth parameters of European children

PARKS, Edward A. (1877–1969): major contributor to the study of bone histology and metabolism in children

PARSONS, Leonard (1879–1950): with Seymour Barling, *Diseases of Infancy and Childhood* (1933)

PATERSON, Donald (b.1890): *Sick Children* (1930)

PEARSON, C. (1857–1936): statistical studies on heredity

PÉHU, Maurice (1874–1945): *L'alimentation des enfants malades* (1908); with A. Dufourt, *Tuberculosis of Infancy* (1927)

PERITZ, George (1870–?): *Die Nervenkrankheiten des Kindesalters* (1912)

PETER, Karl (1870–?): with Joseph Becker, *Handbuch der Anantomie des Kindes* (1938)

PFAUNDLER, Meinhard (1872–1947): *Handbuch der Kinderkrankheiten* (1906)

PIAGET, Jean (1896–1981): pioneer in infant psychosocial development; *La représentation du monde chez l'enfant* (1938)

PISEK, Godfrey (1875–1921): *A Treatise on Diseases of Children* (1909)

PORTER, William (1862–1949): studied socioeconomic impacts on auxology

POTTER, Edith (b.1901): *Pathology of the Fetus and the Newborn* (1952)

POWER, D'Arcy (1855–1941): *An Atlas of the Anatomy and Physiology of the Child* (1901)

POYNTON, Frederick (1869–1943): *Heart Diseases in Childhood*

PRITCHARD, George (1866–?): *Physiological Feeding of Infants and Children*

RAMON, Gaston (1886–1963): conducted research on prophylaxis of diphtheria (1925)

RATNER, Bret (1893–1957): devised an apparatus for puncturing the superior longitudinal sinus of infants

RAUCHFUSS, Karl (1835–1915): established the children's hospital of St. Petersburg

RAUDNITZ, Robert (1856–1921): *Allgemeine Chemie der Milch* (1909)

REUSS, August (1879–1954): *Die Krankheiten des Neugeborenen* (1914)

RIBADEAU-DUMAS, Louis (1876–1950): intravenous correction of dehydration

ROHMER, Paul (1876–1977): *The Infant in Health and Disease* (1931)

ROSSI, Ettore (b.1915): *Herzkrankheiten im Saulingsalter* and *Padiatrie*

ROTHCHILD, Henri (1872–?): *Bibliotheca lactaria* (1902)

ROUX, Emil Pierre Paul (1853–1933): diphtheria toxin

RUBIN, Mitchell (b.1902): studied the maturation of renal function

RUBNER, Max (1854–1932): *Studies of Nutrition in Childhood* (1902); with Heubner, *Treatment of a Nursling* (1905)

RUHRÄH, John (1872–1935): *Diseases of Infancy and Childhood* (1905); *Pediatrics of the Past* (1925); *Pediatric Biographies* (1932)

SACHS, Bernard (1858–1944): father of pediatric neurology; *Nervous Diseases of Children* (1895)

SCHICK, Bela (1877–1967): diphtheria susceptibility test

SCHLOSS, Oscar (1882–1952): contributor to the understanding of acidosis/ dehydration physiology

SCHLOSSMANN, Arthur (1867–1932): demonstrated newborn salivary amylase and fasting ketones in urine; with Meinhard Pfaundler, *Handbuch der Kinderheilkunde* (1906)

SIDBURY, James (1886–1967): devised umbilical vein transfusions

SIGAUD, Claude (1862–1921): described four classes of child somatotypes for genetic studies (1908)

SIWE, S. (1897–1961): researcher in metabolism and reticuloendothelium

SMITH, Carl (1895–1971): *Blood Diseases of Infancy and Childhood*

SOLARES, Aniceto (1886–1972): *Protección a la infancia* (1940)

SPENCE, James (1892–1954): enhanced position of children in the National Health Service

SPITZ, Rene (1887–1974): involutional marasmus research; *La premiere annee de la vie de l'enfant* (1958)

SPITZY, Hans (1872–?): *Surgery and Orthopedics in Children*

SPOCK, Benjamin (1903–1998): best-selling populist pediatrician

STILL, George Frederick (1868–1941): described arthritis in 1896; *Diseases of Children* (1909); *History of Pediatrics* (1931)

STILLMAN, J. Sydney (n.d.): pioneer in pediatric rheumatology

STOKES, Joseph (1896–1972): epidemiologist in child viral diseases

STUART, Harold (1891–1977): conducted studies on growth and development

SUDHOFF, Karl (1853–1938): premier medical historian who translated many medieval texts touching on children

SUTHERLAND, George (1861–?): *The Heart in Early Life* (1914)

TANNER, James (n.d.): with Phyllis Eveleth, *World-Wide Variation in Human Growth* (1976)

TEDESCHI, Vitale (1854–1919): founder of the school of pediatrics in Padua

THOMSON, John (1856–1926): founder of Scottish pediatrics; *Opening Doors* (1923)

TISDALL, Frederick (1893–1949): investigated child nutrition

TISSIER, Henri (1866–1926): studied significance of bacillus bifidus

TOBLER, Ludwig (1877–1915): demonstrated delayed stomach emptying secondary to fat

TRIBOULET, Henri (1864–1920): *Les oeuvres de l'enfance: maternite, premiere enfance, adolescence* (1906)

TRUMPP, Joseph (1867–1945): with Rudolf Hecker, *Atlas of Diseases of Children*
TUGENDREICH, Gustav (1876–?): *Infant Welfare* (1919)
TURPIN, Raymond (1895–1988): early proponent of BCG vaccination

USHER, Robert (b.1934): respiratory distress syndrome of prematurity; studied hypoglycemic syndromes

VAHLQUIST, Bo (1909–1978): Uppsala researcher in cow-milk nutrition; pediatric historian
VALDES-DAPEÑA, Marie (b.1921): research on sudden infant death syndrome
VAN CREVELD, Simon (1894–1971): described glycogen storage disease and coagulation factors of hemophilia
VARIOT, Gaston (1855–1930): *Traite de Hygiene Infantile* (1910)
VEEDER, Borden (1883–1970): studied congenital syphilis and roseola
VEGHELYI, Peter (1908–1986): with Kerpel-Fronius, *Perinatal Medicine*
VON JASCHKE, Rudolph (1881–?): *Physiology, Care and Nutrition of the Newborn* (1927)
VON PIRQUET (1874–1929): described and named the concept of allergy; *Die Serumkrankheit* (1905)

WAARDENBURG, Petrus (1886–1979): clinical geneticist of congenital eye diseases
WALLACE, William (1912–1948): developed rapid electrochemical determination of chloride levels
WALLGREN, Arvid (1889–1973): with Fanconi, *Lehrbuch der Pediatrie* (1950)
WARKANY, Joseph (b.1902): teratologist; *Congenital Malformations* (1971)
WASHBURN, Alfred (1895–1988): auxologist who emphasized longitudinal studies
WEILL, Edmund (1858–1924): *Precis de medecine infantile* (1900)
WEILL-HALLE, Benjamin (1875–1958): proponent of BCG vaccination; with Jerome Lejeune identified trisomy 21
WERNSTEDT, Wilhelm (1872–1962): leader of Karolinska Institute pediatrics
WHIPPLE, Dorothy (1901–1995): *Euthenic Pediatrics*
WICKMAN, Ivar (1872–1914): neuropathologist who defined polio findings
WIELAND, Emil (1867–1947): pioneer in pediatric endocrinology
WILLIAMS, Cicely (1893–1992): descriptions of kwashiorkor
WILLIAMS, Woodridge (1866–1931): emphasized maternal prophylaxis for preventing newborn lues

YLPPÖ, Arvo (1887–?): conducted many facets of research on the premature, focusing particularly on nutrition

ZAHORSKY, John (1871–1963): described roseola infantum and herpangina
ZAPPERT, Julius (1867–?): *Krankheiten des Nervensystems im Kindesalter* (1922); *Die Physikalische Therapie im Kindesalter* (1906)

Appendices

APPENDIX A
Traité akkadien de diagnostics et pronostics médicaux[*]

1. If a baby at birth does not vomit breast milk but his flesh decays: a fit of "dust."

3. If a baby at the time he is held by the nape of the neck becomes frightened and does not extend his arms [Moro reflex?]: a fit of "dust."

4. If a baby after nursing for 3 months, his flesh is wasted and if his hands and feet remain stunted: a fit of "dust."

5. If a baby his flesh is jaundiced, has not fever but his temples are depressed and he rubs his nose vigorously and does not have *upatu*: evil prayers have seized him [spell cast].

6. If a baby of good health has firm flesh but after illness strikes if his flesh collapses, if during 3 or 4 days he has fever and intestinal obstruction but the intestines move normally [peristalsis observed?]: *mehru* has seized him.

8. If a baby in the 1st, 2nd, and 3rd months becomes ill and does not sleep day or night, his flesh collapses, his intestines obstructed but move normally and is always wet: *mehru* has seized him.

10. If a baby has a hot head, if his body is not feverish . . . he does not sweat, hand and feet do not move, if he drools, cries a lot, keeps no food down and vomits: if his teeth fall out; after 15 or 20 days he will experience a painful period and will be prostrated.

13. If a baby is always sick and when you pour water on his abdomen, she does not . . . her abdomen: it is an internal rupture.

14. If a baby although he takes the breast is not satisfied and cries a lot: it is an internal rupture.

---

[*]Labat, R., *Traité akkadien de diagnostics et pronostics médicaux.* Paris: E. J. Brill, 1951.

15. If a baby, his bowels are inflamed and when the breast is offered does not want to eat [suck?]: this baby a wizard has claimed.

16. If a baby after being put to bed turns over, is restless, is afraid; from the bosom of the mother he is bewitched: the witchcraft was woven against him.

17. If a baby after being put to bed awakens, is afraid and cries incessantly; from the bosom of the mother he is bewitched: the witchcraft was woven against him.

18. If a baby, after nursing three months, his hands and feet remain contracted, and his flesh wasted; from the mother's breast he is bewitched: the witchcraft of summer weaves against him.

20. If a baby, at the mother's breast is always afraid and sick; if crying and fever remain constant, evil prayers [a spell] have seized him.

21. If a child, at 1, 2, 3, or 4 years of age is angry, cannot raise himself nor stand, if he cannot eat solids, if his mouth is frozen unable to speak: spell of Sulpaèa; he will not prosper.

24. If a baby at the mother's breast shivers of fright and cries, if he is constantly agitated with fright and leaps from the mother's knees [lap], crying a lot: the daughter of Anu has picked him out.

26. If a baby following birth, at 2 or 3 days stirs but does not accept milk [nurse] and his attack resembles the overwhelming hand of god: hand of Ishtar; his name is "Ravisher"; the infant will die.

28. If a baby does not stop crying; it is the "Ravisher," hand of Ishtar; daughter of Anu.

29. If a baby, his flesh is jaundiced, his intestines blocked, his hands and feet inflamed, is very feverish: it is lung illness; the hand of god; he will heal.

30. If a baby, his bowels are inflamed, cries endlessly, hand of the earth, hand of the daughter of Anu; hand of god; he will heal.

31. If a baby is hot everywhere at the time his abdomen is prominent: hand of Kubu.

32. If a baby, his abdominal muscles are red or yellow: hand of Kubu.

33. If a baby, his bowels are blocked and yellow: hand of Kubu.

34. If a baby is always cold and grinds his teeth, his illness will be long; he has been seized by Kubu.

35. If a baby does not stop shivering and is agitated with fright; hand of Sin; he will recover.

36. If a baby, while nursing, his flesh becomes flabby, even though his wet-

nurse has milk, when offered the breast does not eat [suck]; if he rejects the breast change to the other for his healing [get a new wet nurse?].

38. If a baby is seized by the asu and samanu: is changed to another breast and moreover is chanted over, he will recover.

39. If a baby suffers from cough, grind and mix im-kal-gug with honey and fine fat [light oil?]; the baby will absorb it in fasting; if he will not take it himself, place it on the mother's nipple and he will take it on the same time he nurses: thus, he will recover.

41. If a baby . . . from the neck to the vertebral column, his . . . are loose: he will die.

42. If a baby following an attack from Sin, his intestines are . . . and seems at all extremities[?]: in order to heal, boil down Laurel leaves, grind gum of the pine Alep, sap of the pine, ammonia[?], saffron, green parts, mix it all with galbanum oil: rub it several times on the baby: thus he will recover.

44. If a baby . . . his head is loose the kind of which the skull is dilated and he does not sleep: he will be ill for 7 or 8 days but will recover.

45. If a baby . . . his head is loose the kind of which the skull is dilated; he will die.

46. If a baby shivers and is agitated with fear, weeps, and has fear, and constantly raises his hands and feet; he is seized by Sin. . . .

47. If a baby shivers and is agitated with fear, weeps, and has fear: hand of Ishtar and Sin.

48. If a baby vomiting all he eats, if he has diarrhea, if his hands and feet are paralyzed: you shall petition Sin.

49. If a baby, while having an attack [seizure], appears to improve; this will make the illness last longer, but he will die.

50. Of a baby's appetite, if he constantly opens his mouth, but vomits everything he eats: hand of Mah—, hand of god: he will survive.

51. If a baby presents with warmth and fever, and nevertheless feels constantly cold: he has been seized by Lamastu—the hand of the daughter of Anu.

52. If a baby is hot, is cold, and wants drinking water instantly: he has been seized by Lamastu—the hand of the daughter of Anu.

53. If a baby has a hot and cold abdomen and wants drinking water, and drinks, hand of Lamastu.

54. If a baby's breath from the right nose [nostril] is cold, but hot from the left: hand of Lamastu.

55. If a baby screams, shivers, is agitated with fright and cries of fright, and vomits constantly all he drinks from the breast: hand of Sin and Ishtar.

56. If a baby his hands and feet are all inflamed, and maintains his eyes fixed: rods of Sin and Ishtar.

57. If a baby is constantly feverish, if his . . . from his buttocks and ears are cold: rod of the messenger of Sin.

58. If a baby has a fit like the seizure of Lamastu, comes to regularity each day: hand of Lamastu.

59. If a baby has no fever, but sweats heavily: hand of Ahhazu . . . if the baby (broken _____).

60. If the baby then at the breast has a sudden seizure: hand of. . . .

61. If a baby his flesh is chewed up (_____ depressed _____ [tablet is unreadable]) and he constantly rubs his nose, if tears flow from his eyes: the evil prayer [spell] breaks him.

62. If a baby extends his thumb, his abdomen, his hands and does not stop laughing, if his flesh has a disease [rash]: he shall know the flaccidity of flesh and die.

63. If a baby his intestines are always full [constipated] and his eyes drowsy: hand of god; he will recover.

64. If a baby his intestines are always inflamed and he does not stop crying: hand of god, he will recover.

65. If a baby his intestines are always inflamed: hand of god, he will recover.

66. If a baby his intestines are always clogged: hand of god, he will recover.

67. If a baby the upper part of his nose moves, is red or yellow: hand of god, he will recover.

68. [Incomplete]

69. If a baby . . . and his palate is always dry: hand of god; he will recover.

70. [Incomplete]

71. If a baby his eyes are bathed in tears: hand of Gestin—If the baby, his eyes are. . . .

72. If a baby, his intestines are blocked: hand of Damu. . . .

73. If a baby, when offered the breast, does not eat, his intestines are. . . .

74. If a baby, when offered the breast, does not eat, his intestines are constantly. . . .

75. If a baby his flesh is marked by yellow, his intestines are constantly. . . .

76. If a baby is flesh is marked by yellow: hand of Gula.

77. If a baby his bowels are marked by yellow: hand of Gula.

78. If a baby his stomach is prominent: hand of Gula.

79. If a baby has fever and his bowels are blocked: hand of Gula.

80. If a baby has no fever and his bowels are blocked: hand of Gula.

81. [Incomplete]

82. If a baby turns over constantly and is always sick: hand of Gula.

83. If a baby is endlessly agitated with fear: hand of Gula.

84. If a baby stretches endlessly and his arms are turned: hand of Gula.

85. If a baby his flesh is sometimes flabby and sometimes in good tone: hand of Gula.

86. If a baby is sometimes red and sometimes yellow: hand of Gula.

87. If a baby is sometimes white and sometimes black: hand of Gula.

88. If a baby is sometimes weak and sometimes strong: hand of Gula.

89. If a baby is feverish and his flesh decaying: hand of Gula.

90. If a baby burns of fever: hand of Gula.

91. If a baby his larynx is choked: hand of Gula.

92. If a baby is seized by suffocation and if his flesh is yellow: hand of Gula.

93. If a baby is seized by suffocation, does not drink from the breast and if his body is yellow: hand of Gula.

94. If a baby is seized by suffocation and he does not drink from the breast: hand of Gula.

95. If a baby, his intestines are blocked and if . . . is narrow: hand of Gula.

96. If a baby, his intestines are blocked, and if his body is yellow, and the bad odor seizes him: hand of Gula.

97. If a baby his intestines are blocked and if his mouth is sluggish, the bad odor has seized him.

98. If a baby, has flowing mucous, the bad odor has seized him.

99. If a baby, his mucous contains blood, the bad odor has seized him.

100. If a baby, his skull, chest, and the top of his back are hot: the bad odor has seized him.

101. If a baby, has fever . . . and his intestines are blocked: the bad odor has seized him.

102. If a baby, at the breast of his mother, screams endlessly and his intestines contain bile; he will die.

103. If a baby, at the breast of his mother, is constantly agitated with fear, an evil prayer [spell] has seized him.

104. If a baby, when the breast is offered, drinks, but screams out: a spell has seized him.

105. If a baby, when the breast is offered, does not eat, and his intestines are inflamed: a spell has seized him.

106. If a baby has no fever, but if his intestines are blocked and she cries: seizure by the daughter of Anu.

107. If a baby weeps and remains exhausted: the daughter of Anu has seized him.

108. If a baby weeps day and night: the daughter of Anu has seized him.

109. If a baby grunts and if when the breast is offered does not eat: an evil spell has seized him.

110. If a baby at 1 or 2 months, while nursing has a fit and his hands and feet are spastic: hand of god . . . at his feet, either his father or his mother will die.

111. If a baby, has a fit the kind with spastic hands and feet and his eyes are fogged with tears: at his feet, the house of his father shall collapse.

112. If a baby, in his bed cries without being aware of it [nightmare]; hand of Ishtar.

113. If a baby, in his bed, cries and says all he sees [nightmare]: hand of Ishtar; the evil spell has seized him.

114. If a baby rubs his . . . [?].

115. If a baby, has a feverish body, his head is hot, if drinking at the breast, he screams out; his teeth erupt; for 14 to 20 days, he will know a difficult period, but he will heal.

116. If a baby has no fever and his head is hot; his teeth erupt, for 21 days he will have a difficult period, but he will heal.

117. If a baby his skull is hot; hand of Nusku.

118. If a baby is seized by suffocation and his body is yellow: hand of Gula.

119. If a baby is seized by suffocation, if often feverish, has poor suck at the breast: mamit has seized him.

120. If a baby has no fever, his eyes are blinking, his hands and feet tremble; hand of Sin, he will recover.

121. If a baby has no fever, but trembles: hand of Sin.

122. If a baby has no fever but nevertheless a trembling often takes hold; hand of Sin.

APPENDIX B
Zaubersprüche für Mutter und Kind*

A blue lapis lazuli bead is attached, a green malachite bead is attached, a red jasper bead is attached. You beads fall on the thighs of the torrent, on the scales of the fish in the river, on the feathers of birds in heaven. Run out *nsw*, fall to earth.

   This incantation should be said over three beads, one lapis lazuli, one jasper, and the other one malachite, strung on a thread and hung on the child's neck.

Another incantation: Run out *tmjt*, you bonebreaker, stonebreaker, who enters the vessels [. . .] go out into the fields, in the fields, in the meadows, in the meadows, until the end of [. . .] herbs.

   The voice of Re calls the *Wpt*, while the stomach of this infant, born by Isis, is sick. "How shall he be addressed?" He will be addressed with *itnw n h*, so that he may come down. Look, his fire comes forth. "With what do you put it out?" One puts it out with *itnw n h*.

   Thus I bring the *itnw n h* [. . .] to her, until she is chased away on the head, on the top of the head and on all limbs, created by Chnum for this child, born to his mother.

Another incantation: Depart you demon who comes in the dark, [. . .] who has his nose backwards and face turned missing that for which he came. Depart you demoness who comes in the dark, [. . .] who has her nose backwards and face turned missing that for which she came.

   Came to kiss the child? I will not allow it. Came to calm him? I will not allow it. Came to injure him? I will not allow it. Came to take him away? I will not allow it.

   I have prepared protection against you made of *fzt* herb that makes [. . .], of garlic that harms you, of honey that is sweet for humans but terrible for the dead, of the *zbdw* fish, of the jaw of the [. . .], of the back of the Nile perch.

Sundry [. . .] You, who occupies yourself painting tiles for your father Osiris! You who addresses your father Osiris: "He should live from *dzs* herb and honey!"

---

*Erman, A., *Zaubersprüche für Mutter und Kind* (Papyrus 3027, Berlin Museum) ([. . .] signifies missing or indecipherable text).

Run out, you Asian, who comes from the desert, You black one, who comes from foreign parts. Are you a servant? Then come out in vomit. Are you of superior rank? Then come out in urine. Come out in the sneeze of his nose. Come out in the tail of his limbs.

My hands are on this child, and so are the hands of Isis, as she has them on her son Horus.

To drive away the *nsw* from a child's limbs: You are Horus and you wake up as Horus. Your are the live Horus:

I drive away the sickness that is in your body and the pain that is in your limbs. [. . .] a crocodile fast in the middle of the river and a serpent, fast with poison. You knife in the hands of a brawny butcher. Don't eat his animal, don't fall on his fat; guard yourself from [. . .] their pots will be broken, their knives will [. . .] Run out *nsw*, drop to earth.

You *bnw*, brother of the blood, friend of the pus; father of the tumor! You jackal from the South, come, lie down to sleep, and come where the beautiful women are, those on whose hair myrrh is put and fresh incense on their armpits.

Run out *nsw*, fall to earth. Don't fall on his head, beware of his [. . .] don't fall on the top of his head, beware of his Koth. Don't fall on his forehead beware of his waddling. Don't fall on his eyebrows, beware of his bareness. Don't fall on his eyes, beware of [. . .] beware of his runny eyes, don't fall on his nose, beware of [. . .] don't fall on both his [. . .] they are the [. . .] of Hathor.

Don't fall on his mouth, beware of the occult. Don't fall on his teeth, beware of knocks. Don't fall on his pharynx, beware of bad odor. Don't fall on his tongue, it is the large serpent at the entrance of her cave. Don't fall on his lips, beware of [. . .]

Don't fall on his cranium, it is the back of a goose. Don't fall on his temple, beware of deafness. Don't fall on his ears, beware of being hard of hearing. Don't fall on his neck, beware of [. . .] Don't fall on his shoulders, they are live Sperber birds. Don't fall on his arms, beware of [. . .] Don't fall on his fingers, beware of [. . .] Don't fall on his nipple, beware of destruction. Don't fall on his breast, is the breast of Hathor. Don't fall on [. . .] beware of pain. Don't fall on his belly, it is Nut, who gave birth to the gods. Don't fall on [. . .] beware of union. Don't fall on his navel, it is the morning star. Don't fall on his anus beware of the disgust of the gods [. . .] Don't fall on his phallus, beware of his heat. Don't fall on his flanks, beware the stink. Don't fall on his back, beware [. . .] Don't fall on his spine, it is the soul of Sechmet's son. Don't fall on his behind, beware [. . .] Don't fall on his buttocks, they are ostrich eggs. Don't fall on his legs, beware of the driving back. Don't fall on his foot, beware of breaking. Don't fall on his ankle, beware of his [. . .]

Run out *nsw* drop to the ground. Vomit on the [. . .] his feet. You booty [. . .] from Geb, the [. . .] of the gods. The Nile came to the house of *nsw*. With a cord in his arms on the matter of his [. . .] this Asian. Will you come, you Asian? Do you come in, you Asian? I came to [. . .] the discharge and found sitting with your [. . .] in your hand. [. . .] bread from *nsw* on the twigs of the *hssjt* herb on the tips of the *szj* herb. On the branches of the sycamore. On the [. . .] of the north wind. Run out *snw* drop to the ground.

[. . .] this child from the womb of this woman. Oh Mesechnet, you had a soul and you were armed, oh Mesechnet, [. . .] the hand of Atum, who gave birth to Schu and Tefnet. [. . .] should know in your name Mesechnet, to make a Ka for this child, that is in this woman's womb. I make a royal decree to Keb: "he will make a Ka."

You had a soul and were armed, oh Nut. Swaddlings for this child from this *NN* You will not do [. . .] say something bad [. . .] *Dw-htp*: he drove out the heir and the meals of Nut. You took any god to yourself and their stars are as lamps and they don't move as their stars. Their protection should come so that I can protect *NN*.

To be said over both the tiles of the birth of a Cherheb, and a sacrifice to Nut of meat, geese and incense on the fire. Who performs this incantation should moreover be dressed in a swaddle of the finest linen and carry a country stick.

Another incantation: I was received in *Wrjt* and was borne in *Mr-ntrj* and was bathed in the sight of the Kings. My things belong to you, my things are in [. . .]

To be said when [. . .] the child is born without any mishap. Good!

To drive away the *bcc*. Fruit of the sycamore, fresh dates. Ricinus leaves *smsmt* herb [. . .] *mstz* syrup to be taken by the woman.

Another incantation: Twigs from the *Nbw* herb, ground with water on a pot. Let her drink this.

To drive away the *ssmj*: Oh, you that are in the water. Make fast and this [. . .] who in his chapel, to the Sechmet that follows him, to the glittering [. . .] of the Uto, to lady of Buto: "take this milk to her."

[. . .] One allows the child or the mother to eat a boiled mouse, its bones you hang in a sack of fine linen around his neck and you make seven knots.

You that do not eat the Adufish. Make sure that your corpse is swaddled [. . .] become. You that do not eat the Adufish make sure that your tombs are dug. You that do not eat the Adufish make sure that your coffins come. You that do not eat the Adufish make sure that the death sacrifices are not stolen.

You ate the Adufish, you chewed his [. . .], you adorned yourself with one of his limbs, you know what is up, you know what is down. You ate the entire Adufish? [. . .] NN born to the NN. Protect the rear, protect the one that comes, Protect! You make it from the [. . .] of an Adufish, make a knot on it and hang it on his neck.

Oh Hathor that dwells in the northern sky. Who is given jewels as [. . .] and he hair of [. . .]

About knots for a child and young bird: Are you warm in nest? Is it hot in the bush? Your mother is not with you, there is no sister to fan you, no nurse to protect you.

Thus bring me a golden bullet, amethyst rings, a seal, a crocodile, a hand, in order to fell and drive away these [. . .] in order to warm the body, to fell this demon and demoness from the land of the dead. Run out, you protection.

Incant this over golden bullets, rings of amethyst, a seal, a crocodile and a hand. Draw a thin string of [. . .] and make an amulet and put it on the neck of the child. Good!

To be prayed early in the morning over a child: You rise, oh Re, you rise. When you have seen this dead, as he come to NN, born to NN, and the dead, the woman. So as to throw the mouth under her as she looks around, [. . .] she will not take her child in her arms.

"I am rescued by Re, my lord" says the woman NN. I give up the daughter, I do not give up the son [. . .] My hand lies on you, the seal is your protection.

Re rises, "See, I protect you."

Say this over a seal and over a hand. Make of it an amulet, bind it in seven knots, that is a knot in the morning, another in the evening, until there are seven knots.

You depart oh Re when you have seen the dead, as he comes to NN born to NN and the dead, the woman, so as to throw the mouth under her, as she looks around [. . .] she will not take her child away.

"Lord Re has rescued me," says the NN I do not give you away, I do not give my burden to the demon thief and demoness thief. I lay my hand on you. The seal is your protection. Re leaves, See, I protect you.

Say this in the evening when Re is about to go down from the realm of the living.

To protect the body; to be read over a child when the sun rises: You rise, Re, you rise. Have you seen this dead, as he comes to her, the *NN* born to the *NN*, and the dead, the woman, that on her mouth [. . .] as she looks around.

She wants to take her son in her lap. "You rescue me, my Lord Re," says the *NN* born to the *NN* I do not give you up, I do not give my burden to the demon thief and the demoness thief from the realm of the dead.

My hand lies on you, my seal is your protection. Re rises, run out, you protection.

Say this when Re goes down from the land of the living: You leave, oh Re, you leave. When you have seen this dead, as he comes to her, the *NN* born to the *NN*, and the dead, the woman, that on her mouth [. . .] as she looks around. She will not take her burden in her arms.

"You rescue me, my lord Re," says the *NN* born to the *NN*. I do not give you up, I do not give my burden to the demon thief and the demoness thief from the realm of the dead.

My hand lies on you, my seal is your protection. Re is leaving, run out, you protection.

Medicine done for this child:
Your protection is a protection from heaven, Your protection is a protection from the earth, Your protection is a protection from the night, Your protection is a protection from the day, Your protection is a protection from gold, Your protection is a protection from the *ibhzwtz* stone, Your protection is a protection from Re, Your protection is a protection from these seven gods, who founded the earth and [. . .]

The top of your head is Re, you hail child, your cranium is Osiris, your forehead is Sathis, the lady of the elephants, your temple is Neith, your eyebrows are the lord of the East. Your eyes are the lord of mankind, your nose is the nourisher of gods, your ears are the two royal serpents, your elbows are live birds, Sperbers, your arm is Horus, the other one is Set.

Your [. . .] is Sopd, the other one is Nut the mother of gods, your [. . .] is the box of the clean [. . .] at Heliopolis where everyone is god, your hearth *ib* is Month, your hearth *hotj* is Atum, your lung is Min, your [. . .] resembles Nefertem, your spleen is Sobk, your liver is Harsaphes from Herakleopolis, your entrails are the health, your navel is the morningstar, your leg is Isis, the other one is Nephthys, your feet [. . .] your toes are the [. . .] worm [. . .]

Every god protects your name and everything that is on you, every milk you have fed on, every lap on which you were taken, every leg on which you stand, every garment in which you are dressed, every [. . .] in which you spend your day, every protection which is made for you, everything on which you are laid, every knot that is made for you, every amulet that is hung around your neck.

He protects you with them, he keeps you well with them, he keeps you sound with them, he makes every god and goddess friendly with you.

Sundry for a red woman who [. . .] gave birth: Praise be you. Isis threaded. Nephtys spun the knot of godly thread with seven knots in it, so that you are protected with it, oh child. So that *NN* born to the *NN* be healthy, to make you healthy, to make you strong, to make every god and goddess friendly to you, to fell the demon enemy the [. . .], to fell the demoness enemy the [. . .], to jam the mouth of those that [. . .] like the mouth of those 77 donkeys that were in *Dsds* water.

I know them and know their names, that the one that wants to hit this child does not know, that he should suffer, all in all.

Say this prayer four times over seven rings of *ibhzwtj* stone and seven of gold, and seven threads of linen, which [. . .] two mother-sisters, one threads, the other spins. One makes with this an amulet with seven knots, one hangs it around the child's neck to protect the life of the child.

APPENDIX C
Hippocrates' *On Dentition**

1. Of children, those that be by nature well nourished suck not milk in proportion to their fleshiness.

2. Gross feeders that draw much milk gain not flesh in proportion.

3. Of sucklings, they that pass much water are least inclined to sickness.

4. They that have the belly much moved and good digestion withal are the healthier: they that have scant movement, and being gross feeders are not nourished in proportion, are sickly.

5. In those that vomit much milky-material the belly is confined.

6. They that in teething have the belly much open are less convulsed than he that hath it seldom open.

7. They that in teething have sharp fever come upon them are seldom convulsed.

8. They that whilst teething continue well nourished but are lethargic therewith, are in danger of a convulsive attack.

9. They that teethe in winter, other things being equal, come off best.

10. Not all who are convulsed whilst about teeth, die; many come through it safely.

11. They that teethe with a cough, take long about it; and are the more wasted at the cutting of teeth.

12. They that have stormy times in teething, with proper management bear teething more easily.

13. They that pass water more than stool are correspondingly better nourished.

14. They that pass not water in proper proportion, but their belly from earliest childhood passes constantly undigested matter, are sickly.

15. They that sleep well and are well nourished take much, even though it be set before them not fittingly prepared.

16. They that take other foods during suckling bear weaning the more easily.

17. They that often pass bloody and undigested stools from the belly are specially liable, amongst the symptoms of fever, to drowsiness.

18. Ulcers on the tonsils are less dangerous when they occur without fever.

---

*Hippocrates' *On Dentition*, from the translation of F. Adams (1849).

19. Of infants those that have a cough during suckling usually have the uvula enlarged.

20. They that show rapid onset of spreading sores on the tonsils with persistence of fever and cough are in danger of further occurrence of ulcers.

21. Recurring ulcers on the tonsils are dangerous to little children.

22. When children have considerable ulceration on the tonsils and are able to drink, it points to recovery, and this still more when they have before been unable to drink.

23. With ulcers on the tonsils, much vomiting of bile or its passage from the belly, is dangerous.

24. With ulcers on the tonsils the presence of a sort of spider-web [membrane] is not favorable.

25. With ulcers on the tonsils a flux of phlegm from the mouth after the early stage is beneficial if it has not occurred before; anyway it must be brought up. If the condition begins to slacken it is most satisfactory. When there is no such flux caution is needed.

26. In those with catarrh of the tonsils evacuation downwards from the belly is the best clearance of dry coughs; in little children evacuation upwards of digested matter gives best clearance.

27. Ulcers that remain a long time on the tonsils without extending are free from danger compared with some lasting (only) five or six days.

28. Of sucklings those that take much milk are generally sleepy.

29. Of sucklings those that are not easily nourished are thin and pick up badly.

30. Ulcers on the tonsils occurring in the summer are worse than at other seasons, for they spread more rapidly.

31. Ulcers on the tonsils that spread about the uvula alter the voice in those who recover.

32. The more severe and acute ulcers that spread about the throat usually cause also dyspnea.

APPENDIX D
Table of Contents of Scroll 25, the "Pediatric" of the *Ishimpo**

Yi Xin Fang

Pediatric Protocol 1

Newborn Protocol 2

Protocol for removing blood in the mouth of the newborn 3

Protocol for feeding *gancao* (licorice root) soup 4

Protocol for feeding pearl powder and honey 5

Protocol for feeding *niu huang* (bovine gallstones) 6

Protocol for the first breast feeding of a newborn 7

Protocol for feeding rice 8

Protocol for the first bathing of a baby 9

Protocol for cutting the umbilical cord 10

Protocol for removing *e kao* (goose mouth—thrush?) 11

Protocol for cutting loose the tongue 12

Protocol for piercing *xuan wei* 13

Protocol for *bian zheng* 14

Protocol for choosing a wet-nurse 15

Protocol for naming a child 16

Protocol for first dressing a child 17

Protocol for nurturing a child 18

Forbidden food for small children 19

Protocol for treating *xie lu* (nonclosure of fontanel) 20

Protocol for treating *a bai* (bulging fontanel) 21

Protocol for treating constant head swinging in children 22

Protocol for treating balding in children 23

Protocol for treating *bai tu* (white balding) 24

Protocol for treating *gui tian tau* (ghost-licked head) 25

Protocol for treating head pustules in children 26

Protocol for treating pustules on the head, face and body 27

Protocol for treating white spots on the face of children 28

---

*Translation of Wei Yee Chan, Georgetown University.

Protocol for treating spitting milk 63

Protocol for treating hard to breast feed 64

Protocol for treating hard to breast feed caused by wind 65

Protocol for treating failure of navel closure 66

Protocol for treating navel with exudate 67

Protocol for treating red and swollen navel 68

Protocol for treating sore of the navel 69

Protocol for treating abdominal pain 70

Protocol for treating swollen abdomen 71

Protocol for treating lump in the abdomen 72

Protocol for treating indigestion 73

Protocol for treating urge for eating rice 74

Protocol for treating lump caused by eating dirt 75

Protocol for treating worm in the abdomen 76

Protocol for treating swollen genitalia 77

Protocol for treating painful genitalia 78

Protocol for treating ulcer of the genitalia 79

Protocol for treating bleeding of the vagina 80

Protocol for treating swollen scrotum 81

Protocol for treating hernia 82

Protocol for treating scrotal hernia 83

Protocol for treating prolapse of the anus 84

Protocol for treating itchy anus 85

Protocol for treating sore of the anus 86

Protocol for treating intestinal parasites 87

Protocol for treating infection with *cun bai* worm 88

Protocol for treating epilepsy 89

Protocol for treating ghost child sickness 90

Protocol for treating *ke wu* (scared of people) 91

Protocol for treating crying at night 92

Protocol for treating panic crying during sleep 93

Protocol for treating(?) crying 94

Protocol for treating malaria 95

Protocol for treating disease caused by harmful cold factors 96

Ancient Chinese Pharmacopeia

Ba dou	Croton tiglium bean
Bai ji	Bletilla striata
Bai lian	Ampelopsis japonica
Bai pi	Euomymus tengyuehensis
Bai zi ren	Biota orientalis seed
Black powder tablet	Almond, Da huang, Ma huang
Ceng qing	Copper carbonate (Azurite)
Chan tui	Cryptotympana atrata (insect)
Cheong pu	?
Chen sha	Cinnabar or mercuric sulfide
Chi shi zhi	Aluminum silicate (Halloysite)
Chi xiao dou	Small red bean
Da huang	Rheum officinalem root
Da suan	Allium sativum—garlic
Da zao	Red plum
Dai zhe shi	Ferric oxide (Hematite)
Dang giu san	Angelica sinensis
Fan lu	Stellaria media
Fan si	Chalk
Fang feng	Saposhnikovia divaricata
Fu zi	Aconitum carmichaeli root
Gan di huang	Rehmannia glutinosa
Gancao	Licorice
Ge	Pueraria lobata root
Gou qi gen	Lycium chinensis
Gui xin	Cinnamon
Hu fen	?
Hu man	Linum usitatissimum
Huang bai	Phellodendron amurense bark
Huang lian	Coptis chinensis
Huang qin	Scutellaria baicalensis
Huang qi san	Astragalus membranaceus

Ji shi bai	White chicken dropping (uric acid)
Ji yu	Carassius auratus (freshwater fish)
Ku cai	Sonchus oleraceus
Ku shen	Sophora falvescens root
Li lo	Veratrum nigrum
Lin zi cao	Alternanthera sessilis
Long gu	Dragon bones (fossils)
Ma ji	Cannabis sativa seeds
Moxa	Chinese wormwood Artemisia moxa
Niu huang	Bovine gallstone
Purple pill	Almond, Chi shi zhi, Ba dou, Dai zhe shi
Qiu ye	Catalpa bungei
Rosin	Resin of turpentine
Sang ji sheng	Loranthus parasiticus
Ting li zi	Lepidium apetalum seed
Wu tou	?
Wu zhu yu	Evodia rutaecarpa
Xi xin	Asarum heterotropoides
Yuen hua	Daphne genkwa
Zhu li	Phyllostachys nigra (bamboo sap)
Xiong huang	Arsenic sulfide (Realgar)

Units

Bullet	size of 16 parasol seeds
Fun	500 mg
Liang	50 grams
Sheng	liter

Sources

Ben Cao	Book of Herbals
Bing Yuen Lun	Dissertation on the Source of Illness
Chan Jing	Great Obstetric Classic
Cui Yue Xi Shi Jing	Book of Gourmet by Cui Yue Xi

Da Su Jing	Great Simple Classic
Ge's Fang	Ge's Protocol
Ji Yan Fang	Collected Efficient Protocols
Ji Yiu Fang	Most Important Protocol
Jing Xin Fang	Classic Heart Protocol
Lu Yan Fang	Record of Working Protocols
Luxin Jing	Fontanel Classic
Meng Sen Shi Jing	Book of Gourmet by Meng Sen
Nei Ching Su Wên	Classic on Internal Medicine
Niji	Book of Rites
Pen T'sao	Great Chinese Herbal
Qian Jin Fang	Thousand Gold Protocols or The Most Valuable Protocols
Seng Shen Fang	Buddhist Shen Protocol
Xiao Pin Fang	Treatment Protocol
Yang Shi Leng Yiu Ii	The Book of Important Health Practices
Yue Yi Zhen Jing	Jade Inherited Acupuncture Classic
Zhen Jiu Jing	Acupuncture and Moxibustion Classic
Zi Mu Bi Lu	Child and Mother Secret Record
Xin Lu Fang	New Record Protocol

Glossary

Adenitis swelling and inflammation of the lymph nodes

Anasarca generalized swelling of the body by fluid—dropsy

Anencephaly congenital absence of the brain

Apnea temporary cessation of breathing

Ascaris common roundworm parasite, 30–40-cm long

Ascites accumulated fluid in the peritoneal cavity

Botulism food poisoning causing muscle weakness or paralysis

Bradycardia slow heart rate

Bruxism teeth grinding

Cannabis flowering top of *Cannabis sativa* (hemp)—marijuana

Cardiocentric originating with or determined by heart function

Cephalohematoma blood bump under scalp acquired during birth process

Chlorosis old term for iron-deficiency anemia

Cholestasis sluggish or aberrant bile flow

Chylous pertaining to milklike alkaline product of digestion

Coarctation a narrowing or stricture of a vessel

Dropsy obsolete term for anasarca

Ecchymosis dark hemorrhagic bruising evident under skin

Empyema pus in a cavity, most commonly in lung pleura

Encephalopathy generalized dysfunction of the brain

Enterocolitis infection or inflammation of the bowel

Epistaxis nosebleed

Esophageal atresia congenital absence of an opening in the esophagus

Foramen ovale	an opening between the two upper heart chambers
Gibbus	the hunchback spine curvature
Glomerulonephritis	kidney inflammation marked by blood and protein in the urine and high blood pressure
Glycosuria	sugar in the urine
Helminthes	generic term for worm parasites
Hematemesis	vomiting of blood
Hemiplegia	paralysis of one side of the body
Herniorrhaphy	repair of a hernia
Hydrocele	fluid accumulation in a sac, generally the scrotum
Hydrocephalus	fluid accumulation in the brain ventricles
Hypospadias	congenital abnormality of penile orifice
Hypoxia	temporary deprivation of oxygen
Intussusception	slipping or telescoping of bowel into itself
Ischemia	local and temporary deficiency of blood flow
Koplik spots	oral lesions of measles appearing before rash
Leishmaniasis	protozoal parasite transmitted by flies
Lymphadenopathy	disease of the lymph nodes
Malrotation	failure of viscera to rotate normally in the embryo
Mastitis	infection and/or inflammation of the breast
Mastoiditis	infection of the mastoid process behind the ear
Meconium	first feces of the newborn, greenish black and mucoid
Mediastinum	cavity between the lungs, housing heart, vessels, trachea
Meningococcemia	brain infection by *Neisseria meningitidis*
Necrotizing	a localized process causing tissue death
Nephrosis	degenerative changes in the kidneys
Occiput	back part of the cranium
Opisthotonos	severe spasms of the back causing involuntary arching
Orchiopexy	correction of undescended testicle
Osteomyelitis	infection and inflammation of bone

Otitis media	infection of the middle ear
PDA	patent ductus arteriosus: persistent congenital communication between pulmonary and aortic flow
Pertussis	whooping cough
Petechiae	small purplish hemorrhagic spots
Phimosis	narrowed nonretractile penile foreskin
Postictal	unconscious state following a grand mal seizure
Pulmonary stenosis	narrowing of the pulmonary artery outlet
Ranula	a cystic enlargement under the tongue
Risus sardonicus	spastic involuntary grin seen in tetanus
Rubella	German measles
Schistosomiasis	parasite infection of microscopic blood flukes
Sclerema	hardening of the skin, commonly heralding death
Scoliosis	lateral curvature of the spine
Scrofula	tuberculosis of lymph nodes, commonly of the neck
Sepsis	generalized and serious blood-borne infection
Spina bifida	congenital defect of spine-process fusion
Strabismus	squinting or inability to direct both eyes
Tetanus	*Clostridium tetani* infection causing muscle spasms
Theriac	complex pharmacopeia compound credited with extraordinary properties but no longer in use (see footnote, chapter 4, page 71)
Thoracotomy	operative opening of the chest
Thrush	common fungal infection of babies
Tracheo-esophageal fistula	abnormal congenital connection between the trachea and the esophagus
Trichuriasis	whipworm infection
Vasculitis	inflammation of the blood vessels

Bibliography

PRIMARY SOURCES

Adams, F. 1886. *The Genuine Works of Hippocrates.* New York: William Wood.

Adams. S. S. 1897. The evolution of pediatric literature in the United States. *Transactions of the American Pediatric Society* 9:5–31.

American Practioner. 1826. *The London Practice of Midwifery . . . and Principal Infantile Diseases.* 6th ed. Concord, N.H.: Isaac Hill.

Andry, N. 1743. *Orthopaedia.* London.

Anonymous. 1742. *A Full View of All the Diseases Incident to Children.* London: A. Millar.

Armstrong, G. 1808. *An Account of the Diseases Most Incident to Children.* London: Caldwell and Davies.

Ashby, H. 1889. *The Diseases of Children, Medical and Surgical.* London: Longmans, Green.

Astruc, J. 1746. *A General and Compleat Treatise on All the Diseases Incident to Children, from Their Birth to the Age of Fifteen.* London: John Nourse.

Austrius, S. 1540. *De infantium sive puerorum morborum . . .* Basel: Bartholomaeum Westhemerum.

Avicenna. 1930. *Canon of Medicine.* Translated by O. Cameron. London: Luzac.

———. 1963. *Poem on Medicine (Canticum Avicennae).* Translated by H. Krueger. Springfield, Ill.: Charles Thomas.

Bagellardo, P. 1472. *De Infantium Aegritudinibus et Remediis.* Padua: Valdezoccho and Martinus.

Baker, J. P. 1991. The incubator controversy. *Pediatrics* 87:654–62.

Bard, S. 1771. *An Enquiry into the nature, cause and cure, of the angina suffocativa, or, sore throat distemper, as it is commonly called by the inhabitants of this city and colony.* New York: S. Inslee.

Beck, J. B. 1849. *Essays on Infant Therapeutics; to which are added observations on Ergot and an account of the origin of the use of mercury in inflammatory complaints.* New York: W. E. Dean.

Billard, C. M. 1839. *A Treatise on the Diseases of Infants.* Translated by J. Stewart. New York: George Adlard.

Blankaart, S. 1684. *. . . ziekten der kinderen.* Amsterdam: Hieronymus Sweerts.

Bouchut, E. 1845. *Traite practique des maladies de nouveau-nes, des enfants a la mamelle et de la seconde enfance.* Paris: J. B. Braillière.

Bower, H. 1912. *The Bower Manuscript.* Facsimile leaves of the Nagari Transcript. Collection of the National Library of Medicine.

Boylston, Z. 1726. *An historical account of the small-pox inoculated in New England, upon all sorts of persons, whites, blacks, and of all ages and constitutions.* London: S. Chandler.

Bracken, H. 1737. *The Midwifes's Companion* . . . London: Clarke and Shuchburgh.

Buchan, W. 1807. *Domestic Medicine.* Charleston, S.C.: John Hoff.

————. *Domestic Medicine.* Boston: Phelps and Farnham.

Budin, P. 1907. *The Nursling: The Feeding and Hygiene of Premature and Full-term Infants.* Translated by W. J. Maloney. London: Caxton.

Cadogan, W. 1773. *An Essay upon Nursing, and Management of Children, from Their Birth to Three Years of Age.* London: William and Thomas Bradford.

Chalmers, L. 1776. *An Account of the Weather and Diseases of South Carolina.* Charleston: n.p.

Cheyne, J. 1801. *Essays on the Diseases of Children, with Cases and Discussions.* Edinburgh: Mandell and Sons.

Churchill, F. 1850. *On the Diseases of Infants and Children.* Philadelphia: Lea and Blanchard.

Clark, J. 1815. *Commentaries on Some of the Most Important Diseases of Children.* London: Longman and Hurst.

Cook, J. 1769. *A Plain Account of the Diseases Incident to Children.* London: Edward and Charles Dilly.

Culpeper, N. 1700. *A Directory for Midwives* . . . London: n.p.

Davis, J. B. 1817. *A Cursory Inquiry into Some of the Principal Causes of Mortality among Children* . . . London: Thomas and George Underwood.

Dewees, W. P. 1829. *A Treatise on the Physical and Medical Treatment of Children.* Philadelphia: Carey, Lea and Carey.

Diday, P. 1851/1883. *A Treatise on Syphilis in New-Born Children and Infants at the Breast.* New York: William Wood.

Downes, J. J. 1994. Historic origins and role of pediatric anesthesiology in child health care. *Pediatric Clinics of North America* 41:1–13.

Downman, H. 1802. *Infancy; or, The Management of Children: A Didactic Poem, in Six Books.* Edinburgh: Trewman and Son.

Duffy, J. 1979. *The Healers.* Chicago: University of Illinois Press.

Eberle, J. 1833. *A Treatise on the Diseases and Physical Education of Children* . . . Cincinnati, Ohio: Corey and Fairbanks.

Erman, A. 1901. *Zaubersprüche für Mutter und Kind* (Papyrus 3027 of the Berlin Museum). Berlin: Preuss Akademie der Wissenschaften.

Ferrari, O. 1577. *De arte medica infantium* . . . Verona: Marchettis.

Fleisch, C. B. 1803. *Handbuch uber die Krankheiten der Kinder* . . . Leipzig: Jacobaer.

Fothergill, J. 1748. *An Account of the Sore Throat Attended with Ulcers* . . . London: C. Davis.

Galen. 1951. *De Sanitate Tuenda.* Translated by R. Green. Springfield, Ill.: Charles Thomas.

Gerhardt, C. A. 1861. *Lehrbuch der Kinderkrankheiten.* Berlin.

———. 1877. *Handbuch der Kinderkrankheiten.* Tübingen: H. Laupp'schen Buchandlung.

Germer, R. 1993. *Mummies: Life After Death in Ancient Egypt.* Munich: Prestel.

Gies, F., and J. Gies. 1987. *Marriage and the Family in the Middle Ages.* New York: Harper and Row.

Glass, H. 1762. *The Servants Directory.* Dublin: J. Potts.

Glisson, F. 1650. *De rachitide; sive, morbo puerili . . .* London: Laurentii Sadler.

———. 1668. *A Treatise of the Rickets, Being a Disease Common to Children.* Translated by N. Culpeper. London: John Streater.

Goodhart, J. F. 1885. *A Guide to the Diseases of Children.* Philadelphia: P. Blakiston.

Gower, R. G. 1682. *De le Boe Sylvius of Children's Diseases.* London: George Downs.

Guersant, P. L. 1873. *Surgical Diseases of Infants and Children.* Translated by R. L. Dunglison. Philadelphia: Henry C. Lea.

Harper, R. F. 1904. *The Code of Hammurabi King of Babylon.* Chicago: University of Chicago Press.

Harris, W. 1689. *De Morbis Acutis Infantium.* London: Samuel Smith.

Henoch, E. H. 1882. *Lectures on Disease of Children . . .* New York: William Wood.

Herodotus. 1954. *The Histories.* Translated by A. de Sélincourt. Middlesex, U.K.: Penguin Books.

Hippocrates. 1849. *The Works of Hippocrates Translated from the Greek with a Preliminary Discourse and Annotations.* Translated by F. Adams. London: Sydenham Society.

Holt, L. E., and J. Howland. 1916. *The Diseases of Infancy and Children.* New York: Appelton.

Hunter, J. 1771. *The Natural History of the Human Teeth.* London: J. Johnson.

Hurlock, J. 1742. *A Practical Treatise upon Dentition.* London: C. Rivington.

Ives, E. 1821. *Lectures on the Diseases of Children.* New Haven, Conn.: The Medical Institution of Yale College.

Jacobi, A. 1909. *Collectinae Jacobi.* New York: Critic and Guide.

Jenner, E. 1798. *An Inquiry into the Causes and Effects of the Variolae Vaccinae, a Disease.* London: Sampson Law.

Keating, J. 1890. *Cyclopaedia of the Diseases of Children, Medical and Surgical.* Philadelphia: J. B. Lippincott.

Labat, R. 1951. *Traité akkadien de diagnostics et pronostics médicaux.* Paris: E. J. Brill.

Le Boe Sylvius, Frans de. 1682. *Of childrens diseases, given in a familiar style for weaker capacities.* London: George Downs.

Lobera de Avila, L. 1551. *Libro del regimiento de salud, y de la esterilidad de los hombres y mugeres, y de las enfermedades de los niños . . .* Valladolid, Spain: Sebastian Martinez.

Logan, G. 1825. *Practical Observations on Diseases of Children.* Charleston, S.C.: Archibald E. Miller.

Mather, C. 1724/1972. *The Angel of Bethesda*. Barre, Mass.: American Antiquarian Society.

Mauriceau, F. 1681. *De mulierum praegnantium, parturientium, et puerperarum morbis tractatus . . .* Paris: Author.

———. 1755. *The Diseases of Women with Child . . .* Translated by H. Chamberlen. London: Ware and Longman.

Meigs, J. F. 1848. *A Practical Treatise on the Diseases of Children*. Philadelphia: Lindsay and Blakiston.

Meissner, F. L. 1850. *Grundlage der Literatur de Pädiatrik*. Leipzig: n.p.

Mercuriale, G. 1583. *De morbis puerorum tractatus locupletissimi*. Venice: Paulum Meietum.

Metlinger, B. 1473. *Ein Regiment der junger Kinder*. Augsburg: Gunter Zainer.

Nightingale, F. 1859. *Notes on Nursing*. London: Harrison.

Oribasius. 1876. Synopsis. In *Oeuvres d'Oribase*. Translated by Bussemaker and Daremberg. Paris: J. B. Baillière.

Pare, A. 1585/1968. *The Apologie and Treatise*. Edited by G. Heynes. New York: Dover Publications.

Parrot, J. 1877. *L'athrepsie*. Paris: G. Masson.

Paulus Aegineta. 1844. *The Seven Books*. Translated by Francis Adams. London: The Sydenham Society.

Pliny. 1947. *Natural History*. Translated by H. Rackman. London: William Heinemann.

Pott, P. 1779. *Remarks on That Kind of Palsy of the Lower Limbs*. London: J. Johnson.

Raulin, J. 1770. *De la Conservation des enfans*. Yverdon, Switzerland: n.p.

Razi, Muhammad ibn Zakariya. 1497. *De Aegritudinibus puerorum et Earum Cura*. Venice: Bonetus Locatellus.

Roelans, C. 1925. *Libellus Aegritudinum Infantium*. Facsimile edited by Karl Sudhoff. Munich: Verlag der Munchner Drucke.

Roesslin, E. 1654. *The Byrth of Mankind; otherwise called, the Woman's Book*. Translated by T. Reynald. London: Henry Hood.

Roscoe, W. 1798. *The Nurse: A Poem*. Liverpool: Cadell and Davies.

Rotch, T. M. 1903. *Pediatrics: The Hygienic and Medical Treatment of Children*. Philadelphia: J. B. Lippincott.

Rush, B. 1815. *Medical Inquiries and Observations*. Philadelphia: n.p.

Sainte-Marthe, S. 1797. *Paedotrophia*. Translated by H. W. Tytler. London: John Nichols.

Smith, E. 1884. *A Practical Treatise on Diseases in Children*. New York: William Wood.

Smith, J. L. 1872. *A Treatise on the Diseases of Infancy and Childhood*. Philadelphia: Henry C. Lea.

Snow, J. 1858. *On Chloroform and Other Anaesthetics*. London: John Churchill.

Soranus. 1956. *Gynecology*. Translated by O. Temkin. Baltimore: Johns Hopkins University Press.

Starsmare, J. 1664. *Paidon Nosemata; or Children's Diseases, both Outward and inward . . .* London: Playford and Watkins.

Steuer, R. O., and J. B. de Cusance. 1959. *Ancient Egyptian and Cnidian Medicine.* Berkeley: University of California Press.

Susruta. 1907. *Susruta Samhita.* Translated by K. Bhishagratna. Calcutta: J. M. Bose.

Swyer, P. R. 1991. Energy metabolism. In *History of Pediatrics, 1850–1950.* Edited by B. Nichols, A. Ballabriga, and N. Kretchmer. New York: Raven Press.

Tamba, Y. 982 A.D. *Ishimpo.* Japan: Juntendo University.

Thacher, T. 1677. *A brief rule to guide the common-people of New-England how to order themselves and theirs in the small pocks, or measles.* Boston: John Foster.

Turner, D. 1736. *De Morbis Cutaneis.* London: R. Wilkin.

Underwood, M. 1784. *A Treatise on the Diseases of Children . . .* London: J. Mathews (1842 ed., London: Barrington and Haswell).

Villermé, L. R. 1840. *Tableau de l'etat physique et moral des ouvriers employes dans les manufactures de coton.* Paris: Renouard.

Vogel, C. 1965. *Vagbhata's Astangahrdayasamhita.* Wiesbaden: Deutsche Morgenländische Gesellschaft.

Watt, R. 1813. *Treatise on the history, nature, and treatment of chincough; including a variety of cases and dissections. To which is subjoined an inquiry into the relative mortality of the principal diseases of children.* London: Longman, Hurst, Rees, Orme and Brown.

West, C. 1850. *Lectures on the Diseases of Infancy and Childhood.* Philadelphia: Lea and Blanchard.

Whytt, R. 1768. *Observations on the Dropsy in the Brain.* Edinburgh: Balfour, Auld and Smellie.

Wurtz, F. 1656. *An Experimental Treatise of Surgerie in Four Parts.* London: Gartrude Dawson.

SECONDARY SOURCES

Abt, A. F. 1965. *Abt-Garrison History of Pediatrics.* Philadelphia: W. B. Saunders.

Abt, I. A. 1940. A survey of pediatrics during the past 100 Years. *Illinois Medical Journal* 77:485–95.

———. A history of pediatrics. In *Brennemann's Practice of Pediatrics.* Hagerstown, Md.: W. F. Prior Company.

Acierno, L. J. 1993. *The History of Cardiology.* London: Parthenon.

Ackerknecht, E. 1946. Incubator and taboo. *Journal of the History of Medicine* 1: 144–48.

———. 1982. *A Short History of Medicine.* Baltimore: Johns Hopkins University Press.

Adamson, R. B. 1991. Surgery in ancient Mesopotamia. *Medical History* 35:428–35.

Allis, F. S. Jr. 1980. *Medicine in Colonial Massachusetts 1620–1820.* Charlottesville: University Press of Virginia.

Allsop, K. A., and J. B. Miller. 1996. Honey revisted: a reappraisal of honey in pre-industrial diets. *British Journal of Nutrition* 75:513–20.

Anderson, B. S., and J. P. Zinsser. 1988. *A History of Their Own*, vols. 1 and 2. New York: Harper and Row.

Apple, R. D. 1980. To be used under the direction of a physician: Commerical infant feeding and medical practice, 1870–1940. *Bulletin of the History of Medicine* 54:402–17.

Aries, P. 1965. *Centuries of Childhood.* New York: Vintage.

Aries, P., and G. Duby. 1989. *A History of Private Lives*, vols. 1–5. Cambridge, Mass.: Belknap.

Arriaza, B. T., W. Salo, A. C. Aufderheide, et al. 1995. Pre-Columbian tuberculosis in northern Chile. *American Journal of Physical Anthropology* 98:37–47.

Aspin, R. 1995. *Western Manuscripts Collection: The Wellcome Institute.* London: Empress Litho.

Ballabriga, A. 1991. One century of pediatrics in Europe. In *History of Pediatrics 1850–1950.* Edited by B. Nichols, A. Ballabriga, and N. Kretchmer. New York: Raven Press.

Barlow, A. 1957. Sir Thomas Barlow. In *Pediatric Profiles.* Edited by B. S. Veeder. St. Louis: C. V. Mosby.

Bassett, E. J., M. S. Keith, G. J. Armelagos, et al. 1980. Tetracycline labeled human bone from ancient Sudanese Nubia (A.D. 350). *Science* 209:1532–34.

Baumgartner, L., and E. M. Ramsey. Johann Peter Frank and his "System einer vollständigen medicinischen Polizey." *Annals of Medical History* 6:69–90.

Bayne-Powell, R. 1938. *Eighteenth-Century London Life.* New York: E. P. Dutton.

Beeson, P. B. 1976. Infectious diseases. In *Advances in American Medicine: Essays at the Bicentennial.* Edited by J. Z. Bowers and E. F. Purcell. New York: Josiah Macy Foundation.

Bendiner, E. 1995. Sara Josephine Baker: Crusader for women and children's health. *Hospital Practice* 30(9):68–77.

Bermudez de Castro, J. M., and P. J. Perez. 1995. Enamel hypoplasia in the Middle Pleistocene hominids from Atapuerca. *American Journal of Physical Anthropology* 96:301–14.

Bernard, G. P. 1947. Lithopedion from the case of Dr. William H. H. Parkhurst, 1853. *Bulletin of the History of Medicine* 21:377–89.

Bloch, H. 1993. History of pediatrics (parts 1 and 2). *Southern Medical Journal* 85: 1230–35; 86:85–90.

Boocock, P., C. A. Roberts, and K. Manchester. Maxillary sinusitis in medieval Chichester. *American Journal of Physical Anthropology* 98:483–95.

Bracken, F. 1956. The history of artificial feeding of infants. *Maryland State Medical Journal* 5:40–54.

Braun, W. 1991. German pediatrics. In *History of Pediatrics, 1850–1950.* Edited by B. Nichols, A. Ballabriga, and N. Kretchmer. New York: Raven Press.

Bremner, R. H. 1970–1971. *Children and Youth in America*, 2 vols. Cambridge, Mass.: Harvard University Press.

Brothwell, D., and A. T. Sandison. 1967. *Diseases in Antiquity.* Springfield, Ill.: Charles C. Thomas.

Bryan, C. P. 1931. *The Papyrus Ebers.* New York: Appleton.

———. 1974. *Ancient Egyptian Medicine: The Papyrus Ebers.* Chicago: Ares Publishers.

Budge, E. A. W. 1920/1978. *Egyptian Hieroglyphic Dictionary.* New York: Dover.

Bullough, V. L. 1981. Bottle feeding: An amplification. *Bulletin of the History of Medicine* 55:257–59.

Cable, M. 1972. *The Little Darlings.* New York: Charles Scribner's Sons.

Camp, J. 1973. *Magic, Myth and Medicine.* London: Priory Press.

Caulfield, E. 1930. The infant welfare movement in the eighteenth century. *Annals of Medical History* 2:480–695.

Chadwick, J., and W. N. Mann. 1950. *The Medical Works of Hippocrates.* London: Blackwell.

Chang, J. H. T. 1986. Timelines in the history of pediatric surgery. *Journal of Pediatric Surgery* 21:1068–72.

Chen, T. S., and P. S. Chen. Gastroenterology in ancient Egypt. *Journal of Clinical Gastroenterology* 13:182–87.

Clendening, L. 1960. *Source Book of Medical History.* New York: Dover Publications.

Cockburn, A., and E. Cockburn. 1985. *Mummies, Diseases, and Ancient Cultures.* Cambridge, U.K.: Cambridge University Press.

Cohen, A. 1949. *Everyman's Talmud.* New York: E. P. Dutton.

Colón, A. R. 1987. *The Boke of Children.* Columbus, Ohio: Ross.

———. *A Textbook of Pediatric Hepatology.* Chicago: Yearbook.

Colón, A. R., and P. A. Colón. 1989. The health of America's children. In *Caring for America's Children.* Edited by F. Machiarolla and A. Gartner. New York: American Academy of Political Science.

———. 1992. The psychosocial adaptation of children in space: A speculation. *Journal of Practical Applications in Space* 33:5–20.

Colón, A. R., and M. Ziai. 1985. *Pediatric Pathophysiology.* Boston: Little, Brown.

Cone, T. E. 1961. De pondere infantum recens natorum. *Pediatrics* 27:490–98.

———. 1974. Dr. Henry Pickering Bowditch on the growth of children. *Transactions and Studies of the College of Physicians of Philadelphia* 42:67–76.

———. 1979. *History of American Pediatrics.* Boston: Little, Brown.

———. 1985. *History of the Care and Feeding of the Premature Infant.* Boston: Little, Brown.

Cosnett, J. E. 1989. The origins of intravenous fluid therapy. *Lancet* 1:768–71.

Curtis, R. I. 1991. *Garum and Salsamenta.* Leiden: E. T. Brill.

Dally, A. 1996. The lancet and the gum-lancet: 400 years of teething babies. *Lancet* 348:1710–11.

Denny, F. W. 1990. Infectious diseases and the last 100 years in the American Pediatric Society. *Pediatric Research* 27:S49–S54.

Denny, N., and J. Filmer-Sankey. 1966. *The Bayeux Tapestry.* New York: Atheneum.

de Quadros, C. A., et al. 1992. Polio eradication from the Western Hemisphere. *Annual Review of Public Health* 13:239–52.

Desmond, M. M. 1991. A review of newborn medicine in America: European past and guiding ideology. *American Journal of Perinatology* 8:308–22.

Dettwyler, K. A. 1991. Can paleopathology provide evidence for "compassion"? *American Journal of Physical Anthropology* 84:375–84.

Downes, J. J. 1994. Historic origins and role of pediatric anesthesiology in child
    health care. *Pediatric Clinics of North America* 41:1–13.

Drake, T. G. H. 1935. Infant welfare laws in France in the eighteenth century.
    Annals of Medical History 7:49–61.

Dundes, A. 1992. *The Evil Eye*. Madison: University of Wisconsin Press.

Dunn, P. M. 1994. Dr. Herbert Barker 1814–1865 of Bedford and infant hygiene.
    Archives of Disease in Childhood 70:228–29.

Earle, A. M. 1930. *Child Life in Colonial Days*. New York: Macmillan.

Ebrey, P. B. 1981. *Chinese Civilzation*. New York: Free Press.

Epstein, I. 1948. *The Babylonian Talmud*. London: Soncino Press.

Erman, A. 1901. *Zaubersprüche für Mutter und Kind* (papyrus 3027 of the Berlin
    Museum). Berlin: Preuss Akademie der Wissenschaften.

Faber H. K., and R. McIntosh. 1966. *History of the American Pediatric Society*. New
    York: McGraw-Hill.

Fildes, V. 1986. *Breast, Bottles, and Babies*. Edinburgh: Edinburgh University Press.

Filer, L. J. 1993. Safe foods for infants: The regulation of milk, infant formula and
    other infant foods. *Journal of Nutrition* 123:285–88.

Foote, J. 1919. Ancient poems on infant hygiene. *Annals of Medical History* 2:213–
    27.

Fowke, F. R. 1898. *The Bayeux Tapestry*. London: George Bell & Son.

Garland, R. 1990. *The Greek Way of Life*. Ithaca, N.Y.: Cornell University Press.

Garrison, F. 1929. *An Introduction to the History of Medicine*. Philadelphia: W. B.
    Saunders.

Gartner, L. M., and C. Stone. 1994. Two thousand years of medical advice on
    breastfeeding: Comparison of Chinese and Western texts. *Seminars in Perina-
    tology* 18:532–36.

Gerson, S. 1993. *Ayurveda: The Ancient Indian Healing Art*. Rockport, Mass.:
    Element.

Ghalioungui, P. 1974. *Magic and Medical Science in Ancient Egypt*. Amsterdam: B. M.
    Israel.

Gil'adi, A. 1992. *Children of Islam*. New York: St. Martin's Press.

Glass, H. 1762. *The Servants' Directory*. Dublin: J. Potts.

Gordon, B. L. 1949. *Medicine Throughout Antiquity*. Philadelphia: F. A. Davis.

Gordon, E. C. 1991. Accidents among medieval children as seen from the miracles
    of six English saints and martyrs. *Medical History* 35:145–63.

Griscom, N. T. 1995. History of pediatric radiology in the United States and Can-
    ada. *Radiographics* 15:1399–1422.

Grundbacher, F. J. 1992. Behring's discovery of diphtheria and tetanus antitoxins.
    Immunology Today 13:188–89.

Gudger, E. W. 1925. Stitching wounds with the mandibles of ants and beetles.
    Journal of the American Medical Association 84:1861–64.

Gwei-Djen, L., and J. Needham. 1967. *Clerks and Craftsmen in China and the West*.
    Cambridge, U.K.: Cambridge University Press.

Haggerty, R. J. 1997. Abraham Jacobi, MD, respectable rebel. *Pediatrics* 99:462–
    66.

Hamilton, D. 1981. *The Healers*. Edinburgh: Canongate.

Hare, R. 1967. The antiquity of diseases caused by bacteria and viruses. In *Diseases in Antiquity*. Edited by D. Brothwell and A. T. Sandison. Springfield, Ill.: Charles C. Thomas.

Harper, R. F. 1904. *The Code of Hammurabi, King of Babylon*. Chicago: University of Chicago Press.

Harris, J. E., and K. R. Weeks. 1973. *X-raying the Pharaohs*. New York: Charles Scribner's Sons.

Harrison, H. E. 1991. Rickets. In *History of Pediatrics 1850–1950*. Edited by B. Nichols, A. Ballabriga, and N. Kretchmer. New York: Raven Press.

Hastings, P. 1974. *Medicine: An International History*. London: Ernest Benn.

Hawes, J. M. 1991. *The Children's Rights Movement*. Boston: Twayne Publishers.

Henderson, J. W. 1997. The yellow brick road to penicillin. *Mayo Clinic Proceedings* 72:683–87.

Hendren, W. H. 1994. Pediatric surgery. *Archives of Surgery* 129:345–51.

Hershkovitz, I., B. Ring, M. Speirs, et al. 1991. Possible congenital hemolytic anemia in prehistoric coastal inhabitants of Israel. *American Journal of Physical Anthropology* 85:7–13.

Holden, C. 1995. Did eagle snatch Taung baby? *Science* 269:1675.

Hollander, E. 1921. *Wunder, Wundergeburt und Wundergestalt*. Stuttgart: Verlag von Ferdinand.

Holt, L. E. 1913. Infant mortality, ancient and modern. *Archives of Pediatrics* 30: 885–916.

Howard-Jones, N. 1974. The scientific background of the International Sanitary Conferences, 1851–1938. *WHO Chronicle* 28:159–71.

———. 1979. On the diagnostic term "Down's disease." *Medical History* 23:102–4.

Hsia, E. C. H., I. Veith, and R. H. Geertsma. 1986. *The Essentials of Medicine in Ancient China and Japan*. Leiden: E. J. Brill.

Huard, P., and R. LaPlane. 1981. *Histoire Illustre de la Pediatrie*. Paris: Roger da Costa.

Huard, P., and M. Wong. 1968. *Chinese Medicine*. London: World University Library.

Hunt, D. 1970. *Parents and Children in History*. New York: Basic Books.

Illick, J. E. 1988. Child rearing in seventeenth-century England and America. In *History of Childhood*. Edited by L. deMause. New York: Peter Bedrick.

Jackson, R. 1988. *Doctors and Disease in the Roman Empire*. Norman: University of Oklahoma Press.

Jacob, I., and W. Jacob. 1993. *The Healing Past*. Leiden: E. J. Brill.

Jacobi, A. 1902. History of American pediatrics before 1800. *Janus* 7:460, 518, 590, 626.

Janssens, P. A. 1970. *Paleopathology*. London: John Baker.

Jastrow, M. 1914. *Babylonian–Assyrian Birth Omens and their Cultural Significance*. Giessen, Germany: Opelmann.

Jayne, W. A. 1979. *The Healing Gods of Ancient Civilizations*. New York: AMS Press.

Johanson, D., and M. Edey. 1981. *Lucy*. New York: Simon and Schuster.

Kagan, S. R. 1952. *Jewish Medicine*. Boston: Medico-Historical Press.

King, C. R. 1993. *Children's Health in America*. New York: Twayne Publishers.

King, M. L. 1991. *Women of the Renaissance*. Chicago: University of Chicago Press.

Kneckt-van Eekelen, A., and R. C. Hennekam. 1994. Cornelia de Lange. *American Journal of Medical Genetics* 52:257–66.

Kottek, S. 1991. Citizens! Do you want children's doctors? *Medical History* 35:103–16.

Kramer, S. N. 1959. *History Begins at Sumer*. New York: Doubleday.

———. 1963. *The Sumerians*. Chicago: University of Chicago Press.

Kutumbiah, P. 1959. Pediatrics (Kaumara Bhrtya) in ancient India. *Indian Journal of Pediatrics* 26:328–37.

———. 1962. *Ancient Indian Medicine*. Calcutta: Orient Longmans.

Labat, R. 1951. *Traité akkadien de diagnostics et pronostics médicaux*. Paris: E. J. Brill.

Landsberger, M. 1964. Some pediatric milestones of the 19th century. *American Journal of Diseases of Children* 108:205–10.

Laplane, R. 1991. French pediatrics. In *History of Pediatrics, 1850–1950*. Edited by B. Nichols, A. Ballabriga, and N. Kretchmer. New York: Raven Press.

Leake, C. D. 1952. *The Old Egyptian Medical Papyri*. Lawrence: University of Kansas Press.

Leopold, J. S. 1957. Abraham Jacobi. In *Pediatric Profiles*. Edited by B. S. Veeder. St. Louis: C. V. Mosby.

Levey, M. 1961. Some objective factors of Babylonian medicine in the light of new evidence. *Bulletin of the History of Medicine* 35:61–70.

Lloyd, G. E. R. 1978. *Hippocratic Writings*. Middlesex, U.K.: Penguin Books.

Lomax, E. M. R. 1996. *Small and Special: The Development of Hospitals for Children in Victorian Britain*. London: Wellcome Institute for the History of Medicine.

Lusk, G. 1932. A tribute to the life and work of Max Rubner. *Science* 76:129–35.

Majno, G. 1975. *The Healing Hand*. Cambridge, Mass.: Harvard University Press.

Marks, H. M. 1994. Fatal years. *Bulletin of the History of Medicine* 68:86–94.

Martin-Gil, J., F. J. Martin-Gil, G. Delibes-de-Castro, et al. 1995. The first known use of vermillion. *Experientia* 51:759–61.

Martinez-Lavin, M., J. Mansilla, C. Pineda, et al. 1994. Evidence of hypertrophic osteoarthropathy in human skeletal remains from pre-Hispanic Mesoamerica. *Annals of Internal Medicine* 120:238–41.

McKeon, R. 1941. *The Basic Works of Aristotle*. New York: Random House.

McQuarrie, I. 1954. Pediatrics. In *75 Years of Medical Progress*. Philadelphia: Lea & Febiger.

Medvei, V. C. 1982. *A History of Endocrinology*. Lancaster, U.K.: MTP Press.

Meyerhof, M. 1984. *Studies in Medieval Arabic Medicine*. Edited by P. Johnstone. London: Variorum Reprints.

Michie, C. A., and E. Cooper. 1991. Frankincense and myrrh as remedies in children. *Journal of the Royal Society of Medicine* 84:602–5.

Miller, R. L., G. J. Armelagos, S. Ikram, et al. 1992. Paleoepidemiology of schistosoma infection in mummies. *British Medical Journal* 304:555–56.

Mittler, D. M., and D. P. Van Gerven. 1994. Developmental, diachronic, and demographic analysis of cribra orbitalia. . . . *American Journal of Physical Anthropology* 93:287–97.

Moller, J. H. 1994. Fifty years of pediatric cardiology and challenges for the future. *Circulation* 89:2479–83.

Morse, W. R. 1934. *Chinese Medicine.* New York: P. B. Hoebner.

Mowat, A. 1996. Biliary atresia into the 21st century. *Hepatology* 23:1693–95.

Neal, J. V. 1976. Human genetics. In *Advances in American Medicine: Essays at the Bicentennial.* Edited by J. Z. Bowers and E. F. Purcell. New York: Josiah Macy Foundation.

Needham, J. 1954. *Science and Civilization in China.* Cambridge, U.K.: Cambridge University Press.

Norvenius, S. G., and B. Randers. 1997. 150th Anniversary of the creation of the first chair of paediatrics in the world. *Acta Paediatrica* 86:443–47.

Oppenheim, A. L. 1964. *Ancient Mesopotamia.* Chicago: University of Chicago Press.

———. 1967. *Letters from Mesopotamia.* Chicago: University of Chicago Press.

Osler, W. 1921. *The Evolution of Modern Medicine.* New Haven, Conn.: Yale University Press.

Otori, R. 1986. Preface. In *The Essentials of Medicine in Ancient China and Japan.* Edited by E. C. H. Hsia, I. Veith, and R. H. Geertsma. Leiden: E. J. Brill.

Ozment, S. 1983. *When Fathers Ruled.* Cambridge, Mass.: Harvard University Press.

Park, E., and H. Mason. 1957. Luther Emmet Holt. In *Pediatric Profiles.* Edited by B. S. Veeder. St. Louis: C. V. Mosby.

Pearson, H. A. 1986. *Eli Ives, M.D.: Lectures on the Diseases of Children.* Columbus, Ohio: Ross Laboratories.

———. 1994. The history of pediatrics in the United States. In *Principles and Practice of Pediatrics.* Edited by F. Oski. Philadelphia: J. B. Lippincott.

Ping-Chen, Hsiung. 1995. To nurse the young: Breastfeeding and infant feeding in late imperial China. *Journal of Family History* 20:217–38.

———. 1996a. Newborn care in late imperial China. *Journal of Family History.*

———. 1996b. Treatment of children in traditional China. *Berliner China* 10:73–79.

Pollack, L. A. 1987. *A Lasting Relationship.* Hanover, N.H.: University Press of New England.

Porter, R. 1977. *The Greatest Benefit to Mankind.* London: W. W. Norton.

Prader, A. 1991. Pediatric education. In *History of Pediatrics, 1850–1950.* Edited by B. Nichols, A. Ballabriga, and N. Kretchmer. New York: Raven Press.

Preston, S. H. 1994. After fatal years. *Bulletin of the History of Medicine* 68:124–28.

Radbill, S. X. 1955. A history of children's hospitals. *American Journal of Diseases of Children* 90:411–16.

———. 1963. Pediatrics in the Bible. *Clinical Pediatrics* 2:199–212.

———. 1976. Reared in adversity: Institutional care of children in the 18th century. *American Journal of Diseases of Children* 130:751–61.

Reinhard, K. J., et al. 1987. Helminth remains from prehistoric Indian coprolites on the Colorado plateau. *Journal of Parasitology* 73:630–37.

Richards, G. D., and S. C. Anton. 1991. Craniofacial configuration and postcranial development of a hydrocephalic child. *American Journal of Physical Anthropology* 85:185–200.

Rickham, P. P. 1986. Historical aspects of pediatric surgery. *Progress in Pediatric Surgery* 20:1–105.

Roberts, C., and K. Manchester. 1995. *The Archeology of Disease.* Ithaca, N.Y.: Cornell University Press.

Robinson, A. 1995. *The Story of Writing.* New York: Thames and Hudson.

Rosner, F. 1978. *Julius Preuss' Biblical and Talmudic Medicine.* New York: Sanhedrin Press.

Rothman, K. J. 1996. Lessons from John Graunt. *Lancet* 347:37–39.

Roush, W. 1996. Protein builds second skeletons. *Science* 273:1170.

Ruhräh, J. 1925. *Pediatrics of the Past.* New York: Paul Hoeber.

———. 1938. *Pediatric Biographies.* Chicago: American Medical Association.

Saggs, H. W. F. 1962. *The Greatness That Was Babylon.* New York: Hawthorn Books.

———. 1984. *The Might That Was Assyria.* London: Sigwick and Jackson.

Savage-Smith, E. 1994. *Islamic Culture and the Medical Arts.* Bethesda, Md.: National Library of Medicine.

Scheffel, R. L. 1993. *Discovering America's Past.* Pleasantville, N.Y.: Reader's Digest Association.

Schick, B. 1957. Experiences in pediatrics during the last fifty years. *Medical Clinics of North America* (1049–60).

Seidler, E. 1989. A historical survey of children's hospitals. In *The Hospital in History.* Edited by L. Granshaw and L. Porter. London: Routledge.

Sena, N. 1901. *The Ayurvedic System of Medicine.* Calcutta: Chatterjee.

Silverman, W. A. 1979. Incubator-baby side shows. *Pediatrics* 64:127–41.

———. 1990. Neonatal pediatrics at the century mark. *Pediatric Research* 27:S34–S37.

Silverstein, A. M. 1996. Paul Ehrlich: The founding of pediatric immunology. *Cellular Immunology* 174:1–6.

Singhal G. D., and J. Mitra. 1980. *Pediatric and Gynaecological Considerations and Aphorisms in Ancient Indian Surgery.* Varanasi, India: Banaras Hindu University, Institute of Medical Sciences.

Singleton, E. B. 1995. History of gastrointestinal imaging in pediatrics. *Pediatric Radiology* 25:108–10.

Soren, D., T. Fenton, and W. Birkby. 1995. The late-Roman cemetery near Lugnano in Teverine, Italy. *Journal of Paleopathology* 7:13–42.

Spinks, M. S., and G. L. Lewis. 1973. *Albicasis: On Surgery and Instruments.* London: Wellcome Institute.

Still, G. F. 1931. *The History of Pediatrics.* London: Oxford University Press.

Stillman, J. S. 1987. The history of pediatric rheumatology in the United States. *Rheumatic Disease Clinics in North America* 131:143–47.

Stool, S. E. 1996. A brief history of pediatric otolaryngology. *Otolaryngology and Head and Neck Surgery* 115:278–82.

Strauss, M. B. 1968. *Familiar Medical Quotations.* Boston: Little, Brown.

Strouhal, E. 1992. *Life of the Ancient Egyptians.* Norman: University of Oklahoma Press.

Stumpf, D. A. 1981. The founding of pediatric neurology in America. *Bulletin of the New York Academy of Medicine* 57:804–16.

Sugitatsu, Y. 1984. The scrolls and printed versions of the Ishimpo. In *Ishimpo 1000: Nen no aymi.* Tokyo: Issennen Kinenkai.

Tallmadge, G. K. 1939. Scaevola of Sainte-Marthe and the Paedotrophia. *Bulletin of the History of Medicine* 7:279–314.

Tanner, J. M. 1981. *A History of the Study of Human Growth.* Cambridge, U.K.: Cambridge University Press.

———. 1992. Growth as a measure of the nutritional and hygienic status of a population. *Hormone Research* 38:106–15.

Thwaites, G., M. Taviner, and V. Gant. 1997. The English sweating sickness, 1485 to 1551. *New England Journal of Medicine* 336:580–82.

Touloukian, R. J. 1995. Pediatric surgery between 1860 and 1900. *Journal of Pediatric Surgery* 30:911–16.

Tschanz, D. W. 1997. The Arab roots of European medicine. *Aramco* 48(3):20–31.

Tuttle, E. F. 1976. The trotula and the Old Dame Trot: A note on the Lady of Salerno. *Bulletin of the History of Medicine* 50:61–72.

Vahlquist, B. 1975. Two-century perspective of some major nutritional deficiency diseases in childhood. *Acta Paediatrica Scandinavica* 64:161–71.

Vahlquist, B., and A. Wallgreen. 1964. *Nils Rosen von Rosenstein.* Uppsala: Almquist and Wiksells.

Van Minnen, P. 1955. Medical care in late antiquity. In *Ancient Medicine in Its Socio-Cultural Context.* Edited by van der Eijk, Horstmanshoff, and Schrijvers. Amsterdam: Rodopi.

Vanzan, A. N., and F. Paladin. 1992. Epilepsy and Persian culture. *Epilepsia* 33:1057–64.

Veeder, B. S. 1957. *Pediatric Profiles.* St. Louis: C. V. Mosby.

Veith, I. 1972. *Huang Ti Nei Ching Su Wên.* Berkeley: University of California Press.

Viets, H. R. 1977. *Smallpox in Colonial America.* New York: Arno Press.

Vilaplana Satorre, E. 1934. Bibliographia historica de la pediatria Española. *Pediatria Española* 23:178–89.

Von Staden, H. 1989. *Herophilus.* Cambridge, U.K.: Cambridge University Press.

Vrebos, J. 1992. Harelip surgery in ancient China. *Plastic Reconstructive Surgery* 89:147–50.

Walsh, J. J. 1911. *Old Time Makers of Medicine.* New York: Fordham University Press.

Warkany, J. 1971. *Congenital Malformations.* Chicago: Yearbook.

Waserman, M. J. 1972. Henry Coit and the certified milk movement. *Bulletin of the History of Medicine* 46:359–90.

Wells, C. 1967. A new approach to paleopathology: Harris's lines. In *Diseases in Antiquity.* Edited by D. Brothwell and A. T. Sandison. Springfield, Ill.: Charles C. Tomas.

Wilson, J. A. 1951. *The Culture of Ancient Egypt*. Chicago: Phoenix Books.

Wilson, J. V. K. 1967. Organic diseases of ancient Mesopotamia. In *Diseases in Antiquity*. Edited by D. Brothwell and A. T. Sandison. Springfield, Ill.: Charles C. Tomas.

———. 1996. Diseases of Babylon. *Journal of the Royal Society of Medicine* 89: 135–39.

Wolff, J. A. 1991. History of pediatric oncology. *Pediatric Hematology Oncology* 8: 89–91.

Wong, K. C., and W. Lien-Teh. 1936. *History of Chinese Medicine*. Shanghai: National Quarantine Service.

Ziai, M. 1975. The contributions of Persian medicine to the West. *Clinical Pediatrics* 14:83–85.

Index

About the Authors

A. R. Colón is Professor Emeritus of Pediatrics at Georgetown University School of Medicine. His career in academic medicine spans over thirty years, during which time he taught pediatrics and lectured nationally and internationally on pediatric diseases and child development and health. He has authored several books on pediatric topics, including one on pediatric aphorisms, *The Boke of Children*.

P. A. Colón is a freelance writer who has collaborated with A. R. Colón on several publications of pediatric interest.